Aids to

Radiological Differential Diagnosis

Commissioning Editor: Timothy Horne
Project Development Manager: Siân Jarman
Project Manager: Frances Affleck
Designer: Erik Bigland

Aids to Radiological Differential Diagnosis

Edited by

Stephen Chapman
MBBS, MRCS, FRCP, FRCPCH, FRCR
Consultant Paediatric Radiologist
Birmingham Children's Hospital;
Honorary Senior Clinical Lecturer
University of Birmingham

Richard Nakielny
MA, BM, BCh, FRCR
Consultant Radiologist
CT Body Scan Department
Central Sheffield University Hospitals;
Honorary Senior Clinical Lecturer
University of Sheffield

FOURTH EDITION

Saunders
An Imprint of Elsevier

Aids to Radiological Differential Diagnosis
Chapman & Nakielny

Saunders
An Imprint of Elsevier
90 Tottenham Court Road,
London W1T 4LP

Original ISBN : 0-7020-2650-6

First Printed in India 2003
Reprinted 2004 (Twice)

Indian Reprint ISBN : 81-8147-061-3

Published by Elsevier, a division of Reed Elsevier India Private Limited,
17-A/1, Main Ring Road, Lajpat Nagar-IV, New Delhi - 110 024, INDIA.

Medical knowledge is constantly changing. As new information becomes available, changes in treatment, procedures, equipment and the use of drugs become necessary. The authors, editors, contributors and the publishers have, as far as it is possible, taken care to ensure that the information given in this text is accurate and up to date. However, readers are strongly advised to confirm that the information, especially with regard to drug dose/usage, complies with current legislation and standards of practice.

Printed and bound at
Saurabh Printers Pvt. Ltd., A-16, Sector IV, NOIDA 201 301.

PREFACE TO THE FIRST EDITION

During the period of study prior to taking the final Fellowship of the Royal College of Radiologists, or other similar radiological examinations, many specialist textbooks and the wealth of radiological papers are carefully scoured for lists of differential diagnoses of radiological signs. These will supplement the information already learned and enable that information to be used logically when analysing a radiograph. All this takes precious time when effort is best spent trying to memorize these lists rather than trying to find them within the massive texts or, even worse, trying to construct them oneself.

Consequently we decided to write a book which contains as many useful lists as one might reasonably be expected to know for a postgraduate examination. To make it manageable, we have omitted those lists and conditions which have limited relevance to routine radiological practice. In addition, many of the lists are constructed in terms of a 'surgical sieve' and by using this method we would hope that the lists are easier to remember. We have tried to present the conditions in some order of importance, although we realize that local patient selection and the geographical distribution of diseases will have a great influence in modifying the lists. The lists will, almost certainly, not be acceptable to all radiologists. However, the basic lists are supplemented with useful facts and discriminating features about each condition and these should enable the trainee to give a considered opinion of the radiograph. So that this added information can be kept concise and to avoid unnecessary repetition we have summarized the radiological signs of many important conditions separately in Part 2 of the book.

The book has no radiographs. We have assumed a basic knowledge of radiology in the reader and expect him or her to already be able to recognize the abnormal signs. A limited number of line drawings has been used to emphasize radiographic abnormalities.

The aim of the book is to assist with logical interpretation of the radiograph. It is not intended for use on its own because it is not a complete radiological textbook. Recourse will need to be made to the larger general and specialist texts and journals and the reading of them is still a prerequisite to passing the postgraduate examinations.

More exhaustive lists are to be found in Felson & Reeder's *Gamuts in Radiology* (Oxford: Pergamon Press, 1975) and Kreel's *Outline of Radiology* (London: Heinemann, 1971) and these books are to be commended.

Birmingham and Sheffield

S.C.
R.N.

PREFACE TO THE FOURTH EDITION

This new edition appears 8 years after the last. It has been necessary to bring the further reading up to date and to modernize those chapters which have seen the greatest changes during this time. The chapter on Nuclear Medicine was the only technique-based chapter in the previous edition and its contents, which are still relevant to current practice, have been redistributed to the other organ-based chapters.

As ever, we are extremely grateful to our friends and colleagues who have contributed to the new edition and supported us in our task.

We particularly thank Dr Stuart Coley and Dr Mark Hamilton as new contributors. Stuart Coley, in turn, thanks his colleagues Tim Hodgson, Charles Romanowski and Paul Griffiths for their help in reviewing Chapter 12, and Dr Tom Powell who contributed to the previous version of this chapter.

We hope this new edition continues to provide the sort of information that clinical radiologists will find useful in their day-to-day practice.

Birmingham and Sheffield
2003

S.C.
R.N.

CONTENTS

CONTRIBUTORS

Stuart Coley
MRCP, FRCR
Consultant Neuro-Radiologist, Royal Hallamshire Hospital, Sheffield; Honorary Senior Clinical Lecturer, University of Sheffield

Michael Collins
FRCR
Consultant Radiologist, Royal Hallamshire Hospital, Sheffield; Honorary Senior Clinical Lecturer, University of Sheffield

Mark Davies
FRCR
Consultant Radiologist, The Royal Orthopaedic Hospital, Birmingham; Honorary Senior Clinical Lecturer, University of Birmingham

Mark Hamilton
MRCP, FRCR
Specialist Registrar, Royal Hallamshire Hospital, Sheffield

Josephine McHugo
FRCP, FRCPCH, FRCR
Consultant Radiologist, Birmingham Women's Hospital; Honorary Senior Clinical Lecturer, University of Birmingham

EXPLANATORY NOTES

The 'surgical sieve' classification used in the longer lists is presented in order of commonness, e.g. when 'neoplastic' is listed first then this is the commonest cause as a group. Within the group of neoplastic conditions, number 1 is more common or as common as number 2. However, it does not necessarily follow that all the conditions in the first group are more common than those in subsequent groups, e.g. infective, metabolic, etc.

The groups entitled 'idiopathic' or 'others' are usually listed last even though the disease or diseases within them may be common. This has been done for the sake of neatness only.

In order that the supplementary notes are not unnecessarily repeated in several lists, those conditions which appear in several lists are denoted by an asterisk (*) and a summary of their radiological signs is to be found in Part 2 of the book. In this section conditions are listed alphabetically.

ABBREVIATIONS

ACE	Angiotensin-converting enzyme
ACTH	Adrenocorticotrophic hormone
AD	Autosomal dominant
AFP	Alpha-fetoprotein
AP	Anteroposterior
AR	Autosomal recessive
ASD	Atrial septal defect
AV	Atrioventricular
AVM	Arteriovenous malformation
AXR	Abdomen X-ray
CMCJ	Carpometacarpal joint
CMV	Cytomegalovirus
CNS	Central nervous system
CPA	Cerebellopontine angle
CSF	Cerebrospinal fluid
CT	Computerized tomography
CXR	Chest X-ray
DAI	Diffuse axonal injury
DIC	Disseminated intravascular coagulopathy
DIPJ	Distal interphalangeal joint
EDH	Extradural haemorrhage
FLAIR	Fluid-attenuated inversion recovery
GBM	Glioblastoma multiforme
GE	Gradient echo
HCG	Human chorionic gonadotrophin
HMPAO	Hexamethylpropyleneamineoxime
HOA	Hypertrophic osteoarthropathy
HOCM	Hypertrophic obstructive cardiomyopathy
HRCT	High-resolution CT
HU	Hounsfield units
IAM	Internal auditory meatus
ICA	Internal carotid artery
IUCD	Intrauterine contraceptive device
IVC	Inferior vena cava
IVU	Intravenous urogram
LAT	Lateral
MCA	Middle cerebral artery
MCPJ	Metacarpophalangeal joint
MIBG	Meta-iodo-benzyl-guanidine
MPA	Main pulmonary artery
MPS	Mucopolysaccharidosis
MRI	Magnetic resonance imaging
NEC	Necrotizing enterocolitis

NFT	Neurofibromatosis
PA	Posteroanterior
PAS	Periodic acid–Schiff (stain)
PD	Proton density
PDA	Patent ductus arteriosus
PIPJ	Proximal interphalangeal joint
PMF	Progressive massive fibrosis
PPH	Postpartum haemorrhage
SAH	Subarachnoid haemorrhage
SDH	Subdural haemorrhage
SIJ	Sacroiliac joint
SLE	Systemic lupus erythematosus
SMA	Superior mesenteric artery
SOL	Space-occupying lesion
SPECT	Single photon emission computerized tomography
STIR	Short tau inversion recovery
SVC	Superior vena cava
SXR	Skull X-ray
TAPVD	Total anomalous pulmonary venous drainage
TB	Tuberculosis
TE	Echo time or time to echo
TGA	Transposition of the great arteries
TOF	Tracheo-oesophageal fistula
TR	Repetition time
T_1W	T_1-weighted
T_2W	T_2-weighted
US	Ultrasound
VMA	Vanillylmandelic acid
VSD	Ventricular septal defect
XR	X-linked recessive

Part 1

1 Bones

with contributions by Mark Davies

1.1 RETARDED SKELETAL MATURATION

CHRONIC ILL HEALTH

1. **Congenital heart disease** — particularly cyanotic.
2. **Renal failure.**
3. **Inflammatory bowel disease.**
4. **Malnutrition.**
5. **Rickets*.**
6. **Maternal deprivation.**
7. **Any other chronic illness.**

ENDOCRINE DISORDERS

1. **Hypothyroidism*** — with granular, fragmented epiphyses. This causes severe retardation (five or more standard deviations below the mean).
2. **Steroid therapy and Cushing's disease** — see Cushing's syndrome*.
3. **Hypogonadism** — including older patients with Turner's syndrome.
4. **Hypopituitarism** — panhypopituitarism, growth hormone deficiency and Laron dwarfism.

CHROMOSOME DISORDERS

1. **Trisomy 21.**
2. **Most other chromosome disorders** — severely depressed in trisomy 18.

OTHER CONGENITAL DISORDERS

1. **Most bone dysplasias.**
2. **Most malformation syndromes.**

Further Reading

Poznanski A.K. (1984) *The Hand in Radiologic Diagnosis*, Chapter 3. Philadelphia: Saunders, pp. 67–96.

1.2 GENERALIZED ACCELERATED SKELETAL MATURATION

ENDOCRINE DISORDERS

1. **Idiopathic sexual precocity.**
2. **Intracranial masses in the region of the hypothalamus (hamartoma, astrocytoma and optic chiasm glioma), hydrocephalus and encephalitis.**
3. **Adrenal and gonadal tumours.**
4. **Hyperthyroidism.**

CONGENITAL DISORDERS

1. **McCune–Albright syndrome** — polyostotic fibrous dysplasia with precocious puberty.
2. **Cerebral gigantism (Soto's syndrome).**
3. **Lipodystrophy.**
4. **Pseudohypoparathyroidism.**
5. **Acrodysostosis.**
6. **Weaver (Weaver–Smith) syndrome.**
7. **Marshall (Marshall–Smith) syndrome.**

OTHERS

1. **Large or obese children.**

Further Reading

Poznanski A.K. (1984) *The Hand in Radiologic Diagnosis,* Chapter 3. Philadelphia: Saunders, pp. 67–96.

Rieth K.G., Comite F., Dwyer A.J. *et al.* (1987) CT of cerebral abnormalities in precocious puberty. *Am. J. Roentgenol.*, 148: 1231–8.

1.3 PREMATURE CLOSURE OF A GROWTH PLATE

1. **Local hyperaemia** — juvenile idiopathic arthritides, infection, haemophilia or arteriovenous malformation.
2. **Trauma.**
3. **Vascular occlusion** — infarcts and sickle-cell anaemia.
4. **Radiotherapy.**
5. **Thermal injury** — burns, frostbite.
6. **Multiple exostoses and enchondromatosis (Ollier's disease).**

1.4 ASYMMETRICAL MATURATION

1. **Normal children** — minor differences only.

HEMIHYPERTROPHY OR LOCALIZED GIGANTISM

1. **Vascular anomalies**
   (a) Haemangioma and AVM.
   (b) Klippel–Trenaunay–Weber syndrome — hypertrophy of the skeleton and soft tissues of one limb or one side of the body in association with an angiomatous malformation.
   (c) Maffucci's syndrome — enchondromas + haemangiomas.
2. **Chronic hyperaemia** — e.g. chronic arthritides (juvenile chronic arthritis or haemophilia).
3. **Hemihypertrophy** — M > F. R > L. May be a presenting feature of Beckwith–Wiedemann syndrome (hemihypertrophy, macroglossia and umbilical hernia). Increased incidence of Wilms' tumour.
4. **Neurofibromatosis*.**
5. **Macrodystrophia lipomatosa.**
6. **Russell–Silver dwarfism** — evident from birth. Triangular face with down-turned corners of the mouth, frontal bossing, asymmetrical growth and skeletal maturation.

HEMIATROPHY OR LOCALIZED ATROPHY

1. **Paralysis** — with osteopenia and overtubulation of long bones.
2. **Radiation treatment in childhood.**

1.5 SHORT LIMB SKELETAL DYSPLASIAS

RHIZOMELIC (PROXIMAL LIMB SHORTENING)

1. **Hypochondroplasia** — resembles a mild form of achondroplasia.
2. **Achondroplasia*.**
3. **Chondrodysplasia punctata** — see 1.46.
4. **Pseudoachondroplasia** — see 1.6.

MESOMELIC (MIDDLE SEGMENT LIMB SHORTENING)

1. **Dyschondrosteosis (Leri–Weil disease)** — limb shortening with a Madelung deformity.
2. **Mesomelic dysplasia**
   (a) Type Langer.
   (b) Type Reinhardt–Pfeiffer.

ACROMESOMELIC (MIDDLE AND DISTAL SEGMENT LIMB SHORTENING)

1. **Chondroectodermal dysplasia (Ellis–van Creveld syndrome)** — similar to asphyxiating thoracic dysplasia but: (a) hexadactyly is a constant finding, (b) there is severe hypoplasia of the fingers and nails, (c) congenital heart disease is common and (d) hypoplastic lateral tibial plateau is characteristic in childhood.
2. **Acromesomelic dysplasia.**
3. **Mesomelic dysplasia**
   (a) Type Nievergelt.
   (b) Type Robinow.
   (c) Type Werner.

ACROMELIC (DISTAL SEGMENT SHORTENING)

1. **Asphyxiating thoracic dysplasia (Jeune's syndrome)** — narrow thorax with short ribs leading to respiratory distress. Spur-like projections of the acetabular roof. Premature ossification of the femoral capital epiphyses. Occasional postaxial hexadactyly. Cone-shaped epiphyses in childhood.
2. **Peripheral dysostosis.**

1.6 SHORT SPINE SKELETAL DYSPLASIAS

1. **Pseudoachondroplasia** — short limb and short spine dwarfism, marked joint laxity, platyspondyly with exaggerated grooves for the ring apophyses, C1/2 dislocation.
2. **Spondyloepiphyseal dysplasia** — ovoid or 'pear-shaped' vertebral bodies in infancy → severe platyspondyly in later life; normal metaphyses; retarded development of the symphysis pubis and femoral heads; coxa vara, which may be severe; ± odontoid hypoplasia and C1/2 instability.
3. **Spondylometaphyseal dysplasias**
   (a) Type Kozlowski.
   (b) Other types.
4. **Diastrophic dwarfism** — progressive kyphoscoliosis, hitch-hiker thumb, delta-shaped epiphyses, interpedicular narrowing of the lumbar spine.
5. **Metatropic dwarfism** — short-limbed dwarfism in infancy → short spine dwarfism in later childhood, severe progressive scoliosis, dumbbell-shaped long bones, hypoplastic odontoid.
6. **Kniest syndrome** — dumbbell-shaped long bones, irregular epiphyses, kyphoscoliosis, platyspondyly, interpedicular narrowing of the lumbar spine, limited and painful joint movements.

1.7 LETHAL NEONATAL DYSPLASIA

1. **Osteogenesis imperfecta*** — usually type II.
2. **Thanatophoric dwarfism** — small thorax, severe platyspondyly with 'H'-shaped or 'inverted U'-shaped vertebral bodies, 'telephone handle'-shaped long bones ± 'clover-leaf' skull deformity.
3. **Chondrodysplasia punctata** — rhizomelic form. See 1.46.
4. **Asphyxiating thoracic dysplasia (Jeune's syndrome)** — see 1.5.
5. **Campomelic dwarfism** — bowed long bones.
6. **Achondrogenesis** — types I and II.
7. **Short rib syndromes ± polydactyly**
   (a) Type I (Saldino–Noonan).
   (b) Type II (Majewski).
   (c) Type III (lethal thoracic dysplasia).
8. **Homozygous achondroplasia*.**
9. **Hypophosphatasia*** — lethal type.

1.8 DUMBBELL-SHAPED LONG BONES

Short narrow diaphyses with marked metaphyseal widening.

1. **Metatropic dwarfism** — see 1.6.
2. **Pseudoachondroplasia** — see 1.6.
3. **Kniest syndrome** — see 1.6.
4. **Diastrophic dwarfism** — see 1.6.
5. **Osteogenesis imperfecta (type III)*.**
6. **Chondroectodermal dysplasia (Ellis–van Creveld syndrome)** — see 1.5.

1.9 CONDITIONS EXHIBITING DYSOSTOSIS MULTIPLEX

Dysostosis multiplex is a constellation of radiological signs which are exhibited, in total or in part, by a number of conditions caused by defects of complex carbohydrate metabolism. These signs include: (a) abnormal bone texture, (b) widening of diaphyses, (c) tilting of distal radius and ulna towards each other, (d) pointing of the proximal ends of the metacarpals, (e) large skull vault with calvarial thickening, (f) anterior beak of upper lumbar vertebrae, and (g) 'J-shaped' sella.

MUCOPOLYSACCHARIDOSES

Type	*Eponym*	*Inheritance*	*Onset*	*Osseous and visceral abnormalities*	*Neurological features*
IH	Hurler*	AR	By 1–2 years	Marked. Severe dwarfism. Skeletal abnormalities ++. Corneal clouding	Severe
IS	Scheie	AR	Childhood	Carpal tunnel syndrome	Mild
II	Hunter	XR	2–4 years	Marked. Severe dwarfism. Dysostosis multiplex similar to Hurler but less severe. No corneal clouding	Mild to moderate
III	Sanfilippo	AR	Childhood	Mild	Severe
IV	Morquio*	AR	1–3 years	Severe skeletal abnormalities	Absent (but may be neurological complications of spinal abnormalities)
VI	Maroteaux-Lamy	AR	Childhood	Severe dwarfism and skeletal abnormalities	Absent (except as a complication of meningeal involvement)
VII	Sly	AR		Mild to severe	Absent to severe

MUCOLIPIDOSES

1. **MLS I (neuraminidase deficiency).**
2. **MLS II (I – Cell disease).**
3. **MLS III (pseudopolydystrophy of Maroteaux).**

OLIGOSACCHARIDOSES

1. **Fucosidosis I.**
2. **Fucosidosis II.**
3. **GM_1 gangliosidosis.**
4. **Mannosidosis.**
5. **Aspartylglucosaminuria.**

1.10 GENERALIZED INCREASED BONE DENSITY – CHILDREN

NB. Infants in the first few months of life can exhibit 'physiological' bone sclerosis which regresses spontaneously.

DYSPLASIAS

1. **Osteopetrosis*.**
2. **Pyknodysostosis** — short stature, hypoplastic lateral ends of clavicles, hypoplastic terminal phalanges, bulging cranium and delayed closure of the anterior fontanelle. AR.
3. **The craniotubular dysplasias** — abnormal skeletal modelling ± increased bone density.
   (a) Metaphyseal dysplasia (Pyle).
   (b) Craniometaphyseal dysplasia.
   (c) Craniodiaphyseal dysplasia.
   (d) Frontometaphyseal dysplasia.
   (e) Osteodysplasty (Melnick–Needles).
4. **The craniotubular hyperostoses** — overgrowth of bone with alteration of contours and increased bone density.
   (a) Endosteal hyperostosis, Van Buchem type.
   (b) Endosteal hyperostosis, Worth type.
   (c) Sclerosteosis.
   (d) Diaphyseal dysplasia (Camurati–Engelmann).

METABOLIC

1. **Renal osteodystrophy*** – rickets + osteosclerosis.

POISONING

1. **Lead** — dense metaphyseal bands. Cortex and flat bones may also be slightly dense. Modelling deformities later, e.g. flask-shaped femora.
2. **Fluorosis** — more common in adults. Usually asymptomatic but may present in children with crippling stiffness and pain. Thickened cortex at the expense of the medulla. Periosteal reaction. Ossification of ligaments, tendons and interosseous membranes.
3. **Hypervitaminosis D** — slightly increased density of skull and vertebrae early, followed later by osteoporosis. Soft-tissue calcification. Dense metaphyseal bands and widened zone of provisional calcification.

4. **Chronic hypervitaminosis A** — not before 1 year of age. Failure to thrive, hepatosplenomegaly, jaundice, alopecia and haemoptysis. Cortical thickening of long and tubular bones, especially in the feet. Subperiosteal new bone. Normal epiphyses and reduced metaphyseal density. The mandible is not affected (cf. Caffey's disease).

IDIOPATHIC

1. **Caffey's disease (infantile cortical hyperostosis)** — see 1.14.
2. **Idiopathic hypercalcaemia of infancy** — probably a manifestation of hypervitaminosis D. Elfin facies, failure to thrive and mental retardation. Generalized increased density or transverse dense metaphyseal bands. Increased density of the skull base.

Further Reading

Beighton P. & Cremin B.J. (1980) *Sclerosing Bone Dysplasias*. Berlin: Springer-Verlag.
Herman T.E. & McAlister W.H. (1991) Inherited diseases in bone density in children. *Radiol. Clin. North Am.*, 29(1): 149–64.
Vanhoenacker F.M., De Beuckeleer L.H., Van Hul W., *et al.* (2000) Sclerosing bone dysplasias: genetic and radioclinical features. *Eur. Radiol.*, 10: 1423–33.

1.11 GENERALIZED INCREASED BONE DENSITY – ADULTS

MYELOPROLIFERATIVE

1. **Myelosclerosis** — marrow cavity is narrowed by endosteal new bone. Patchy lucencies due to persistence of fibrous tissue. (Generalized osteopenia in the early stages due to myelofibrosis.) Hepatosplenomegaly.

METABOLIC

1. **Renal osteodystrophy*.**

POISONING

1. **Fluorosis** — with periosteal reaction, prominent muscle attachments and calcification of ligaments and interosseous membranes. Changes are most marked in the innominate bones and lumbar spine.

NEOPLASTIC (more commonly multifocal than generalized)

1. **Osteoblastic metastases** — most commonly prostate and breasts — see 1.18.
2. **Lymphoma*.**
3. **Mastocytosis** — sclerosis of marrow containing skeleton with patchy areas of radiolucency. Urticaria pigmentosa. Can have symptoms and signs of carcinoid syndrome.

IDIOPATHIC (more commonly multifocal than generalized)

1. **Paget's disease*** — coarsened trabeculae, bony expansion and thickened cortex.

THOSE CONDITIONS WITH ONSET IN THE PAEDIATRIC AGE GROUP (see 1.10)

1.12 SOLITARY SCLEROTIC BONE LESION

DEVELOPMENTAL

1. **Bone island (enostosis).**
2. **Fibrous dysplasia*.**

NEOPLASTIC

1. **Metastasis** — most commonly prostate or breast.
2. **Lymphoma*.**
3. **Osteoma/osteoid osteoma/osteoblastoma*.**
4. **Healed or healing benign or malignant bone lesion** — e.g. lytic metastasis following radiotherapy or chemotherapy, bone cyst, fibrous cortical defect, eosinophilic granuloma or brown tumour.
5. **Primary bone sarcoma.**

VASCULAR

1. **Bone infarct.**

TRAUMATIC

1. **Callus** — especially a transverse density around a healing stress fracture.

INFECTIVE

1. **Sclerosing osteomyelitis of Garré.**

IDIOPATHIC

1. **Paget's disease*.**

1.13 MULTIPLE SCLEROTIC BONE LESIONS

DEVELOPMENTAL

1. **Fibrous dysplasia.***
2. **Osteopoikilosis** — asymptomatic. 1–10 mm, round or oval densities in the appendicular skeleton and pelvis. Ribs, skull and spine are usually exempt. Tend to be parallel to the long axis of the affected bones and are especially numerous near the ends of bones.
3. **Osteopathia striata (Voorhoeve's disease)** — asymptomatic. Linear bands of dense bone parallel with the long axis of the bone. The appendicular skeleton and pelvis are most frequently affected; skull and clavicles are spared.
4. **Tuberous sclerosis*.**

NEOPLASTIC

1. **Metastases** (see 1.18) — most commonly prostate or breast.
2. **Lymphoma*.**
3. **Mastocytosis.**
4. **Multiple healed or healing benign or malignant bone lesions** — e.g. lytic metastases following radiotherapy or chemotherapy, eosinophilic granuloma and brown tumours.
5. **Multiple myeloma*** — sclerosis in up to 3% of cases.
6. **Osteomata** — e.g. Gardner's syndrome.
7. **Multifocal osteosarcoma*.**

IDIOPATHIC

1. **Paget's disease*.**

VASCULAR

1. **Bone infarcts.**

TRAUMATIC

1. **Callus** — around numerous fractures.

1.14 BONE SCLEROSIS WITH A PERIOSTEAL REACTION

TRAUMATIC

1. **Healing fracture with callus.**

NEOPLASTIC

1. **Metastasis.**
2. **Lymphoma*.**
3. **Osteoid osteoma/osteoblastoma*.**
4. **Osteosarcoma*.**
5. **Ewing's sarcoma*.**
6. **Chondrosarcoma*.**

INFECTIVE

1. **Osteomyelitis** — including Garré's sclerosing osteomyelitis and Brodie's abscess.
2. **Syphilis** — congenital or acquired.

IDIOPATHIC

1. **Infantile cortical hyperostosis** (Caffey's disease) — in infants up to 6 months of age. Multiple bones involved at different times, most frequently mandible, ribs and clavicles; long bones less commonly; spine, hands and feet are spared. Increased density of bones is caused by massive periosteal new bone. In the long bones the epiphyses and metaphyses are spared.
2. **Melorheostosis** — cortical and periosteal new bone giving the appearance of molten wax flowing down a burning candle. The hyperostosis tends to extend from one bone to the next. Usually affects one limb but both limbs on one side may be affected. Sometimes it is bilateral but asymmetrical. Skull, spine and ribs are seldom affected.

Further Reading

Freyschmidt J. (2001) Melorheostosis: a review of 23 cases. *Eur. Radiol.*, 11: 474–9.

1.15 SOLITARY SCLEROTIC BONE LESION WITH A LUCENT CENTRE

NEOPLASTIC

1. **Osteoid osteoma*.**
2. **Osteoblastoma*.**

INFECTIVE

1. **Brodie's abscess.**
2. **Syphilis, yaws and tuberculosis.**

1.16 CONDITIONS INVOLVING SKIN AND BONE

OSTEOLYTIC BONE LESIONS

1. **Congenital**
   (a) Neurofibromatosis*.
   (b) Basal cell naevus syndrome.
   (c) Angiodysplasias.
2. **Acquired**
   (a) Scleroderma*.
   (b) Rheumatoid arthritis*.
   (c) Gout*.
   (d) Leprosy.
   (e) Syphilis.
   (f) Actinomycosis.
   (g) Langerhans cell histiocytosis*.
   (h) Sarcoidosis*.
   (i) Mastocytosis.
   (j) Pancreatitis with osteonecrosis.

OSTEOSCLEROTIC BONE LESIONS

1. **Congenital**
   (a) Osteopoikilosis.
   (b) Osteopathia striata.
   (c) Melorrheostosis.
   (d) Gardner's syndrome.

2. **Acquired**
   (a) Reiter's syndrome*.
   (b) SAPHO* (Synovitis, Acne, Pustulosis, Hyperostosis, Osteitis) — also termed pustulotic arthro-osteitis (PAO).
   (c) Lymphoma*.
   (d) Sarcoidosis*.
   (e) Haemangiomatosis.
   (f) Lipoatrophic diabetes mellitus.

MIXED OSTEOLYTIC/OSTEOSCLEROTIC BONE LESIONS

1. **Gaucher's disease.**
2. **Psoriatic arthritis*.**
3. **SAPHO*.**
4. **Reiter's syndrome*.**
5. **Sarcoidosis*.**
6. **Pancreatic bone lesions.**

TUMOROUS LESIONS

1. **Maffucci's syndrome** — enchondromatosis + haemangiomas.
2. **Fibrous dysplasia*.**
3. **Haemangioma.**

Further Reading

Cotton A., Flipo R.-M., Mentre A. *et al.* (1995) SAPHO syndrome. *RadioGraphics*, 15: 1147–54.

Freyschmidt J. & Freyschmidt-Paul P. (2001) SKIBO diseases: a concept to avoid bloody diagnostic procedures in ambiguous lesions. *Eur. Radiol.*, 11: 1729–42.

1.17 COARSE TRABECULAR PATTERN

1. **Paget's disease*** — an enlarged bone with a thickened cortex. If only part of the bone is affected the demarcation between normal and pagetoid bone is clear cut.
2. **Osteoporosis** (see 1.32) } Resorption of secondary trabeculae accentuates the remaining primary trabeculae.
3. **Osteomalacia*** } Resorption of secondary trabeculae accentuates the remaining primary trabeculae.
4. **Haemoglobinopathies** — especially thalassaemia*.
5. **Haemangioma** — especially in a vertebral body.
6. **Gaucher's disease.**

1.18 SKELETAL METASTASES – MOST COMMON RADIOLOGICAL APPEARANCES

LUNG

1. **Carcinoma**	lytic
2. **Carcinoid**	sclerotic

BREAST

lytic or mixed

GENITO-URINARY

1. **Renal cell carcinoma**	lytic, expansile
2. **Wilms' tumour**	lytic
3. **Bladder (transitional cell)**	lytic, occasionally sclerotic
4. **Prostate**	sclerotic

REPRODUCTIVE ORGANS

1. **Cervix**	lytic or mixed
2. **Uterus**	lytic
3. **Ovary**	lytic
4. **Testis**	lytic; occasionally sclerotic

THYROID

lytic, expansile

GASTROINTESTINAL TRACT

1. **Stomach**	sclerotic or mixed
2. **Colon**	lytic; occasionally sclerotic
3. **Rectum**	lytic

ADRENAL

1. **Phaeochromocytoma**	lytic, expansile
2. **Carcinoma**	lytic
3. **Neuroblastoma**	lytic; occasionally sclerotic

SKIN

1. **Squamous cell carcinoma**	lytic
2. **Melanoma**	lytic, expansile

Further Reading

Gold R.I., Seeger L.L., Bassett L.W. *et al.* (1990) An integrated approach to the evaluation of metastatic bone disease. *Radiol. Clin. North Am.*, 28(2): 471–83.

Kagan R.A., Steckel R.J., Bassett L.W. *et al.* (1986) Radiologic contributions to cancer management. Bone metastases. *Am. J. Roentgenol.*, 147: 305–12.

Pagani J.J. & Libshitz H.I. (1982) Imaging bone metastases. *Radiol. Clin. North Am.*, 20 (3): 545–60.

Thrall J.H. & Ellis B.I. (1987) Skeletal metastases. *Radiol. Clin. North. Am.*, 25(6): 1155–70.

1.19 PAEDIATRIC TUMOURS THAT METASTASIZE TO BONE

1. **Neuroblastoma.**
2. **Leukaemia** — although not truly metastases.
3. **Lymphoma*.**
4. **Clear cell sarcoma (Wilms' variant).**
5. **Rhabdomyosarcoma.**
6. **Retinoblastoma.**
7. **Ewing's sarcoma** — lung metastases much more common.
8. **Osteosarcoma*** — lung metastases much more common.

Further Reading

Parker B.R. (1997) Leukaemia and lymphoma in childhood. *Radiol. Clin. North Am.*, 35(6): 1495–516.

1.20 SITES OF ORIGIN OF PRIMARY BONE NEOPLASMS

(A composite diagram modified from Madewell *et al.*, 1981.)

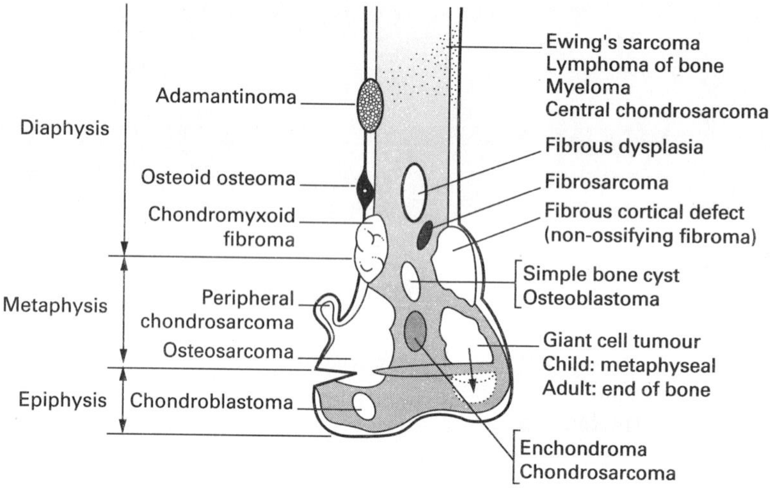

Further Reading

Madewell J.E., Ragsdale B.D. & Sweet D.E. (1981) Radiologic and pathologic analysis of solitary bone lesions. *Radiol. Clin. North Am.*, 19: 715–48.

1.21 PEAK AGE INCIDENCE OF PRIMARY BONE NEOPLASMS

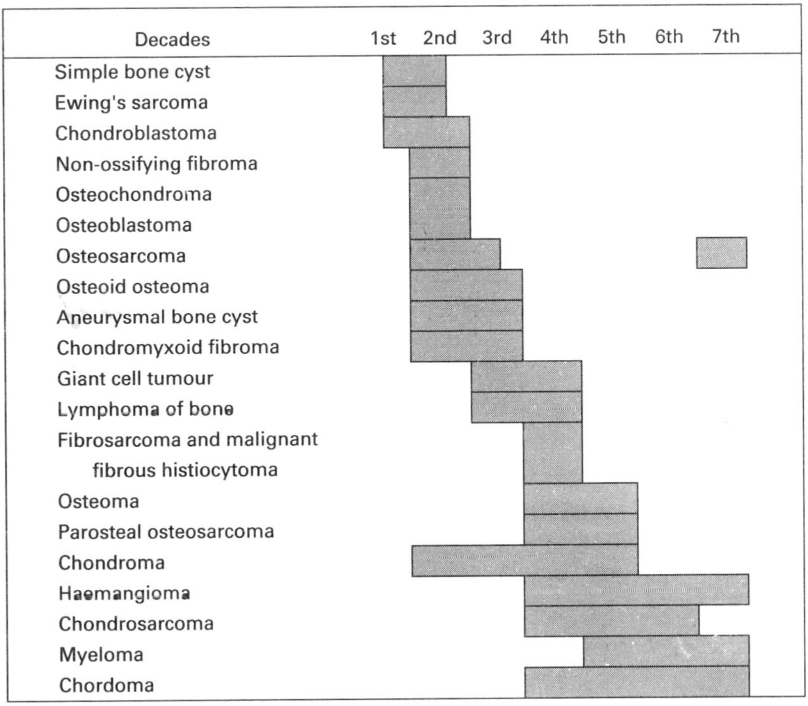

1.22 LUCENT BONE LESION IN THE MEDULLA – WELL-DEFINED, MARGINAL SCLEROSIS, NO EXPANSION

Indicates a slowly progressing lesion.

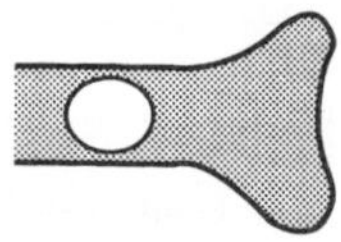

1. **Geode** — a subarticular cyst. Other signs of arthritis. See 1.27.
2. **Healing benign or malignant bone lesion** — e.g. metastasis, eosinophilic granuloma or brown tumour.
3. **Brodie's abscess.**
4. **Benign bone neoplasms**
   (a) Simple bone cyst* — 75% arise in the proximal humerus and femur.
   (b) Enchondroma* — more than 50% are found in the tubular bones of the hands. ± Internal calcification.
   (c) Chondroblastoma* — in an epiphysis. Most common sites are proximal humerus, distal femur and proximal tibia. Internal hazy calcification.
5. **Fibrous dysplasia*.**

1.23 LUCENT BONE LESION IN THE MEDULLA – WELL-DEFINED, NO MARGINAL SCLEROSIS, NO EXPANSION

The absence of reactive bone formation implies a fast growth rate.

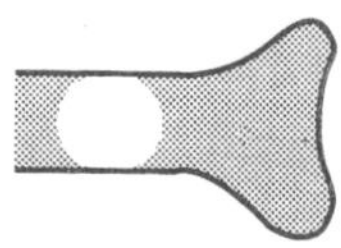

1. **Metastasis** — especially from breast, bronchus, kidney or thyroid.
2. **Multiple myeloma*.**
3. **Eosinophilic granuloma*.**
4. **Brown tumour of hyperparathyroidism*.**
5. **Benign bone neoplasms**
   (a) Enchondroma*.
   (b) Chondroblastoma*.

1.24 LUCENT BONE LESION IN THE MEDULLA – ILL-DEFINED

An aggressive pattern of destruction.

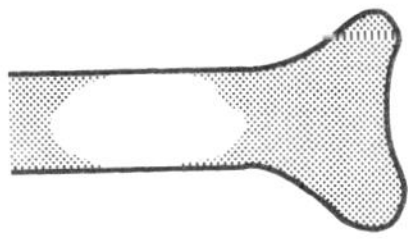

1. **Metastasis.**
2. **Multiple myeloma*.**
3. **Osteomyelitis.**
4. **Lymphoma of bone.**
5. **Long bone sarcomas**
   (a) Osteosarcoma*.
   (b) Ewing's sarcoma*.
   (c) Central chondrosarcoma*.
   (d) Fibrosarcoma and malignant fibrous histiocytoma.

Further Reading

Mulligan M.E., McRae G.A. & Murphey M.D. (1999) Imaging features of primary lymphoma of bone. *Am. J. Roentgenol.*, 173: 1691–7.

Oudjhane K. & Azouz E.M. (2001) Imaging of osteomyelitis in children. *Radiol. Clin. North Am.*, 39(2): 251–66.

Tehranzadeh J., Wong E., Wang F. *et al.* (2001) Imaging of osteomyelitis in the mature skeleton. *Radiol. Clin. North Am.*, 39(2): 223–50.

1.25 LUCENT BONE LESION IN THE MEDULLA – WELL-DEFINED, ECCENTRIC EXPANSION

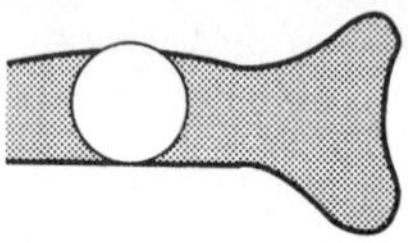

1. **Giant cell tumour*** — typically subarticular after epiphyseal fusion (3% are metaphyseal prior to fusion). Ill-defined endosteal margins. Septa. ± Soft-tissue extension and destroyed cortex. Mostly long bones.
2. **Aneurysmal bone cyst*** — in the unfused metaphysis or metaphysis and epiphysis following fusion of the growth plate. Intact but thin cortex. Well-defined endosteal margin. ± thin internal strands of bone. Fluid–fluid levels on CT and MRI.
3. **Enchondroma*** — diaphyseal. Over 50% occur in the tubular bones of the hands and feet. Internal ground glass appearance ± calcification within it. May be multilocular in long bones.
4. **Non-ossifying fibroma (fibrous cortical defect)*** — frequently in the distal tibia or femur and produces an eccentric expanded cortex. (In a thin bone such as the fibula central expansion is observed.) Metaphyseal. Smooth, sharp margins with a thin rim of surrounding sclerosis.
5. **Chondromyxoid fibroma*** — 75% in the lower limbs (50% in the proximal tibia). Metaphyseal and may extend into the epiphysis. Frequently has marginal sclerosis.

1.26 LUCENT BONE LESION – GROSSLY EXPANSILE

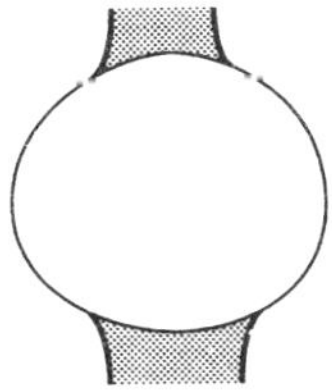

MALIGNANT BONE NEOPLASMS

1. **Metastases** — renal cell carcinoma and thyroid; less commonly melanoma, bronchus, breast and phaeochromocytoma.
2. **Plasmacytoma*** — ± soft tissue extension. ± Internal septa.
3. **Central chondrosarcoma/lymphoma of bone/ fibrosarcoma** — when slow growing may have this appearance.
4. **Telangiectatic osteosarcoma*** — rare. Uncommon vascular variant that mimics aneurysmal bone cyst.

BENIGN BONE NEOPLASMS

1. **Aneurysmal bone cyst*** — in the unfused metaphysis or metaphysis and epiphysis following fusion of the growth plate. ± Internal septa. Fluid–fluid levels on CT and MRI.
2. **Giant cell tumour*** — typically subarticular after epiphyseal fusion. Ill-defined endosteal margin. ± Soft-tissue extension and destroyed cortex.
3. **Enchondroma*** — ground-glass appearance ± internal calcifications.

NON-NEOPLASTIC

1. **Fibrous dysplasia*** — ground-glass appearance ± internal calcification. Modelling deformities of affected bone.
2. **Haemophilic pseudotumour** (see Haemophilia*) — especially in the iliac wing and lower limb bones. Soft-tissue swelling. ± Haemophilic arthropathy.
3. **Brown tumour of hyperparathyroidism*** — the solitary skeletal sign of hyperparathyroidism in 3% of patients. Most commonly in the mandible, followed by pelvis, ribs and femora. Usually unilocular.
4. **Hydatid.**

Further Reading

Lewall D.B. (1998) Hydatid disease: biology, pathology, imaging and classification. *Clin. Radiol.*, 53: 863–74.

1.27 SUBARTICULAR LUCENT BONE LESION

ARTHRITIDES

1. **Osteoarthritis** — may be multiple 'cysts' in the load-bearing areas of multiple joints. Surrounding sclerotic margin. Joint-space narrowing, subchondral sclerosis and osteophytes.
2. **Rheumatoid arthritis*** — no sclerotic margin. Begins periarticularly near the insertion of the joint capsule. Joint-space narrowing and juxta-articular osteoporosis.
3. **Calcium pyrophosphate arthropathy** (see Calcium pyrophosphate dihydrate deposition disease*) — similar to osteoarthritis but frequently larger and with more collapse and fragmentation of the articular surface.
4. **Gout** — ± erosions with overhanging edges and adjacent soft-tissue masses.
5. **Haemophilia*.**

NEOPLASTIC

1. **Metastases/multiple myeloma*** — single or multiple. Variable appearance.
2. **Aneurysmal bone cyst*** — solitary. Expansile. Narrow zone of transition.
3. **Giant cell tumour*** — solitary. Eccentric. Ill-defined endosteal margin.
4. **Chondroblastoma*** — solitary. Predilection for the proximal ends of the humerus, femur and tibia. Contains amorphous or spotty calcification in 50%.

5. **Pigmented villonodular synovitis*** — mainly the lower limb, especially the knee. Soft-tissue mass. Cyst-like defects with sharp sclerotic margins. May progress to joint destruction.

OTHERS

1. **Post-traumatic** — particularly in the carpal bones. Well-defined.
2. **Osteonecrosis** — with bone sclerosis, collapse and fragmentation. Preservation of joint space.
3. **Tuberculosis** — wholly epiphyseal or partly metaphyseal. Well-defined or ill-defined. No surrounding sclerosis.

Further Reading

Bullough P.G. & Bansal M. (1988) The differential diagnosis of geodes. *Radiol. Clin. North Am.*, 26: 1165–84.

Resnick D., Niwayama G. & Coutts R.D. (1977) Subchondral cysts (geodes) in arthritic disorders: pathologic and radiographic appearance of the hip joint. *Am. J. Roentgenol.*, 128: 799–806.

1.28 LUCENT BONE LESION – CONTAINING CALCIUM OR BONE

NEOPLASTIC

1. **Metastases** — especially from breast.
2. **Cartilage neoplasms**
   (a) Benign — enchondroma, chondroblastoma and chondromyxoid fibroma.
   (b) Malignant — chondrosarcoma.
3. **Bone (osteoid) neoplasms**
   (a) Benign — osteoid osteoma and osteoblastoma.
   (b) Malignant — osteosarcoma.
4. **Fibrous-tissue neoplasms**
   (a) Malignant — fibrosarcoma and malignant fibrous histiocytoma.

OTHERS

1. **Fibrous dysplasia*.**
2. **Osteoporosis circumscripta** (Paget's disease*).
3. **Avascular necrosis and bone infarction.**
4. **Osteomyelitis** — with sequestrum.
5. **Eosinophilic granuloma*.**
6. **Intraosseous lipoma.**

1.29 'MOTH-EATEN BONE'

Multiple scattered lucencies of variable size with no major central lesion. Coalescence may occur later. Cancellous and/or cortical bone is involved.

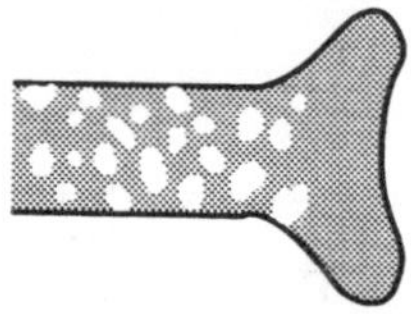

NEOPLASTIC

1. **Metastases** — including neuroblastoma in a child.
2. **Multiple myeloma*.**
3. **Leukaemia** — consider when there is involvement of an entire bone or a neighbouring bone with low signal on T_1W and high signal on T_2W and short tau inversion recovery (STIR) MRI.
4. **Long-bone sarcomas**
   (a) Ewing's sarcoma*.
   (b) Lymphoma of bone.
   (c) Osteosarcoma*.
   (d) Chondrosarcoma*.
   (e) Fibrosarcoma and malignant fibrous histiocytoma.
5. **Langerhans cell histiocytosis*.**

INFECTIVE

1. **Acute osteomyelitis.**

Further Reading

Sammak B., Abd El Bagi M., Al Shahed M. *et al.* (1999) Osteomyelitis: a review of currently used imaging techniques. *Eur. Radiol.*, 9: 894–900.

1.30 REGIONAL OSTEOPENIA

Decreased bone density confined to a region or segment of the appendicular skeleton.

1. **Disuse** — during the immobilization of fractures, in paralysed segments and in bone and joint infections. Usually appears after 8 weeks of immobilization. The patterns of bone loss may be uniform (commonest), spotty (mostly periarticular), band-like (subchondral or metaphyseal) or endosteal cortical scalloping and linear cortical lucencies.

2. **Sudeck's atrophy (reflex sympathetic dystrophy syndrome)** — is mediated via a neurovascular mechanism and associated with post-traumatic and postinfective states, myocardial infarction, calcific tendinitis and cervical spondylosis. It most commonly affects the shoulder and hand and develops rapidly. Pain and soft-tissue swelling are clinical findings.
3. **Transient osteoporosis of the hip** — a severe, progressive osteoporosis of the femoral head and, to a lesser degree, of the femoral neck and acetabulum. Full recovery is seen in 6 months.
4. **Regional migratory osteoporosis** — pain, swelling and osteoporosis affect the joints of the lower limbs in particular. The migratory nature differentiates it from other causes. Marrow oedema in affected areas is seen as low signal on T_1W and high signal on T_2W MRI.

1.31 GENERALIZED OSTEOPENIA

1. **Osteoporosis** — diminished quantity of normal bone.
2. **Osteomalacia*** — normal quantity of bone but it has an excess of uncalcified osteoid.
3. **Hyperparathyroidism*** — increased bone resorption by osteoclasts.
4. **Diffuse infiltrative bone disease** — e.g. multiple myeloma and leukaemia.

Further Reading

Mayo-Smith W. & Rosenthal D.I. (1991) Radiographic appearance of osteopenia. *Radiol. Clin. North Am.*, 29(1): 37–47.

1.32 OSTEOPOROSIS

1. Decreased bone density.
2. Cortical thinning with a relative increase in density of the cortex and vertebral end-plates. Skull sutures are relatively sclerotic.
3. Relative accentuation of trabecular stress lines because of resorption of secondary trabeculae.
4. Brittle bones with an increased incidence of fractures, especially compression fractures of vertebral bodies, femoral neck and wrist fractures.

ENDOCRINE

1. **Hypogonadism**
   (a) Ovarian — postmenopausal, Turner's syndrome*.
   (b) Testicular — eunuchoidism.
2. **Cushing's syndrome*.**
3. **Diabetes mellitus.**
4. **Acromegaly*.**
5. **Addison's disease.**
6. **Hyperthyroidism.**
7. **Mastocytosis** — mast cells produce heparin.

DISUSE

IATROGENIC

1. **Steroids*.**
2. **Heparin.**

DEFICIENCY STATES

1. **Vitamin C (scurvy*).**
2. **Protein.**

IDIOPATHIC

1. **In young people** — a rare self-limiting condition occurring in children of 8–12 years. Spontaneous improvement is seen.

CONGENITAL

1. **Osteogenesis imperfecta*.**
2. **Turner's syndrome*.**
3. **Homocystinuria*.**
4. **Neuromuscular diseases.**
5. **Mucopolysaccharidoses.**
6. **Trisomy 13 and 18.**
7. **Pseudohypoparathyroidism and pseudopseudohypoparathyroidism*.**
8. **Glycogen storage diseases.**
9. **Progeria.**

Further Reading

Herman T.E. & McAlister W.H. (1991) Inherited diseases in bone density in children. *Radiol. Clin. North Am.*, 29(1): 149–64.

1.33 OSTEOMALACIA AND RICKETS*

VITAMIN D DEFICIENCY

1. **Dietary.**
2. **Malabsorption.**

RENAL DISEASE

1. **Glomerular disease (renal osteodystrophy*).**
2. **Tubular disease**
   (a) Renal tubular acidosis
      (i) Primary — sporadic or hereditary.
      (ii) Secondary.
         Inborn errors of metabolism, e.g. cystinosis, galactosaemia, Wilson's disease, tyrosinosis, hereditary fructose intolerance.
         Poisoning, e.g. lead, cadmium, beryllium.
         Drugs, e.g. amphotericin B, lithium salts, outdated tetracycline, ifosfamide.
         Renal transplantation.
   (b) Fanconi syndrome — osteomalacia or rickets, growth retardation, renal tubular acidosis (RTA), glycosuria, phosphaturia, aminoaciduria and proteinuria. It is most commonly idiopathic in aetiology but may be secondary to those causes of RTA given above.
   (c) Vitamin D-resistant rickets (familial hypophosphataemia, X-linked hypophosphataemia) — short stature developing after the first 6 months of life, genu varum or valgum, coxa vara, waddling gait. Radiographic changes are more severe in the legs than the arms.

HEPATIC DISEASE

1. **Parenchymal failure.**
2. **Obstructive jaundice** — especially biliary atresia.

VITAMIN D-DEPENDENT RICKETS — see below

ANTICONVULSANTS

1. **Phenytoin and phenobarbitone.**

TUMOUR-ASSOCIATED

1. **Soft tissues** — haemangiopericytoma.
2. **Bone** — non-ossifying fibroma, giant cell tumour, osteoblastoma, osteosarcoma (and fibrous dysplasia, neurofibromatosis and melorrheostosis).

CONDITIONS WHICH MIMIC RICKETS/OSTEOMALACIA

1. **Hypophosphatasia*** — low serum alkaline phosphatase.
2. **Metaphyseal chondrodysplasia (type Schmid)** — normal serum phosphate, calcium and alkaline phosphatase differentiate it from other rachitic syndromes.

If the patient is less than 6 months of age then consider:

1. **Biliary atresia.**
2. **Metabolic bone disease of prematurity** — combined dietary deficiency and hepatic hydroxylation of vitamin D.
3. **Hypophosphatasia*.**
4. **Vitamin D-dependent rickets** — rachitic changes are associated with a severe myopathy in spite of adequate dietary intake of vitamin D.

Further Reading

Herman T.E. & McAlister W.H. (1991) Inherited diseases in bone density in children. *Radiol. Clin. North Am.*, 29(1): 149–64.

Sundaram M. & McCarthy E.F. (2000) Oncogenic osteomalacia. *Skeletal Radiol.*, 29: 117–24.

1.34 PERIOSTEAL REACTIONS — TYPES

(Modified from Ragsdale *et al*., 1981.)

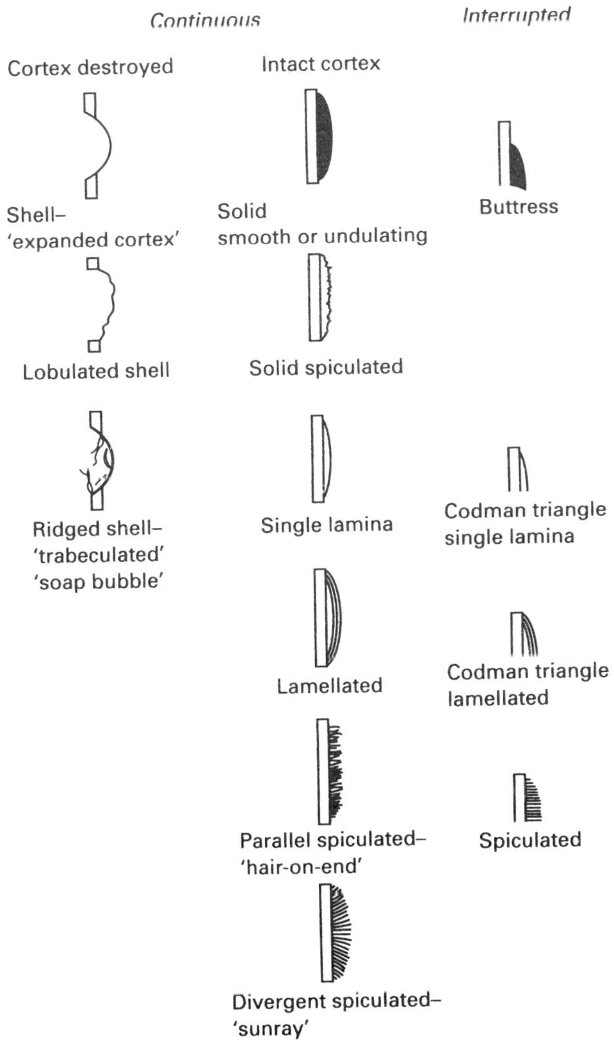

The different types are, in general, non-specific, having multiple aetiologies. However, the following comments can be made.

CONTINUOUS WITH DESTROYED CORTEX

This is the result of an expanding lesion. See 1.25 and 1.26.

PARALLEL SPICULATED ('HAIR-ON-END')

1. **Ewing's sarcoma*.**
2. **Syphilis.**
3. **Infantile cortical hyperostosis** (Caffey's disease).

See 12.72 for causes in the skull vault.

DIVERGENT SPICULATED ('SUNRAY')

1. **Osteosarcoma*.**
2. **Metastases** — especially from sigmoid colon and rectum.
3. **Ewing's sarcoma*.**
4. **Haemangioma*.**
5. **Meningioma.**
6. **Tuberculosis.**
7. **Tropical ulcer.**

CODMAN ANGLE (SINGLE LAMINA OR LAMELLATED)

1. **Aggressive malignant tissue extending into soft tissue.**
2. **Infection** — occasionally.

Further Reading

Ragsdale B.D., Madewell J.E. & Sweet D.E. (1981) Radiologic and pathologic analysis of solitary bone lesions. Part II: Periosteal reactions. *Radiol. Clin. North Am.*, 19: 749–83.

1.35 PERIOSTEAL REACTIONS – SOLITARY AND LOCALIZED

1. **Traumatic.**
2. **Inflammatory.**
3. **Neoplastic**
   (a) Malignant
      i primary.
      ii secondary.
   (b) Benign — an expanding shell or complicated by a fracture.

1.36 PERIOSTEAL REACTIONS – BILATERALLY SYMMETRICAL IN ADULTS

1. **Hypertrophic osteoarthropathy (HOA)** — clinically there is clubbing of the fingers and painful swelling of knees, ankles, wrists, elbows and metacarpophalangeal joints. The periosteal reaction occurs in the metaphysis and diaphysis of the radius, ulna, tibia, fibula and, less commonly, the humerus, femur and tubular bones of the hands and feet. It can be a single lamina, lamellated or solid and undulating. The thickness of the periosteal reaction correlates with the duration of disease activity. Periarticular osteoporosis, soft-tissue swelling and joint effusions are other features. The condition can be caused by the conditions in section 1.37 (q.v.).
2. **Pachydermoperiostosis** — a rare, self-limiting and familial condition, usually affecting boys at puberty and with a predilection for blacks. Clinically there is an insidious onset of thickening of the skin of the extremities (including the face), hyperhidrosis and clubbing. Compared with HOA it is relatively pain-free. The bones most commonly affected are the tibia, fibula, radius and ulna (less

commonly the carpus, tarsus and tubular bones of the hands and feet). The periosteal reaction is similar to HOA but is more solid and spiculated and also involves the epiphysis to produce outgrowths around joints. The concavity of the diaphysis may be filled in. ± Ligamentous calcification.

3. **Vascular insufficiency (venous, lymphatic or arterial)** — the legs are almost exclusively affected with involvement of tibia, fibula, metatarsals and phalanges. There is a solid undulating periosteal reaction, which is, initially, separated from the cortex but later merges with it. No definite relationship to soft-tissue ulceration. Phleboliths may be associated with venous stasis. Soft-tissue swelling is a feature whatever the aetiology. Arterial insufficiency due to polyarteritis nodosa or other arteritides may also be associated with a mild periostitis and is also usually confined to the lower limbs.
4. **Thyroid acropachy** — in 0.5–10% of patients following thyroidectomy for thyrotoxicosis and who may now be euthyroid, hypothyroid or hyperthyroid. Clinically there is soft-tissue swelling, clubbing, exophthalmos and pretibial myxoedema. A solid, spiculated, almost lace-like periosteal reaction affects the diaphysis of the metacarpals and phalanges of the hands, especially the radial side of the thumbs and index fingers. Less commonly the feet, lower legs and forearms are involved.
5. **Fluorosis** — solid, undulating periosteal reaction with osteosclerosis. The long bones and tubular bones are most frequently affected. Ligamentous calcification.
6. **Diffuse idiopathic skeletal hyperostosis (DISH; Forestier Disease)** — bone proliferation at sites of tendon and ligament insertions. Predominantly affects the spine but also seen at sacroiliac joints, symphysis pubis, coracoclavicular ligament, tibial tuberosity and interosseous membranes.

Further Reading

Pineda C.J., Sartoris D.J., Clopton P. *et al.* (1987) Periostitis in hypertrophic osteoarthropathy: relationship to disease duration. *Am. J. Roentgenol.*, 148: 773–8.

Vanhoenacker F.M. (2001) Thyroid acropachy: correlation of imaging and pathology. *Eur. Radiol.*, 11: 1058–62.

1.37 PERIOSTEAL REACTIONS – BILATERALLY ASYMMETRICAL

1. **Metastases.**
2. **Osteomyelitis.**
3. **Arthritides** — especially Reiter's syndrome* and psoriatic arthropathy*.
4. **Osteoporosis** (q.v.) } because of the increased
5. **Osteomalacia** (q.v.) } liability to fractures.
6. **Non-accidental injury*.**
7. **Bleeding diatheses.**
8. **Hand–foot syndrome** (sickle-cell dactylitis) — see Sickle-cell anaemia*.

Further Reading

Jurriaans E., Singh N.P., Finlay K. *et al.* (2001) Imaging of chronic recurrent multifocal osteomyelitis. *Radiol. Clin. North Am.*, 39(2): 305–27.

1.38 HYPERTROPHIC OSTEOARTHROPATHY

PULMONARY

1. **Carcinoma of bronchus.**
2. **Lymphoma*.**
3. **Abscess.**
4. **Bronchiectasis** — frequently due to cystic fibrosis*.
5. **Metastases.**

PLEURAL

1. **Pleural fibroma** — has the highest incidence of accompanying HOA, although it is itself a rare cause.
2. **Mesothelioma.**

CARDIOVASCULAR

1. **Cyanotic congenital heart disease** — produces clubbing but only rarely a periosteal reaction.

GASTROINTESTINAL

1. **Ulcerative colitis*.**
2. **Crohn's disease*.**
3. **Dysentery** — amoebic or bacillary.
4. **Lymphoma*.**
5. **Whipple's disease.**
6. **Coeliac disease.**
7. **Cirrhosis** — especially primary biliary cirrhosis.
8. **Nasopharyngeal carcinomas (Schmincke's tumour).**
9. **Juvenile polyposis.**

1.39 PERIOSTEAL REACTIONS – BILATERALLY SYMMETRICAL IN CHILDREN

1. **Normal infants** — diaphyseal, not extending to the growth plate, bilaterally symmetrical and a single lamina. Very unusual beyond 4 months of age.
2. **Juvenile idiopathic arthritis*** — in approximately 25% of cases. Most common in the periarticular regions of the phalanges, metacarpals and metatarsals. When it extends into the diaphysis it will eventually result in enlarged, rectangular tubular bones.
3. **Acute leukaemia** — associated with prominent metaphyseal bone resorption ± a dense zone of provisional calcification. Osteopenia. Periosteal reaction is due to cortical involvement by tumour cells. Metastatic neuroblastoma can look identical.
4. **Rickets*** — the presence of uncalcified subperiosteal osteoid mimics a periosteal reaction because the periosteum and ossified cortex are separated.
5. **Caffey's disease** — first evident before 5 months of age. Mandible, clavicles and ribs show cortical hyperostosis and a diffuse periosteal reaction. The scapulae and tubular bones are less often affected and tend to be involved asymmetrically.

6. **Scurvy*** — subperiosteal haemorrhage is most frequent in the femur, tibia and humerus. Periosteal reaction is particularly evident during the healing phase. Age 6 months or older.
7. **Prostaglandin E_1 therapy** — in infants with ductus-dependent congenital heart disease. Severity is related to duration of therapy. Other features include fever, flushing, diarrhoea, skin oedema, pseudowidening of cranial sutures and bone-in-bone appearance.
8. **Congenital syphilis** — an exuberant periosteal reaction can be due to infiltration by syphilitic granulation tissue or the healing (with callus formation) of osteochondritis. The former is essentially diaphyseal and the latter around the metaphyseal/ epiphyseal junction.

Further Reading

Matzinger M.A., Briggs V.A., Dunlap H.J. *et al.* (1992) Plain film and CT observations in prostaglandin-induced bone changes. *Pediatr. Radiol.*, 22: 264–6.

Shopfner C.E. (1966) Periosteal bone growth in normal infants. *Am. J. Roentgenol.*, 97: 154–63.

Swischuk L.E. & John S.D. (1995) *Differential Diagnosis in Pediatric Radiology*, 2nd edn. Baltimore: Williams and Wilkins, pp. 318–26.

1.40 DIFFERENTIAL DIAGNOSIS OF SKELETAL LESIONS IN NON-ACCIDENTAL INJURY*

Disease	*Shaft fractures*	*Abnormal metaphysis*	*Osteopenia*	*Periosteal reaction*	*Comments*
Non-accidental injury*	+	+	–	+	
Accidental trauma	+	–	–	callus	
Birth trauma	+	±	–	±	Clavicle, humerus and femur are most frequent fractures
Osteogenesis imperfecta*	+	±	+	–	Highly unlikely in the absence of osteopenia, wormian bones dentinogenesis imperfecta and a relevant family history
Osteomyelitis	–	+	localized	+	May be multifocal

Disease	*Shaft fractures*	*Abnormal metaphysis*	*Osteopenia*	*Periosteal reaction*	*Comments*
Rickets*	+	+	+	+	↑ Alkaline phosphatase
Scurvy*	–	+	+	+	Not before 6 months age
Congenital syphilis	–	+	–	+	
Congenital insensitivity to pain	+	+	–	+	
Paraplegia	+	+	+	with fractures	Lower limb changes only
Prostaglandin E_1 therapy	–	–	–	+	
Menke's syndrome	–	+	+	+	Males only. Abnormal hair. Retardation. Wormian bones
Copper deficiency	+	+	+	±	See note 1

[1]*Copper deficiency*. Rare. Unlikely in the absence of at least one risk factor — prematurity, total parenteral nutrition, malabsorption or a low copper diet. Unlikely in full term infants less than 6 months age. Microcytic, hypochromic anaemia. Leukopenia. Normal serum copper and caeruloplasmin does not exclude the diagnosis. Skull fracture never recorded in copper deficiency. Rib fractures only recorded in premature infants.

Further Reading

Chapman S. & Hall C.M. (1997) Non-accidental injury or brittle bones. *Pediatr. Radiol.*, 27: 106–10.

Kleinman P. (1998) *Diagnostic Imaging of Child Abuse,* 2nd edn. St Louis: Mosby.

Shaw J.C.L. (1988) Copper deficiency and non-accidental injury. *Arch. Dis. Childhood,* 63: 448–55.

1.41 SYNDROMES AND BONE DYSPLASIAS WITH MULTIPLE FRACTURES AS A FEATURE

WITH REDUCED BONE DENSITY

1. **Osteogenesis imperfecta*.**
2. **Achondrogenesis.**
3. **Hypophosphatasia.**
4. **Mucolipidosis II (I-cell disease).**
5. **Cushing's syndrome.**

WITH NORMAL BONE DENSITY

1. **Cleidocranial dysplasia.**
2. **Fibrous dysplasia.**

WITH INCREASED BONE DENSITY

1. **Osteopetrosis*.**
2. **Pyknodysostosis** — see 1.10.

1.42 EXCESSIVE CALLUS FORMATION

1. **Steroid therapy and Cushing's syndrome*.**
2. **Neuropathic arthropathy*** — including congenital insensitivity to pain.
3. **Osteogenesis imperfecta*.**
4. **Non-accidental injury*.**
5. **Paralytic states.**
6. **Renal osteodystrophy*.**
7. **Multiple myeloma*.**

1.43 STRESS FRACTURES – SITES AND CAUSATIONS

(Modified from Daffner, 1978.)

Site	*Activity*
Lower cervical/upper thoracic spinous processes	Clay shovelling
Pars interarticularis	Ballet; heavy lifting; scrubbing floors
Obturator ring	Stooping; bowling; gymnastics
Ribs	Carrying heavy pack; coughing; golf
Coracoid process of scapula	Trap shooting
Humerus — distal shaft	Throwing a ball
Hamate	Golf; tennis; baseball
Ulna — coronoid — shaft	Pitching a ball Pitchfork worker; propelling a wheelchair
Femur — neck — shaft	Ballet; marching; long-distance running; gymnastics Ballet; long distance running
Patella	Hurdling
Fibula — proximal shaft — distal shaft	Jumping; parachuting Long distance running
Tibia — proximal shaft — mid and distal shaft	Running Ballet; long distance running
Calcaneus	Jumping; parachuting; prolonged standing
Navicular	Marching; long distance runing
Metatarsal – shaft	Marching; prolonged standing; ballet
Sesamoids of metatarsals	Prolonged standing

Further Reading

Anderson M.W. & Greenspan A. (1996) Stress fractures. *Radiology,* 199: 1–12.
Daffner R.H. (1978) Stress fractures: current concepts. *Skeletal Radiol.,* 2: 221–9.

1.44 PSEUDARTHROSIS

1. **Non-union of a fracture** — including pathological fracture.
2. **Congenital** — in the middle to lower third of the tibia ± fibula. 50% present in the first year. Later there may be cupping of the proximal bone end and pointing of the distal bone end.
3. **Neurofibromatosis*.**
4. **Osteogenesis imperfecta*.**
5. **Cleidocranial dysplasia*** — congenitally in the femur.
6. **Fibrous dysplasia*.**
7. **Ankylosing spondylitis*** — in the fused bamboo spine.

Further Reading

Boyd H.B. & Sage F.P. (1958) Congenital pseudarthrosis of the tibia. *J. Bone Joint Surg.*, 40A; 1245–70.

Park W.M., Spencer D.G., McCall I.W. *et al.* (1981) The detection of spinal pseudarthrosis in ankylosing spondylitis. *Br. J. Radiol.*, 54: 467–72.

1.45 'BONE WITHIN A BONE' APPEARANCE

1. **Normal neonate** — especially in the spine.
2. **Growth arrest/recovery lines.**
3. **Paget's disease*.**
4. **Sickle-cell anaemia*.**
5. **Osteopetrosis*.**
6. **Acromegaly*.**
7. **Gaucher's disease.**
8. **Heavy metal poisoning.**
9. **Prostaglandin E_1 therapy** — see 1.39.

Further Reading

Brill P.W., Baker D.H. & Ewing M.L. (1973) Bone within bone in the neonatal spine. *Radiology,* 108: 363–6.

Frager D.H. & Subbarao K. (1983) The 'bone within a bone'. *J. Am. Med. Assoc.*, 249: 77–9.

Matzinger M.A., Briggs V.A., Dunlap H.J. *et al.* (1992) Plain film and CT observations in prostaglandin-induced bone changes. *Pediatr. Radiol.*, 22: 264–6.

O'Brien J.P. (1969) The manifestations of arrested bone growth: the appearance of a vertebra within a vertebra. *J. Bone Joint Surg.* 51A: 1376–8.

1.46 IRREGULAR OR STIPPLED EPIPHYSES

1. **Normal** — particularly in the distal femur.
2. **Avascular necrosis** (q.v.) — single, e.g. Perthes' disease (although 10% are bilateral), or multiple, e.g. sickle-cell anaemia.
3. **Congenital hypothyroidism*** — not present at birth. Delayed appearance and growth of ossification centres. Appearance varies from slightly granular to fragmentation. The femoral capital epiphysis may be divided into inner and outer halves.
4. **Morquio's syndrome*** — irregular ossification of the femoral capital epiphyses results in flattening.
5. **Multiple epiphyseal dysplasia** — onset 5–14 years. May be familial. Delayed appearance and growth of epiphyses but the time of fusion is normal. ± Metaphyseal irregularity. Carpal and tarsal bones, hips, knees and ankles are most commonly affected. Tibio–talar slant. Short, stubby digits and metacarpals. Spine usually, but not always, normal. Early and severe osteoarthritis.
6. **Meyer dysplasia** — an epiphyseal dysplasia resembling MED but confined to the femoral heads.
7. **Chondrodysplasia punctata** — autosomal dominant and (rarer) autosomal recessive types are recognized.
   (a) Autosomal dominant type (Conradi–Hünerman) — in the newborn stippling is evident in the long bone epiphyses, spine and larynx. ± Malsegmentation of vertebral bodies. Stippling disappears by 2 years of age. Asymmetrical shortening of limbs. Usually survive to adulthood.
   (b) Autosomal recessive (severe rhizomelic) type — marked symmetrical rhizomelia with humeri more severely affected than femora. Spinal stippling is mild. Stillborn or perinatal death.
8. **Trisomy 18 and 21.**
9. **Prenatal infections.**
10. **Warfarin embryopathy** — stippling of uncalcified epiphyses, particularly of the axial skeleton, proximal femora and calcanei. Disappears after first year.
11. **Zellweger syndrome** (cerebrohepatorenal syndrome).
12. **Fetal alcohol syndrome** — mostly calcaneum and lower extremities.

1.47 AVASCULAR NECROSIS

TOXIC

1. **Steroids*** — probably does not occur with less than 2 years of treatment.
2. **Anti-inflammatory drugs** — indomethacin and phenylbutazone.
3. **Alcohol** — possibly because of fat emboli in chronic alcoholic pancreatitis.
4. **Immunosuppressives.**

TRAUMATIC

1. **Idiopathic** — e.g. Perthes' disease and other osteochondritides.
2. **Fractures** — especially femoral neck, talus and scaphoid.
3. **Radiotherapy.**
4. **Heat** — burns.
5. **Fat embolism.**

INFLAMMATORY

1. **Rheumatoid arthritis*** } in the absence of drugs
2. **Systemic lupus erythematosus*** } probably due to a vasculitis.
3. **Scleroderma*.**
4. **Infection** — e.g. following a pyogenic arthritis
5. **Pancreatitis.**

METABOLIC AND ENDOCRINE

1. **Pregnancy.**
2. **Diabetes.**
3. **Cushing's syndrome*.**
4. **Hyperlipidaemias.**
5. **Gout*.**

HAEMOPOIETIC DISORDERS

1. **Haemoglobinopathies** — especially sickle-cell anaemia*.
2. **Polycythaemia rubra vera.**
3. **Gaucher's disease.**
4. **Haemophilia*.**

THROMBOTIC AND EMBOLIC

1. **Dysbaric osteonecrosis.**
2. **Arteritis.**

MRI detects changes earlier than CT or radionuclide scanning. These are:

	T_1W	T_2W	*Comment*
Margin	↓	↓	Well-delineated dark band
Central region			
Grade 1	↑ (= fat)	↑ (= fat)	Viable marrow fat due to revascularization. Haemorrhage
Grade 2	↑ or ↓	↑ or ↓	Oedema
Grade 3	↓	↑	Established sclerotic bone
Grade 4	↓	↓	

Further Reading

Boles C.A. & El-Khoury G.Y. (1997) Slipped capital femoral epiphysis. *RadioGraphics,* 17: 809–23.

1.48 SOLITARY RADIOLUCENT METAPHYSEAL BAND

Apart from point 3, this is a non-specific sign which represents a period of poor endochondral bone formation.

1. **Normal neonate.**
2. **Any severe illness.**
3. **Metaphyseal fracture** — especially in non-accidental injury*. Depending on the radiographic projection there may be the additional appearance of a 'corner' or 'bucket-handle' fracture.
4. **Healing rickets.**
5. **Leukaemia, lymphoma* or metastatic neuroblastoma.**
6. **Congenital infections.**
7. **Intrauterine perforation.**
8. **Scurvy*.**

Further Reading

Kleinman P.K., Marks S.C. & Blackbourne B. (1986) The metaphyseal lesion in abused infants: a radiologic-histopathologic study. *Am. J. Roentgenol.,* 146: 895–905.
Wolfson J.J. & Engel R.R. (1969) Anticipating meconium peritonitis from metaphyseal bands. *Radiology,* 92: 1055–60.

1.49 ALTERNATING RADIOLUCENT AND DENSE METAPHYSEAL BANDS

1. **Growth arrest or Park's lines.**
2. **Rickets*** — especially those types that require prolonged treatment such as vitamin D-dependent rickets.
3. **Osteopetrosis*.**
4. **Chemotherapy.**
5. **Chronic anaemias** — sickle-cell and thalassaemia.
6. **Treated leukaemia.**

Further Reading

Follis R.H. & Park E.A. (1952) Some observations on bone growth, with particular respect to zones and transverse lines of increased density in the metaphysis. *Am. J. Roentgenol;* 68: 709–24.

Roebuck D.J. (1999) Skeletal complications in pediatric oncology patients. *RadioGraphics,* 19: 873–85.

1.50 SOLITARY DENSE METAPHYSEAL BAND

1. **Normal infants.**
2. **Lead poisoning** — dense line in the proximal fibula is said to differentiate from normal. Other poisons include bismuth, arsenic, phosphorus, mercury fluoride and radium.
3. **Radiation.**
4. **Congenital hypothyroidism*.**
5. **Osteopetrosis*.**
6. **Hypervitaminosis D.**

Further Reading

Mitchell M.J. & Logan P.M. (1998) Radiation induced changes in bone. *RadioGraphics,* 18: 1125–36.

Raber S.A. (1999) The dense metaphyseal band sign. *Radiology,* 211: 773–4.

1.51 DENSE VERTICAL METAPHYSEAL LINES

1. **Congenital rubella** — celery stalk appearance. Less commonly in congenital CMV.
2. **Osteopathia striata** — ± exostoses.
3. **Hypophosphatasia*.**
4. **Localized metaphyseal injury.**

1.52 FRAYING OF METAPHYSES

1. **Rickets*.**
2. **Hypophosphatasia*.**
3. **Chronic stress (in the wrists of young gymnasts)** — with wide, irregular, asymmetrical widening of the distal radial growth plate and metaphyseal sclerosis.
4. **Copper deficiency.**

Further Reading

Carter S.R., Aldridge M.J., Fitzgerald R. *et al.* (1988) Stress changes of the wrist in adolescent gymnasts. *Br. J. Radiol.*, 61: 109–12.

Grünebaum M., Horodniceanu C. & Steinherz R. (1980) The radiographic manifestations of bone changes in copper deficiency. *Paed. Radiol.*, 9: 101–4.

1.53 CUPPING OF METAPHYSES

Often associated with fraying.

1. **Normal** — especially of the distal ulna and proximal fibula of young children. No fraying.
2. **Rickets*** — with widening of the growth plate and fraying.
3. **Trauma** — to the growth plate and/or metaphysis. Asymmetrical and localized changes.
4. **Bone dysplasias** — a sign in a large number, e.g. achondroplasia*, pseudoachondroplasia, metatropic dwarfism, diastrophic dwarfism, the metaphyseal chondrodysplasias and hypophosphatasia*.
5. **Scurvy*** — usually after fracture.

1.54 ERLENMEYER FLASK DEFORMITY

An Erlenmeyer flask is a wide-necked glass container used in chemical laboratories and named after the German chemist Richard August Carl Emil Erlenmeyer (1825–1907). The shape of the flask is also used to describe the distal expansion of the long bones, particularly the femora, that is observed in a number of the sclerosing skeletal dysplasias and in other afflictions of bone.

1. **Pyle's disease (metaphyseal dysplasia)** — rare. AR. Individuals have good health and normal life span. Genu valgum is associated with limited elbow extension. Cranial nerve compression and impairment of marrow function are not features of this sclerosing dysplasia. Radiologically there is sclerosis of the skull vault and base, widening of the medial ends of the clavicles and expansion of the pubic and ischial bones. The long bone metaphyses are grossly expanded, this expansion being most marked in the distal femora but also present in the proximal humeri, distal radii and ulnae, and proximal tibiae and fibulae. The expanded portions are relatively lucent and the mid-diaphyses show endosteal sclerosis.
2. **Craniometaphyseal dysplasia** — AD (common) or AR (rare). It is confused with Pyle's disease but unlike that condition Vth and VIIIth cranial nerve palsies do occur. The long bone modelling abnormalities are not as severe as Pyle's disease and although the distal femora are flask-shaped in childhood they are more club-shaped in adulthood.
3. **Osteodysplasty (Melnick–Needles syndrome)** — nearly all the reported cases have been females. Clinically these patients have bulging eyes, prominent cheeks, high forehead, malaligned teeth and micrognathia. Radiologically, the ribs are distorted and irregular and the clavicles are sigmoid-shaped. In addition to the metaphyseal flaring, the long bones show cortical irregularity, patchy sclerosis and an S-shape or bowing of the longitudinal axis. 'Osteodysplasty' means 'bones which are badly formed'.
4. **Osteopetrosis***.
5. **Thalassaemia** — coarse trabecular pattern, thickened calvarium with a spiculated or 'hair-on-end' appearance.
6. **Gaucher's disease** — three forms are recognized and are all due to a defect in the activity of the enzyme beta-glucosidase. AR. Infantile and juvenile types are lethal, due to accumulation of cerebrosides in the brain; the adult type is compatible with a

normal life span. This form has its maximal prevalence in Ashkenazi Jews, with an incidence as high as 1 in 2500. Presentation is usually with splenomegaly but orthopaedic problems and bone pain are important features. Skeletal involvement is evident by late childhood and includes patchy sclerosis and lysis, pathological fractures and avascular necrosis of femoral heads.

7. **Niemann–Pick Disease** — a rare disorder characterized by the accumulation of lipid in the body. Because the pathogenesis of this and Gaucher's disease are similar the skeletal manifestations are also similar but, unlike the latter condition, there is no epiphyseal osteonecrosis.
8. **Lead poisoning** — thick transverse dense metaphyseal bands are the classic manifestation of chronic infantile and juvenile lead poisoning. Additionally there may be flask-shaped femora which may persist for years before resolving.

Further Reading

Beighton P. & Cremin B.J. (1980) *Sclerosing Bone Dysplasias.* Berlin: Springer-Verlag.

Goldblatt J., Sacks S. & Beighton P. (1978) Orthopaedic aspects of Gaucher disease. *Clin. Orthop. Rel. Res.,* 137: 208–14.

Myer H.S., Cremin B.J., Beighton P. *et al.* (1975) Chronic Gaucher's disease: radiological findings in 17 South African cases. *Br. J. Radiol.,* 48: 465–9.

Pease C.N. & Newton G.G. (1962) Metaphyseal dysplasia due to lead poisoning in children. *Radiology,* 79: 233.

1.55 EROSIONS OF THE MEDIAL METAPHYSIS OF THE PROXIMAL HUMERUS

1. **Normal variant.**
2. **Leukaemia.**
3. **Metastatic neuroblastoma.**
4. **Gaucher's disease.**
5. **Hurler's syndrome*.**
6. **Glycogen storage disease.**
7. **Niemann–Pick disease.**
8. **Hyperparathyroidism.**
9. **Rheumatoid arthritis.**

Further Reading

Li J.K., Birch P.D. & Davies A.M. (1988) Proximal humerus defects in Gaucher's disease. *Br. J. Radiol.*, 61: 579–83.

1.56 EROSION OR ABSENCE OF THE OUTER END OF THE CLAVICLE

1. **Rheumatoid arthritis*.**
2. **Hyperparathyroidism*.**
3. **Multiple myeloma*.**
4. **Metastasis.**
5. **Post-traumatic osteolysis.**
6. **Cleidocranial dysplasia*.**
7. **Pyknodysostosis.**

1.57 FOCAL RIB LESION (SOLITARY OR MULTIPLE)

NEOPLASTIC

Secondary more common than primary. Primary malignant more common than benign.

1. **Metastases**
   (a) **Adult male** — bronchus, kidney or prostate most commonly.
   (b) **Adult female** — breast.
   (c) **Child** — neuroblastoma.
2. **Primary malignant**
   (a) **Multiple myeloma/plasmacytoma*.**
   (b) **Chondrosarcoma*.**
   (c) **Ewing's sarcoma*** — in a child.
   (d) **Askin tumour** — uncommon tumour of an intercostal nerve causing rib destruction.
3. **Benign**
   (a) **Osteochondroma*.**
   (b) **Enchondroma*.**
   (c) **Langerhans cell histiocytosis*.**

NON-NEOPLASTIC

1. **Healed rib fracture.**
2. **Fibrous dysplasia.**
3. **Paget's disease*.**
4. **Brown tumour of hyperparathyroidism*.**
5. **Osteomyelitis** — bacterial, tuberculous or fungal.

Further Reading

Guttentag A.R. & Salwen J.K. (1999) Keep your eyes on the ribs: the spectrum of normal variants and diseases that involve the ribs. *RadioGraphics,* 19: 1125–42.

Omell G.H., Anderson L.S. & Bramson R.T. (1973) Chest wall tumours. *Radiol. Clin. North Am.,* 11: 197–214.

1.58 RIB NOTCHING – INFERIOR SURFACE

ARTERIAL

1. **Coarctation of the aorta** — rib signs are unusual before 10 years of age. Affects 4–8th ribs bilaterally; not the upper two if conventional. Unilateral and right-sided if the coarctation is proximal to the left subclavian artery. Unilateral and left-sided if associated with an anomalous right subclavian artery distal to the coarctation. Other signs include a prominent ascending aorta and a small descending aorta with an intervening notch, left ventricular enlargement and possibly signs of heart failure.
2. **Aortic thrombosis** — usually the lower ribs bilaterally.
3. **Subclavian obstruction** — most commonly after a Blalock operation (either subclavian-to-pulmonary artery anastomosis) for Fallot's tetralogy. Unilateral rib notching of the upper three or four ribs on the operation side.
4. **Pulmonary oligaemia** — any cause of decreased pulmonary blood supply.

VENOUS

1. **Superior vena caval obstruction.**

ARTERIOVENOUS

1. **Pulmonary arteriovenous malformation.**
2. **Chest wall arteriovenous malformation.**

NEUROGENIC

1. **Neurofibromatosis*** — 'ribbon ribs' may also be a feature.

Further Reading

Boone M.L., Swenson B.E. & Felson B. (1964) Rib notching: its many causes. *Am. J. Roentgenol.*, 91: 1075–88.

1.59 RIB NOTCHING – SUPERIOR SURFACE

CONNECTIVE TISSUE DISEASES

1. **Rheumatoid arthritis*.**
2. **Systemic lupus erythematosus*.**
3. **Scleroderma*.**
4. **Sjögren's syndrome.**

METABOLIC

1. **Hyperparathyroidism*.**

MISCELLANEOUS

1. **Neurofibromatosis*.**
2. **Restrictive lung disease.**
3. **Poliomyelitis.**
4. **Marfan's syndrome*.**
5. **Osteogenesis imperfecta*.**
6. **Progeria.**

Further Reading

Boone M.L., Swenson B.E. & Felson B. (1964) Rib notching: its many causes. *Am. J. Roentgenol.*, 91: 1075–88.

1.60 WIDE OR THICK RIBS

1. **Chronic anaemias** — due to marrow hyperplasia.
2. **Fibrous dysplasia*.**
3. **Paget's disease*.**
4. **Healed fractures with callus.**
5. **Achondroplasia*.**
6. **Mucopolysaccharidoses.**

1.61 MADELUNG DEFORMITY

A deformity which comprises: (a) short distal radius which shows a dorsal and ulnar curve; (b) triangular shape of the distal radial epiphysis; (c) premature fusion of the ulnar side of the distal radial epiphysis; (d) dorsal subluxation of the distal ulna; (e) enlarged and distorted ulnar head; and (f) wedging of the triangular-shaped carpus between the distal radius and ulna.

1. **Isolated** — bilateral > unilateral. Asymmetrical. Predominantly adolescent or young adult women.
2. **Dyschondrosteosis (Leri–Weil disease)** — bilateral with mesomelic limb shortening. AD. Predominantly men.
3. **Diaphyseal aclasis.**
4. **Turner's syndrome*.**
5. **Post-traumatic.**
6. **Postinfective.**

1.62 CARPAL FUSION

ISOLATED

Tends to involve bones in the same carpal row (proximal or distal). More common in Afro-Caribbeans than Caucasians.

1. **Triquetral–lunate** — the most common site. Affects 1% of the population.
2. **Capitate–hamate.**
3. **Trapezium–trapezoid.**

SYNDROME-RELATED

Tends to exhibit massive carpal fusion affecting bones in different rows (proximal and distal).

1. **Acrocephalosyndactyly (Apert's syndrome).**
2. **Arthrogryposis multiplex congenita.**
3. **Ellis–van Creveld syndrome.**
4. **Holt–Oram syndrome.**
5. **Turner's syndrome*.**
6. **Symphalangism.**

ACQUIRED

1. **Inflammatory arthritides** — especially juvenile idiopathic arthritis* and rheumatoid arthritis*.
2. **Pyogenic arthritis.**
3. **Chronic tuberculous arthritis.**
4. **Post-traumatic.**
5. **Post-surgical.**

Further Reading

Cope J.R. (1974) Carpal coalition. *Clin. Radiol.*, 25: 261–6.

1.63 SHORT METACARPAL(S) OR METATARSAL(S)

As the sole or predominant abnormality.

1. **Idiopathic.**
2. **Post-traumatic** — iatrogenic, fracture, growth plate injury, thermal or electrical.
3. **Postinfarction** — e.g. sickle-cell anaemia*.
4. **Turner's syndrome*** — 4th ± 3rd and 5th metacarpals.
5. **Pseudohypoparathyroidism and pseudopseudohypoparathyroidism*** — 4th and 5th metacarpals.

Further Reading

Bell J. (1951) On brachydactyly and symphalangism. In: Penrose L.S. (ed.) *The Treasury of Human Inheritance*, Vol. 5, Part 1. Cambridge: Cambridge University Press, pp. 1–31.
Poznanski A.K. (1984) *The Hand in Radiologic Diagnosis*, 2nd edn, Vol. 1, Chapter 9. Philadelphia: Saunders, pp. 209–62.

1.64 ARACHNODACTYLY

Elongated and slender tubular bones of the hands and feet. The metacarpal index is an aid to diagnosis and is estimated by measuring the lengths of the 2nd, 3rd, 4th and 5th metacarpals and dividing by their breadths taken at the exact mid-points. These four figures are then added together and divided by 4.
Normal range 5.4–7.9.
Arachnodactyly range 8.4–10.4.
The metacarpal index is a poor discriminator between Marfan's syndrome and constitutional tall stature.

1. **Marfan's syndrome*** — although arachnodactyly is not necessary for the diagnosis.
2. **Homocystinuria*** — morphologically resembles Marfan's syndrome but 60% are mentally handicapped, they have a predisposition to arterial and venous thromboses and the lens of the eye dislocates downward rather than upward.

Further Reading

Eldridge R. (1964) The metacarpal index: a useful aid in the diagnosis of the Marfan syndrome. *Arch. Intern. Med.*, 113: 14–16.
Nelle M, Tröger J., Rupprath G. *et al.* (1994) Metacarpal index in Marfan's syndrome and in constitutional tall stature. *Arch. Dis. Child.*, 70: 149–50.

1.65 ABNORMAL THUMBS – CONGENITAL

BROAD

1. **Acrocephalopolysyndactyly (Carpenter type)** — two ossification centres for the proximal phalanx in childhood → duplication in adulthood.
2. **Acrocephalosyndactyly (Apert type)** — partial or complete duplication of the proximal phalanx. Complete syndactyly of digits II–V — 'mitten hand' and 'sock foot'.
3. **Diastrophic dysplasia** — short, ovoid thumb metacarpal with proximally located thumb.
4. **Rubinstein–Taybi syndrome** — terminal phalanx + 'hitch-hiker thumb'.
5. **Oto-palato-digital syndrome** — large cone epiphysis of the distal phalanx.

LARGE

1. **Klippel–Trenaunay–Weber syndrome.**
2. **Macrodystrophia lipomatosa.**
3. **Maffucci's syndrome.**
4. **Neurofibromatosis*.**

SHORT OR SMALL

1. **Fanconi's anaemia** — ± other radial ray abnormalities. Onset of pancytopaenia at 5–10 years of age.
2. **Holt–Oram syndrome** — finger-like, absent, hypoplastic or triphalangeal thumb + congenital heart disease (ASD, VSD).
3. **Brachydactyly C or D.**
4. **Cornelia de Lange syndrome** — hypoplastic metacarpal.
5. **Fetal hydantoin** — finger-like thumb with hypoplasia of all the distal phalanges.
6. **Fibrodysplasia ossificans progressiva.**

ABSENT

1. **Fanconi's anaemia.**
2. **Poland syndrome** — partial or complete absence of pectoralis muscles + abnormalities of the ipsilateral upper limb.
3. **Thalidomide.**
4. **Trisomy chromosome 18.**

TRIPHALANGEAL

1. **Fanconi's anaemia.**
2. **Holt–Oram syndrome.**
3. **Blackfan–Diamond syndrome** — pure red cell aplasia. Musculoskeletal abnormalities in 30%.
4. **Poland syndrome.**
5. **Trisomy chromosome 13 and 21.**
6. **Thalidomide.**

ABNORMALLY POSITIONED

1. **Cornelia de Lange syndrome** — proximally placed.
2. **Diastrophic dysplasia** — 'hitch-hiker thumb'.
3. **Rubinstein–Taybi syndrome** — 'hitch-hiker thumb' + broad terminal phalanx.

Further Reading

De Kerviler E., Guermazi A., Zagdanski A.-M. *et al.* (2000) The clinical and radiological features of Fanconi's anaemia. *Clin. Radiol.*, 55: 340–5.

Taybi H. & Lachman R.S. (1996) *Radiology of Syndromes, Metabolic Disorders and Skeletal Dysplasias,* 4th edn. St Louis: Mosby, pp. 1042–3.

1.66 DISTAL PHALANGEAL DESTRUCTION

NB. Because of reinforced Sharpey's fibres periosteal reaction is rare at this site.

RESORPTION OF THE TUFT

1. **Scleroderma*.**
2. **Raynaud's disease.**
3. **Psoriatic arthropathy*** — can precede the skin changes.
4. **Neuropathic diseases** — diabetes mellitus, leprosy, myelomeningocoele, syringomyelia and congenital indifference to pain.
5. **Thermal injuries** — burns, frostbite and electrical.
6. **Trauma.**
7. **Hyperparathyroidism*.**
8. **Epidermolysis bullosa.**
9. **Porphyria** — due to cutaneous photosensitivity leading to blistering and scarring.
10. **Phenytoin toxicity** — congenitally in infants of epileptic mothers.
11. **Snake and scorpion venom** — due to tissue breakdown by proteinases.

RESORPTION OF THE MID-PORTION

1. **Polyvinyl chloride tank cleaners.**
2. **Acro-osteolysis of Hajdu and Cheney.**
3. **Hyperparathyroidism*.**

PERIARTICULAR — i.e. erosion of the distal interphalangeal joints

1. **Psoriatic arthropathy*.**
2. **Erosive osteoarthritis.**
3. **Hyperparathyroidism*.**
4. **Thermal injuries.**
5. **Scleroderma*.**
6. **Multicentric reticulohistiocytosis.**

POORLY DEFINED LYTIC LESIONS

1. **Osteomyelitis** — mostly staphylococcal with diabetics at particular risk. Periosteal reaction is infrequent.

2. **Metastases** — bronchus is the most common primary site. Bone metastases to the hand are commonest in the terminal phalanx and may be the only metastasis to bone. The subarticular cortex is usually the last to be destroyed.
3. **Multiple myeloma*.**
4. **Aneurysmal bone cyst*** — rare at this site. Marked thinning and expansion of cortex.
5. **Giant cell tumour*** — usually involving the base of the phalanx.
6. **Leprosy** — at any age, but 30% present before 15 years of age.

WELL-DEFINED LYTIC LESIONS

1. **Implantation dermoid/epidermoid cyst** — an expanding lesion. 1–20 mm, with minimal sclerosis ± soft-tissue swelling.
2. **Enchondroma*.**
3. **Sarcoidosis*** — associated 'lace-like' destruction of phalangeal shaft, subperiosteal erosion leading to resorption of terminal tufts and endosteal sclerosis.
4. **Glomus tumour** — soft-tissue swelling with disuse osteoporosis because of pain. Bone involvement is uncommon but there may be pressure erosion or a well-defined lytic lesion.
5. **Osteoid osteoma*.**
6. **Fibrous dysplasia*.**

Further Reading

Jones S.N. & Stoker D.J. (1988) Radiology at your fingertips; lesions of the terminal phalanx. *Clin. Radiol.*, 39: 478–85.

Qteishat W.A., Whitehouse G.H. & Hawass N.E.D. (1985) Acroosteolysis following snake and scorpion envenomation. *Br. J. Radiol.*, 58: 1035–9.

1.67 FLUID–FLUID LEVELS IN BONE LESIONS ON CT AND MRI

BENIGN

1. **Aneurysmal bone cyst*.**
2. **Chondroblastoma*.**
3. **Giant cell tumour*.**
4. **Simple bone cyst*.**
5. **Fibrous dysplasia*.**

MALIGNANT

1. **Telangiectatic osteosarcoma*.**
2. **Malignant fibrous histiocytoma.**
3. **Any necrotic bone tumour.**

1.68 MRI OF NORMAL BONE MARROW

	T_1W	T_2W	*Comments*
Red marrow (haemopoietic)	↓	↑	Usually symmetrical in distribution but can mimic metastases in metaphyses of long bones. Reconversion to red marrow can occur due to increased demand (e.g. chronic anaemia, cardiac failure) or malignant infiltrate elsewhere in the skeleton.
Yellow marrow (fat)	↑	↑	Variable quantity, increases with age, can be focal in spine. Radiotherapy causes marked increase in fat.
Trabecular bone	↓	↓	Produces an inhomogeneous ripple in the applied magnetic field which produces a susceptibility artefact (signal loss due to dephasing). This is most marked on gradient echo images as there is no 180 degree rephasing pulse.
Epiphyseal plate	↓	↓	If the plate is at an angle to the scan plane it can appear as a patchy signal loss on T_1W and mimic a metastasis.

NB. Chemical shift artefact can interfere with visualization of the vertebral end-plates (particularly at high field strength). It occurs along the frequency encoded direction which is usually along the axis of the spine because the phase encoded axis is along the short axis of the image in order to decrease the time of the examination.

Further Reading

Hosten N., Schorner W., Neuman K. *et al.* (1993) MR imaging of bone marrow — review of the literature and possible indications for contrast enhanced studies. *Adv. MR Contrast,* 1: 84–98.

1.69 MRI OF ABNORMAL BONE MARROW

NB. Fat suppression/saturation techniques may be required to highlight the T_2 component of the lesion.

	T_1W	*T_2W*	*Comments*
Metastases			
– lytic	↓	±↑	
– sclerotic	↓	↓	Discs appear higher in signal intensity than adjacent vertebra on T_1W — normally they appear lower in signal intensity.
Myeloma	↓	±↑ (↓ after treatment)	
Lymphoma	↓	iso	
Osteoporotic vertebral collapse	±↓ due to oedema	±↑	Osteoporotic collapse is said not to have an associated epidural soft-tissue mass. However, discrimination from metastatic collapse is only possible if there is no oedema and the normal marrow signal is preserved. Osteoporotic and metastatic collapse can both show gadolinium enhancement.
Radiotherapy	↑++	±↑	The striking increase in signal on T_1W is due to fat deposition. There is a sharp cut off at the edge of the radiotherapy field. The increase in signal can be observed from 3 weeks after the radiotherapy.
Haemangioma	↑+	↑	Rounded in shape, relatively common.
Discitis	↓	↑	Vertebral end-plates destroyed.
Vertebral end-plate reaction to a degenerative disc:			
Type 1	↓	↑	Vascularised fibrous tissue. Intact vertebral end plate distinguishes it from discitis.
Type 2	↑	↑	Conversion of red to yellow marrow.
Gaucher's disease	↓	iso	
Bone marrow transplantation	↑ in centre with bands of ↓ around this due to regeneration of red marrow		

Further Reading

Deely D.M. & Schweitzer M.E. (1997) MR imaging of bone marrow disorders. *Radiol. Clin. North Am.*, 35(1): 193–212.

Vanel D., Dromain C. & Tardivon A. (2000) MRI of bone marrow disorders. *Eur. Radiol.*, 10: 224–9.

1.70 INCREASED UPTAKE ON BONE SCANS

1. **Metastatic disease** — multiple, randomly scattered lesions especially in the axial skeleton.
2. **Joint disease** — commonly degenerative in the cervical spine, hips, hands and knees. Also inflammatory joint disease.
3. **Traumatic fractures**
   (a) Aligned fractures in ribs are traumatic.
   (b) Single lesions elsewhere — always ask if history of trauma.
   (c) Stress fractures.
4. **Post surgery** — after joint replacement. Increased uptake lasts 1 year.
5. **Paget's disease*** — diffuse involvement with much increased uptake. Commonly affects the pelvis, skull, femur and spine. Involvement of the whole of the vertebra is typical.
6. **Superscan** — high uptake throughout the skeleton often due to disseminated secondary disease with poor or absent renal images but often with bladder activity. Look carefully at the skull and ribs where the inhomogeneity may be apparent.
7. **Metabolic bone disease** — high uptake in the axial skeleton, proximal long bones, with prominent calvarium and mandible. Faint or absent kidney images.
8. **Dental disease** — inflammation, recent extraction.
9. **Infection** — increased uptake in vascular and blood pool phases also.
10. **See 1.71.**

1.71 INCREASED UPTAKE ON BONE SCANS NOT DUE TO SKELETAL ABNORMALITY

ARTEFACTS

These are common.

1. **Patient**
   (a) Beware spots of urine in the pelvic area and urine on handkerchiefs.
   (b) Sweat — axillae.
   (c) Injection site.
   (d) Scars of recent operations.
   (e) Breast — accentuation of ribs at the lower border of the breast due to small angle scatter.
2. **Equipment**
   (a) Edge effect — increase in intensity at the edge of the field of view, especially in vertebrae.
   (b) Contamination of the collimator or crystal — check using a uniformity source.

PHYSIOLOGICAL VARIANTS

1. **Epiphyses in children.**
2. **Inferior angle of the scapula.**
3. **Calcification of cartilages** — especially those in the ribs and anterior neck.
4. **Bladder diverticulum.**
5. **Nipples** — especially confusing if at different heights.
6. **Renal pelvis.**

SOFT-TISSUE UPTAKE

1. **Calcification**
   (a) Myositis ossificans.
   (b) Soft-tissue osseous metaplasia.
   (c) Soft-tissue tumours with calcification.
   (d) Vascular calcification.
   (e) Calcific tendonitis.
   (f) Abscess.
2. **Others**
   (a) Acute infarction of the myocardium, cerebrum, skeletal muscle.
   (b) Malignant pleural effusion.

(c) Inflammatory carcinoma of the breast.
(d) Hepatic necrosis.
(e) Hepatic metastases — colon, breast, oat-cell carcinoma.
(f) Tumour uptake.

VISUALIZATION OF NORMAL ORGANS

1. **Free pertechnetate** — thyroid, stomach, salivary glands.
2. **Colloid formation** — liver, spleen and sometimes lung.
3. **Study on the previous day.**

1.72 PHOTOPENIC AREAS (DEFECTS) ON BONE SCANS

1. **Artefacts** — the commonest cause.
   (a) External — metal objects such as coins, belts, lockets, buckles.
   (b) Internal — joint prosthesis, pacemakers.
2. **Avascular lesions** — for example cysts.
3. **Multiple myeloma*** — may show increased uptake.
4. **Leukaemia** — may show increased uptake.
5. **Haemangiomas of the spine** — occasionally slightly increased uptake.
6. **Radiotherapy fields** — usually oblong in shape.
7. **Advanced cancer** — especially breast. Possibly related to chemotherapy.
8. **Spina bifida.**

Further Reading

Fogelman I. (ed.) (1987) *Bone Scanning in Clinical Practice.* London: Springer-Verlag.

1.73 ABNORMAL BONE SCAN WITH NORMAL OR MINIMAL RADIOGRAPHIC CHANGES

1. **Early disease**
   (a) Metastatic.
   (b) Paget's.
   (c) Osteomyelitis.
   (d) Asceptic necrosis.
   (e) Arthritides.
2. **Fractures**
   (a) Ribs.
   (b) Hands or feet.
3. **Lymphoma*.**
4. **Myelofibrosis.**
5. **Primary hyperparathyroidism*.**
6. **Osteodystrophy**
   (a) Renal.
   (b) Pulmonary.

Further Reading

Silberstein E.B. & McAfee J.G. (eds) (1984) *Differential Diagnosis in Nuclear Medicine.* New York: McGraw-Hill.

1.74 POSITIVE RADIOGRAPH WITH NORMAL BONE SCAN

1. **Benign conditions**
   (a) Bone cyst.
   (b) Bone island.
   (c) Exostoses.
2. **Recent fractures** — within 48 h.
3. **Multiple myeloma*.**
4. **Osteoporosis** — see 1.32.
5. **Metastases** — very rare but occurs if there is no osteoblastic reaction.

Further Reading

Silberstein E.B. & McAfee J.G. (eds) (1984) *Differential Diagnosis in Nuclear Medicine.* New York: McGraw-Hill.

2 Spine

2.1 IMAGING OF SPINAL ABNORMALITIES

1. **Plain Radiography (with tomography)** — still valuable for acute trauma and for long-term sequelae, congenital and other causes of spinal deformity, suspected spondylolisthesis, spinal (as opposed to radicular) pain, and survey views for metastases. Limited role in degenerative diseases (rarely contributes to management), and suspected spinal tumours (may show remodelling in slow-growing tumours such as neurofibroma and ependymoma).
2. **Myelography** — a largely obsolescent method, but widely used in the absence of sufficient availability of MRI. Certain attributes remain of considerable diagnostic value:
   (a) Suspected disc herniation: sensitive and specific, limited only by inability to show very laterally placed intraforaminal disc fragments.
   (b) Suspected spinal vascular malformation. More sensitive and more specific than MRI, which is sometimes equivocal due to flow-related artefacts.
   (c) Intraspinal mass lesions: sensitive, and specific in terms of the compartment involved by the tumour. In most cases it is possible to predict tumour type on the basis of the myelogram.
3. **CT** — of less overall usefulness compared with MRI, but having advantages in its better definition of bone and joint abnormalities.
   (a) Suspected disc herniation: of little value in the cervical region, but still regarded as sensitive in the detection of prolapsed lumbar disc. Sensitivity further enhanced by postmyelogram CT. Time and dose considerations usually confine the examination to three levels, and this can be a problem in atypical presentations. In the thoracic region, the lack of level-specific clinical information prevents the

effective use of CT, other than as a postmyelographic method, and where further assessment of previously detected calcification is required.

(b) Suspected fractures and dislocations: CT has great advantages in its potential for detailed study without additional trauma to the patient, and in its excellent definition of bone abnormalities. However, transversely-oriented fractures and mild wedge compression fractures are difficult to visualize.

(c) Facet joint disease: technique of choice in most cases, though MRI is not without usefulness in this area.

(d) Congenital abnormalities: spondylolisthesis, dysraphism, diastematomyelia, and foramen magnum anomalies require CT for full assessment.

(e) Bone tumours of the spine require CT for full assessment, particularly to identify and quantify any calcific components. Intraspinal tumours are not well shown, though calcific components may be shown in meningiomas, and fatty elements in dermoid and teratomatous lesions.

(f) Spinal infection: CT is sensitive in the demonstration of epidural and subdural abscess, though a high volume of intravenous contrast may be required. The extraspinal components are also well known.

4. **MRI** — the high soft-tissue contrast, the better tissue characterization, and the freedom from artefact make MRI the optimal technique in many types of spinal pathology. The lack of bone signal is an occasional disadvantage.

(a) Suspected disc herniation: sensitive and specific in the detection of disc herniation in cervical, thoracic and lumbar regions. Partial volume averaging and soft-tissue contrast problems sometimes limit the demonstration of laterally placed cervical disc fragments. Sagittal scanning allows for multilevel demonstrations, thereby avoiding errors due to over-reliance on clinical findings: this is particularly important in suspected thoracic disc.

(b) Spinal stenosis: sagittal sections allow for multilevel displays, which are invaluable in the detection of cervical and lumbar canal stenosis.

(c) Spinal tumours: the sensitivity of tumour detection is very high, and the good tissue characterization allows confident histological diagnosis in many cases. Gadolinium enhancement often useful: almost all tumours enhance; other expanding lesions such as infarcts, and acute plaques may not. The non-invasive nature of MRI avoids disturbance of CSF flow dynamics in the potentially unstable situation of total or near total spinal block. By contrast, myelography may precipitate the need for surgery.

(d) Vascular malformations: MRI will show the distended veins characteristic of spinal (usually dural) vascular malformations as flow voids, best shown on spin-echo T_2W sections. Sensitivity probably a little inferior to myelography.

(d) Arachnoiditis: adhesion of the nerves of the cauda equina to the theca and to themselves is best shown by MRI. Given that myelography has a causal role in many cases, it is undesirable to use this for its demonstration.

(e) Trauma: MRI will show ligamentous injury, particularly oedema and haemorrhage, whereas CT may appear normal or equivocal. Bone marrow oedema secondary to incremental fractures is also shown. Intraspinal complications of trauma (haemorrhage into the epidural or subdural space, or into the cord) are optimally shown by MRI.

(f) Spinal infection: MRI is rather more sensitive than CT for showing both the intraspinal and extraspinal components, and will demonstrate the rare intramedullary abscess, which CT is unlikely to show.

(g) Vascular and inflammatory lesions, including MS. MRI will show spinal cord infarction and haemorrhage, and also acute and chronic plaques in demyelinating disease.

Further Reading

Brant-Zawadzki M.N., Dennis S.C., Gade G.F. *et al.* (2000) Low back pain. *Radiology,* 217: 321–30.

Corr P. & Govender S. (1999) The role of magnetic resonance imaging on spinal trauma. *Clin. Radiol.,* 54: 629–35.

Harvey C.J., Richenberg J.L., Saifuddin A. *et al.* (1998) Pictorial review: the radiological investigation of lumbar spondylolysis. *Clin. Radiol.,* 53: 723–8.

Jevtic V. (2001) Magnetic resonance imaging appearances of different disc vertebral lesions. *Eur. Radiol.,* 11: 1123–35.

Laredo J.-D. (ed.) (2000) Imaging of low back pain I. *Radiol. Clin. North Am.,* 38(6).

Laredo J.-D. (ed.) (2001) Imaging of low back pain II. *Radiol. Clin. North Am.,* 39(1).

Morgan S. & Saifuddin A (1999) MRI of the lumbar intervertebral disc. *Clin. Radiol.,* 54: 703–23.

Nizard R.S., Wybier M. & Laredo J.-D. (2001) Radiologic assessment of lumbar intervertebral instability and degenerative spondylolisthesis. *Radiol. Clin. North Am.,* 39: 55–70.

Saifuddin A. (2000) The imaging of lumbar spinal stenosis. *Clin. Radiol.,* 55: 581–94.

Schonstrom N. & Willen J. (2001) Imaging lumbar spinal stenosis. *Radiol. Clin. North Am.,* 39: 31–53.

Wilmink J.T. (1999) MR imaging of the spine: trauma and degenerative disease. *Eur. Radiol.,* 9: 1259–66.

2.2 SCOLIOSIS

IDIOPATHIC

2% prevalence for curves > 10°.

1. **Infantile** — diagnosed before the age of 4 years. 90% are thoracic and concave to the right. More common in boys. 90% resolve spontaneously.
2. **Juvenile** — diagnosed between 4 and 9 years. More common in girls. Almost always progressive.
3. **Adolescent** — diagnosed between 10 years and maturity. More common in females. Majority are concave to the left in the thoracic region.

CONGENITAL

Prognosis is dependent on the anatomical abnormality and a classification (see figure opposite) is, therefore, important.

Failure of Formation. A. Incarcerated hemivertebra. A straight spine with little tendency to progression. **B.** Free hemivertebra. May be progressive. **C.** Wedge vertebra. Better prognosis than a free hemivertebra. **D.** Multiple hemivertebrae. Failure of formation on the same side results in a severe curve. Hemivertebrae on opposite sides may compensate each other. **E.** Central defect. Butterfly vertebra.

Failure of Segmentation. A. Bilateral → block vertebra and a short spine, e.g. Klippel–Feil. **B.** Unilateral unsegmented bar. Severely progressive curve with varying degrees of kyphosis or lordosis depending on the position of the bar.

Mixed defects. A. Unilateral unsegmented bar and a hemivertebra. Severely progressive. **B.** Partially segmented incarcerated hemivertebra. **C.** Bilateral failure of segmentation incorporating a hemivertebra.

Indicators of serious progression are:

(a) Deformity present at birth.
(b) Severe deformity of the chest wall.
(c) Unilateral unsegmented bars.
(d) Thoracic abnormality.

Associated abnormalities may occur — urinary tract (18%), congenital heart disease (7%), undescended scapulae (6%) and diastematomyelia (5%).

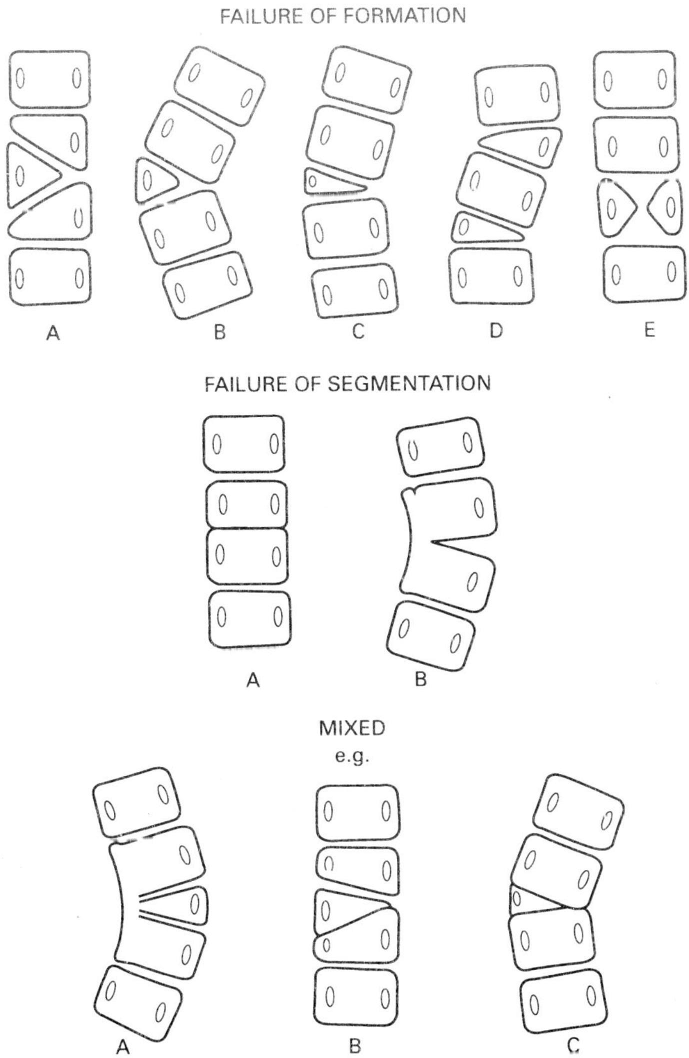

FAILURE OF FORMATION
A
B
C
D
E
FAILURE OF SEGMENTATION
A
B
MIXED
e.g.
A
B
C

NEUROPATHIC DISORDERS

1. **Tethered cord.**
2. **Syringomyelia.**
3. **Chiari malformations.**
4. **Diastematomyelia.**
5. **Meningocoele/myelomeningocoele.**

NEUROMUSCULAR DISEASES

1. **Myelomeningocoele.**
2. **Spinal muscular atrophy.**
3. **Friedreich's ataxia.**
4. **Poliomyelitis.**
5. **Cerebral palsy.**
6. **Muscular dystrophy.**

MESODERMAL AND NEUROECTODERMAL DISEASES

1. **Neurofibromatosis*** — in up to 40% of patients. Classically a sharply angled short segment scoliosis with a severe kyphosis. The apical vertebrae are irregular and wedged with adjacent dysplastic ribs. 25% have a congenital vertebral anomaly.
2. **Marfan's syndrome*** — scoliosis in 40–60%. Double structural curves are typical.
3. **Homocystinuria*** — similar to Marfan's syndrome.
4. **Other skeletal dysplasias** — spondyloepiphyseal dysplasia congenita, spondyloepimetaphyseal dysplasia, pseudoachondroplasia, metatropic dwarfism, diastrophic dwarfism, Kniest disease, spondylocostal dysostosis.

POST RADIOTHERAPY

Wedged and hypoplastic vertebrae ± unilateral pelvic or rib hypoplasia.

LEG LENGTH DISCREPANCY

A flexible lumbar curve, convex to the side of the shorter leg. Disparity of iliac crest level.

PAINFUL SCOLIOSIS

1. **Osteoid osteoma*** — 10% occur in the spine. A lamina or pedicle at the apex of the curve will be sclerotic or overgrown.

2. **Osteoblastoma*.**
3. **Intraspinal tumour** (see 2.21).
4. **Infection.**

Further Reading

Kim F.M., Poussaint T.Y. & Barnes P.D. (1999) Neuroimaging of scoliosis in childhood. *Neuroimaging Clin. North Am.*, 9(1): 195–221.

Redla S., Sikdar T. & Saifuddin A. (2001) Magnetic resonance imaging of scoliosis. *Clin. Radiol.*, 56: 360–71.

Winter R.B. (1983) *Congenital Deformities of the Spine.* New York: Thieme-Stratton.

2.3 SOLITARY COLLAPSED VERTEBRA

1. **Neoplastic disease**
   (a) Metastasis — breast, bronchus, prostate, kidney and thyroid account for the majority of patients with a solitary spinal metastasis. The disc spaces are preserved until late. The bone may be lytic, sclerotic or mixed. ± destruction of a pedicle.
   (b) Multiple myeloma/plasmacytoma* — a common site, especially for plasmacytoma. May mimic an osteolytic metastasis or be expansile and resemble an aneurysmal bone cyst.
   (c) Lymphoma*.
2. **Osteoporosis** (q.v.) — generalized osteopenia. Coarsened trabecular pattern in adjacent vertebrae due to resorption of secondary trabeculae.
3. **Trauma.**
4. **Infection** — with destruction of vertebral end-plates and adjacent disc spaces.
5. **Langerhans cell histiocytosis*** — eosinophil granuloma is the most frequent cause of a solitary vertebra plana in childhood. The posterior elements are usually spared.
6. **Benign tumours** — haemangioma, giant cell tumour and aneurysmal bone cyst.
7. **Paget's disease*** — diagnosis is difficult when a solitary vertebra is involved. Neural arch is affected in most cases. Sclerosis and expansion. If other non-collapsed vertebrae are affected then diagnosis becomes much easier.

Further Reading

Laredo J.-D., el Quessar A., Bossard P. *et al.* (2001) Vertebral tumours and pseudotumours. *Radiol. Clin. North Am.*, 39(1): 137–63.

Varma R., Lander P. & Assaf A. (2001) Imaging of pyogenic infectious spondylodiskitis. *Radiol. Clin. North Am.*, 39(2): 203–13.

2.4 MULTIPLE COLLAPSED VERTEBRAE

1. **Osteoporosis** (q.v.) — reduced bone density. Vertebral bodies may be wedged or biconcave (fish-shaped).
2. **Neoplastic disease** — wedge fractures are particularly related to osteolytic metastases and osteolytic marrow tumours, e.g. multiple myeloma, leukaemia and lymphoma. Altered or obliterated normal trabeculae. Disc spaces are usually preserved until late. Paravertebral soft-tissue mass is more common in myeloma than metastases.
3. **Trauma** — discontinuity of trabeculae, sclerosis of the fracture line due to compressed and overlapped trabeculae. Disc space usually preserved. The lower cervical, lower dorsal and upper lumbar spine are most commonly affected. Usually no soft-tissue mass. MRI usually shows the end-plates to be spared, c.f. pyogenic infection.
4. **Scheuermann's disease** — irregular end-plates and numerous Schmorl's nodes in the thoracic spine of children and young adults. Disc-space narrowing. Often progresses to a severe kyphosis. Secondary degenerative changes later.
5. **Infection** — destruction of end-plates adjacent to a destroyed disc. Although it is usually not possible to differentiate radiologically between pyogenic and tuberculous spondylitis in white patients the following signs are said to be helpful.

Pyogenic	*Tuberculous*
Rapidly progressive	Slower progression
Marked osteoblastic response	Less sclerosis
Less collapse	Marked collapse
Small or no paravertebral abscess	Large paravertebral abscess ± calcification
Early bridging of affected vertebrae	

In the acute phase of pyogenic spondylodiscitis, MRI typically shows low signal on T_1W, with loss of definition of the adjacent vertebral end-plates and high signal on T_2W of the disc and adjacent vertebral bodies. The disc shows a variable pattern of enhancement with gadolinium.

6. **Langerhans cell histiocytosis*** — the spine is more frequently involved in eosinophilic granuloma and Hand–Schüller–Christian disease than in Letterer–Siwe disease. Most common in young people. The thoracic and lumbosacral spine are the usual sites of disease. Disc spaces are preserved.

7. **Sickle-cell anaemia*** — characteristic step-like depression in the central part of the end-plate.

Further Reading

Laredo J.-D., el Quessar A., Bossard P. *et al.* (2001) Vertebral tumours and pseudotumours. *Radiol. Clin. North Am.*, 39(1): 137–63.
Mahboubi S. & Morris M.C. (2001) Imaging of spinal infections in children. *Radiol. Clin. North Am.*, 39(2): 215–22.
Moore S.L. & Rafii M. (2001) Imaging of musculoskeletal and spinal tuberculosis. *Radiol. Clin. North Am.*, 39(2): 329–42.
Varma R., Lander P. & Assaf A. (2001) Imaging of pyogenic infectious spondylodiskitis. *Radiol. Clin. North Am.*, 39(2): 203–13.

2.5 PLATYSPONDYLY IN CHILDHOOD

This sign describes a decrease in the distance between the upper and lower vertebral end-plates and should be differentiated from wedge-shaped vertebrae. Platyspondyly may be generalized, affecting all the vertebral bodies, multiple, affecting some of the vertebral bodies, or localized, involving one vertebral body (also termed vertebra plana).

CONGENITAL PLATYSPONDYLY

1. **Thanatophoric dwarfism** — inverted 'U'- or H-shaped vertebrae with a markedly increased disc space: body height ratio. Telephone handle-shaped long bones.
2. **Metatropic dwarfism.**
3. **Osteogenesis imperfecta*** — type IIA.

PLATYSPONDYLY IN LATER CHILDHOOD

1. **Morquio's disease*.**
2. **Spondyloepiphyseal dysplasia congenita.**
3. **Spondyloepiphyseal dysplasia tarda.**
4. **Kniest syndrome.**

ACQUIRED PLATYSPONDYLY — see 2.4

Further Reading

Kozlowski K. (1974) Platyspondyly in childhood. *Paed. Radiol.*, 2: 81–8.

2.6 EROSION, DESTRUCTION OR ABSENCE OF A PEDICLE

1. **Metastasis**
2. **Multiple myeloma***

} metastatic carcinoma involves the pedicle relatively early and contrasts with the late preservation of the pedicle in multiple myeloma.

3. **Neurofibroma** — often causes erosion of adjacent pedicle or pedicles. Chronic intramedullary tumours, typically ependymoma, cause flattening of both pedicles at affected levels, with a widened interpedicular distance.
4. **Tuberculosis** — uncommonly. With a large paravertebral abscess.
5. **Benign bone tumour** — aneurysmal bone cyst or giant cell tumour.
6. **Congenital absence** — ± sclerosis of the contralateral pedicle.

Further Reading

Bell D. & Cockshott W.P. (1971) Tuberculosis of the vertebral pedicle. *Radiology,* 99: 43–8.

2.7 SOLITARY DENSE PEDICLE

1. **Osteoblastic metastasis** — no change in size.
2. **Osteoid osteoma*** — some enlargement of the pedicle ± radiolucent nidus.
3. **Osteoblastoma*** — larger than osteoid osteoma and more frequently a lucency with a sclerotic margin rather than a purely sclerotic pedicle.
4. **Secondary to spondylolysis** — ipsilateral or contralateral.
5. **Secondary to congenitally absent or hypoplastic contralateral posterior elements.**

Further Reading

Laredo J.-D., el Quessar A., Bossard P. *et al.* (2001) Vertebral tumours and pseudotumours. *Radiol. Clin. North Am.,* 39(1): 137–63.

Pettine K. & Klassen R. (1986) Osteoid osteoma and osteoblastoma of the spine. *J. Bone Joint Surg.,* 68A: 354–61.

Wilkinson R.H. & Hall J.E. (1974) The sclerotic pedicle: tumour or pseudotumour? *Radiology,* 111: 683–8.

2.8 ENLARGED VERTEBRAL BODY

GENERALIZED

1. **Gigantism.**
2. **Acromegaly*.**

LOCAL (SINGLE OR MULTIPLE)

1. **Paget's disease*.**
2. **Benign bone tumour**
   (a) Aneurysmal bone cyst* — typically purely lytic and expansile. Involves the anterior and posterior elements more commonly than the anterior or posterior elements alone. Rapid growth.
   (b) Haemangioma* — with a prominent vertical trabecular pattern.
   (c) Giant cell tumour* — involvement of the body alone is most common. Expansion is minimal.
3. **Hydatid** — over 40% of cases of hydatid disease in bone occur in vertebrae.

Further Reading

Beabout J.W., McLeod R.A. & Dahlin D.C. (1979) Benign tumours. *Semin. Roentgonol.*, 14: 33–43.

Dahlin D.C. (1977) Giant cell tumour of vertebrae above the sacrum. A review of 31 cases. *Cancer*, 39: 1350–6.

Laredo J.-D., el Quessar A., Bossard P. *et al.* (2001) Vertebral tumours and pseudotumours. *Radiol. Clin. North Am.*, 39(1): 137–63.

Mohan V., Gupta S.K., Tuli S.M. *et al.* (1980) Symptomatic vertebral haemangiomas. *Clin. Radiol.*, 31: 575–9.

Koeller K.K., Rosenblum R.S. & Morrison A.L. (2000) Neoplasms of the spinal cord and filum terminale: radiologic-pathologic correlation. *RadioGraphics*, 20: 1721–49.

2.9 SQUARING OF ONE OR MORE VERTEBRAL BODIES

1. **Ankylosing spondylitis*.**
2. **Paget's disease*.**
3. **Psoriatic arthropathy*.**
4. **Reiter's syndrome*.**
5. **Rheumatoid arthritis*.**

2.10 BLOCK VERTEBRAE

1. **Klippel–Feil syndrome** — segmentation defects in the cervical spine, short neck, low hairline and limited cervical movement, especially rotation. The radiological appearance of the cervical spine resembles (1) above. C2–C3 and C5–C6 are most commonly affected. Other anomalies are frequently associated, the most important being
   (a) Scoliosis > 20° in more than 50% of patients.
   (b) Sprengel's shoulder in 30%, ± an omovertebral body.
   (c) Cervical ribs.
   (d) Genito-urinary abnormalities in 66%; renal agenesis in 33%.
   (e) Deafness in 33%.
2. **Isolated congenital** — a failure of segmentation. Most common in the lumbar spine but also occurs in the cervical and thoracic regions. The ring epiphyses of adjacent vertebrae do not develop and thus the AP diameter of the vertebrae at the site of the segmentation defect is decreased. The articular facets, neural arches or spinous processes may also be involved. A faint lucency representing a vestigial disc may be observed.
3. **Rheumatoid arthritis*** — especially juvenile onset rheumatoid arthritis and juvenile chronic arthritis with polyarticular onset. There may be angulation at the fusion site and this is not a feature of the congenital variety. The spinous processes do not fuse.
4. **Ankylosing spondylitis*** — squaring of anterior vertebral margins and calcification in the intervertebral discs and anterior and posterior longitudinal ligaments.
5. **Tuberculosis** — vertebral body collapse and destruction of the disc space, paraspinal calcification. There may be angulation of the spine.
6. **Operative fusion.**
7. **Post-traumatic.**

2.11 IVORY VERTEBRAL BODY

Single or multiple very dense vertebrae. The list excludes those causes where increased density is due to compaction of bone following collapse. If there is generalized involvement of the spine see 1.11.

1. **Metastases** — sclerotic metastases or an initially lytic metastasis which, after treatment, has become sclerotic. Usually no alteration in vertebral body size. Disc spaces preserved until late.
2. **Paget's disease*** — usually a single vertebral body is affected. Expanded body with a thickened cortex and coarsened trabeculation. Disc space involvement is uncommon.
3. **Lymphoma*** — more frequent in Hodgkin's disease than the other reticuloses. Normal size vertebral body. Disc spaces intact.
4. **Low-grade infection** — with end-plate destruction, disc-space narrowing and a paraspinal soft-tissue mass.
5. **Haemangioma** — sclerosis is accompanied by a coarsened trabecular pattern, predominantly vertical in orientation. ± expansion.

2.12 ATLANTOAXIAL SUBLUXATION

When the distance between the posterior aspect of the anterior arch of the atlas and the anterior aspect of the odontoid process exceeds 3 mm in adults and older children, or 5 mm in younger children, or an interosseous distance that changes considerably between flexion and extension.

TRAUMA

ARTHRITIDES

1. **Rheumatoid arthritis*** — in 20–25% of patients with severe disease. Associated erosion of the odontoid may be severe enough to reduce it to a small spicule of bone.
2. **Psoriatic arthropathy*** — in 45% of patients with spondylitis.
3. **Juvenile idiopathic arthritis*** — most commonly in seropositive juvenile onset adult rheumatoid arthritis.
4. **Systemic lupus erythematosus*.**
5. **Ankylosing spondylitis*** — in 2% of cases. Usually a late feature.

CONGENITAL

1. **Down's syndrome*** — in 20% of cases. ± odontoid hypoplasia. May, rarely, have atlanto–occipital instability.
2. **Morquio's syndrome*.**
3. **Spondyloepiphyseal dysplasia.**
4. **Congenital absence/hypoplasia of the odontoid process** — many have a history of previous trauma (NB. In children < 9 years it is normal for the tip of the odontoid to fall well below the top of the anterior arch of the atlas.

INFECTION

1. **Retropharyngeal abscess in a child.**

Further Reading

Elliott S. (1988) The odontoid process in children – is it hypoplastic? *Clin. Radiol.*, 39: 391–3.

Martel W. (1961) The occipito-atlanto-axial joints in rheumatoid arthritis and ankylosing spondylitis. *Am. J. Roentgenol.*, 86: 223–40.

Rosenbaum D.M., Blumhagen J.D. & King H.A. (1986) Atlanto-occipital instability in Down syndrome. *Am. J. Roentgenol.*, 146: 1269–72.

2.13 INTERVERTEBRAL DISC CALCIFICATION

1. **Degenerative spondylosis** — in the nucleus pulposus. Usually confined to the dorsal region. With other signs of degenerative spondylosis — disc-space narrowing, osteophytosis and vacuum sign in the disc. A frequent finding in the elderly.
2. **Alkaptonuria*** — symptoms of arthropathy first appear in the 4th decade. Widespread disc calcification, osteoporosis, disc-space narrowing and osteophytosis. The disc calcification is predominantly in the inner fibres of the annulus fibrosus but may be diffuse throughout the disc. Severe changes progress to ankylosis and may mimic ankylosing spondylitis.
3. **Calcium pyrophosphate dihydrate deposition disease*** — predominantly in the outer fibres of the annulus fibrosus.
4. **Ankylosing spondylitis*** — in the nucleus pulposus. Ankylosis, square vertebral bodies and syndesmophytes.
5. **Juvenile idiopathic arthritis*** — may mimic ankylosing spondylitis.
6. **Haemochromatosis*** — in the outer fibres of the annulus fibrosus.
7. **Diffuse idiopathic skeletal hyperostosis (DISH)** — may mimic ankylosing spondylitis.
8. **Gout*.**
9. **Idiopathic** — a transient phenomenon in children. The cervical spine is most often affected. Clinically associated with neck pain and fever but may be asymptomatic. Persistent in adults.
10. **Following spinal fusion.**

Further Reading

Weinberger A. & Myers A.R. (1978) Intervertebral disc calcification in adults: a review. *Semin. Arthritis Rheum.*, 18: 69–75.

2.14 BONY OUTGROWTHS OF THE SPINE

SYNDESMOPHYTES

Ossification of the annulus fibrosus. Thin, vertical and symmetrical. When extreme results in the 'bamboo spine'.

1. **Ankylosing spondylitis*.**
2. **Alkaptonuria.**

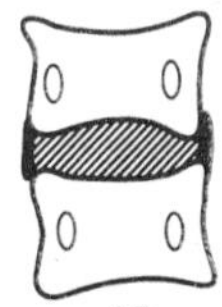

PARAVERTEBRAL OSSIFICATION

Ossification of paravertebral connective tissue which is separated from the edge of the vertebral body and disc. Large, coarse and asymmetrical.

1. **Reiter's syndrome*.**
2. **Psoriatic arthropathy*.**

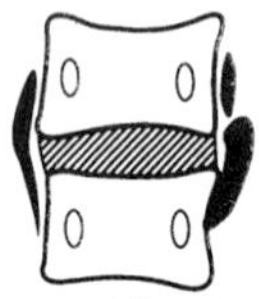

CLAW OSTEOPHYTES

Arising from the vertebral margin with no gap and having an obvious claw appearance.

1. **Stress response** — but in the absence of disc-space narrowing does not indicate disc degeneration.

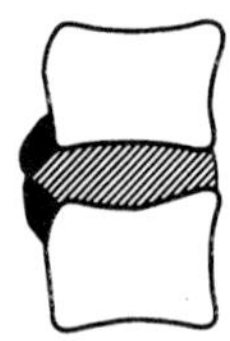

TRACTION SPURS

Osteophytes with a gap between the end-plate and the base of the osteophyte and with the tip not protruding beyond the horizontal plane of the vertebral end-plate.

1. **Shear stresses across the disc** — more likely to be associated with a degenerative disc.

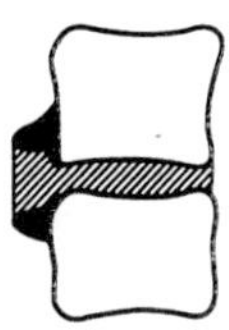

UNDULATING ANTERIOR OSSIFICATION

Undulating ossification of the anterior longitudinal ligament, intervertebral disc and paravertebral connective tissue.

1. **Diffuse idiopathic skeletal hyperostosis (DISH).**

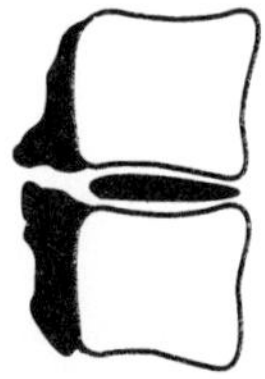

Further Reading

Jones M.D., Pais M.J. & Omiya B. (1988) Bony overgrowths and abnormal calcifications about the spine. *Radiol. Clin. North Am.*, 26: 1213–34.

2.15 CORONAL CLEFT VERTEBRAL BODIES

NORMAL VARIANT

Fusion of the anterior and posterior ossification centres of the vertebral body normally occurs before the 16th week of intrauterine life. Persisting notochordal remnants in the lower thoracic and lumbar region may prevent fusion but the condition usually resolves without sequelae in the first few months of life.

AS A FEATURE OF BONE DYSPLASIAS

1. **Chondrodysplasia punctata** — rhizomelic type.
2. **Kniest syndrome.**
3. **Metatropic dwarfism.**

ACQUIRED

As a result of herniation of a normal intervertebral disc into an osteoporotic vertebral body or secondary to trauma.

Further Reading

Fielden P. & Russell J.G. (1970) Coronally cleft vertebrae. *Radiology,* 21: 327–8.

Wilson A.R., Wastie M.L., Preston B.J. *et al.* (1989) Acquired coronal cleft vertebra. *Clin. Radiol.,* 40: 167–73.

2.16 ANTERIOR VERTEBRAL BODY BEAKS

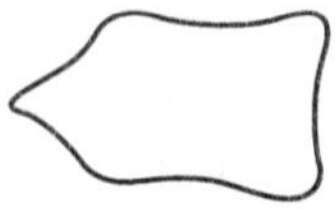

Central

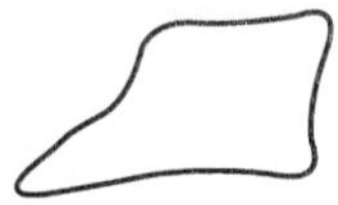

Lower third

Involves 1–3 vertebral bodies at the thoracolumbar junction and usually associated with a kyphosis. Hypotonia is probably the common denominator which leads to an exaggerated thoracolumbar kyphosis, anterior herniation of the nucleus pulposus and subsequently an anterior vertebral body defect.

CENTRAL

1. **Morquio's syndrome*.**

LOWER THIRD

1. **Hurler's syndrome*.**
2. **Achondroplasia*.**
3. **Pseudoachondroplasia.**
4. **Cretinism*.**
5. **Down's syndrome*.**
6. **Neuromuscular diseases.**

Further Reading

Swischuk L.E. (1970) The beaked, notched or hooked vertebra. Its significance in infants and young children. *Radiology*, 95: 661–4.

2.17 POSTERIOR SCALLOPING OF VERTEBRAL BODIES

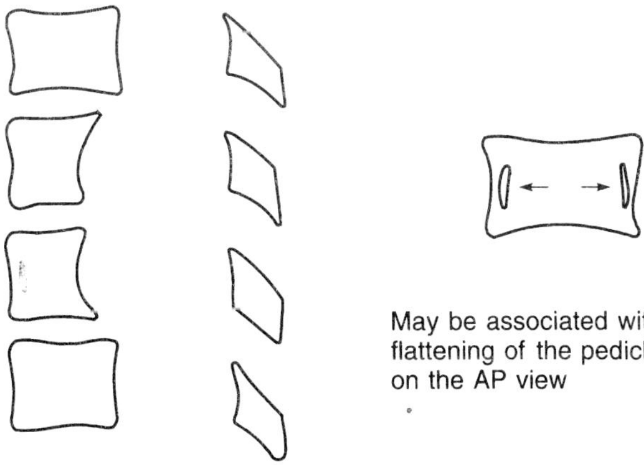

May be associated with flattening of the pedicles on the AP view

Scalloping is most prominent: (a) at either end of the spinal canal; (b) with large and slow growing lesions; and (c) with those lesions which originate during the period of active growth and bone modelling.

1. **Tumours in the spinal canal** — ependymoma (especially of the filum terminale and conus), dermoid, lipoma, neurofibroma and, less commonly, meningioma. Chronic raised intraspinal pressure distal to a tumour producing spinal block also causes extensive vertebral scalloping.
2. **Neurofibromatosis*** — scalloping is due to a mesodermal dysplasia and is associated with dural ectasia. Localized scalloping can also result from pressure resorption by a neurofibroma, in which case there may also be enlargement of an intervertebral foramen and flattening of one pedicle ('dumbbell tumour'). However, multiple wide thoracic intervertebral foramina are more likely owing to lateral meningocoeles than to local tumours.
3. **Acromegaly*** — other spinal changes include increased AP and transverse diameters of the vertebral bodies giving a spurious impression of decreased vertebral height, osteoporosis, spur formation and calcified discs.
4. **Achondroplasia*** — with spinal stenosis and anterior vertebral body beaks.
5. **Communicating hydrocephalus** — if severe and untreated.

6. **Syringomyelia** — especially if the onset is before 30 years of age.
7. **Other congenital syndromes**
   (a) Ehlers–Danlos
   (b) Marfan's*
   } both associated with dural ectasia.
   (c) Hurler's*.
   (d) Morquio's*.
   (e) Osteogenesis imperfecta*.

Further Reading

Mitchell G.E., Lourie H. & Berne A.S. (1967) The various causes of scalloped vertebrae and notes on their pathogenesis. *Radiology*, 89: 67–74.

2.18 ANTERIOR SCALLOPING OF VERTEBRAL BODIES

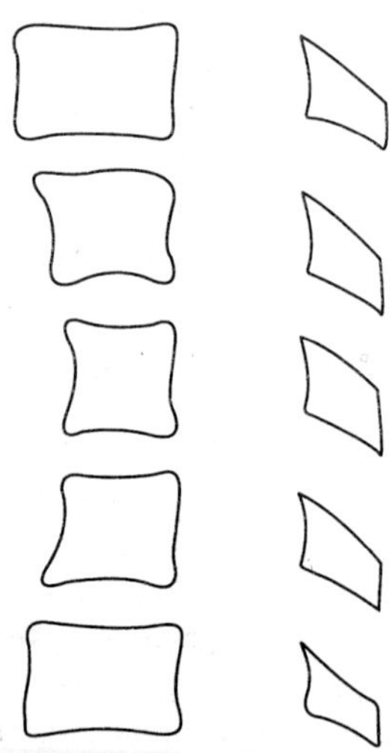

1. **Aortic aneurysm** — intervertebral discs remain intact. Well-defined anterior vertebral margin. ± Calcification in the wall of the aorta.
2. **Tuberculous spondylitis** — with marginal erosions of the affected vertebral bodies. Disc-space destruction. Widening of the paraspinal soft tissues.
3. **Lymphadenopathy** — pressure resorption of bone results in a well-defined anterior vertebral body margin unless there is malignant infiltration of the bone.
4. **Delayed motor development** — e.g. Down's syndrome.

2.19 SYNDROMES WITH A NARROW SPINAL CANAL

1. **Achondroplasia***.
2. **Hypochondroplasia** — AD. Large calvarium, short stature and long fibula.
3. **Pseudohypoparathyroidism* and pseudopseudohypoparathyroidism***.
4. **Diastrophic dwarfism.**
5. **Kniest syndrome.**
6. **Acrodysostosis.**

2.20 WIDENED INTERPEDICULAR DISTANCE

Most easily appreciated by comparison with adjacent vertebrae. ± Flattening of the inner side of the pedicles.

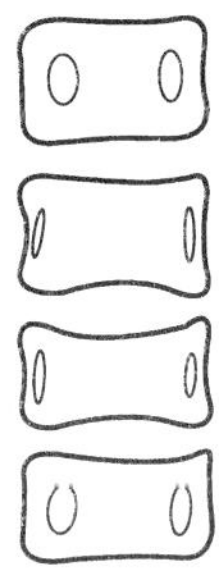

1. **Meningomyelocoele** — fusiform distribution of widened interpedicular distances with the greatest separation at the mid-point of the involved segment. Disc spaces are narrowed and bodies appear to be widened. Spinous processes and laminae are not identifiable. Facets may be fused into a continuous mass. Scoliosis (congenital or developmental) in 50–70% of cases ± kyphosis.
2. **Intraspinal mass** (see 2.21) — especially ependymoma.
3. **Diastematomyelia** — 50% occur between L1 and L3; 25% between T7 and T12. Widened interpedicular distances are common but not necessarily at the same level as the spur. The spur is visible in 33% of cases and extends from the neural arch forward. Laminar fusion associated with a neural arch defect at the same or adjacent level are important signs in predicting the presence of diastematomyelia. ± Associated meningocoele, neurenteric cyst or dermoid.

2.21 INTRASPINAL MASSES

Mass lesions in the spinal canal are classified as extradural, intradural and intramedullary in situation. Techniques for demonstration include plain radiography (to show secondary bony changes), myelography (obsolescent but much used in areas of inadequate MRI provision), CT (of limited value but may show bone changes, calcification and contrast uptake), and MRI, which is the definitive method at the present time.

The nature of an intraspinal mass may be partly elucidated by myelography, which allows the above subclassification to be made:

Extradural mass	Intradural mass (extramedullary)	Intramedullary mass

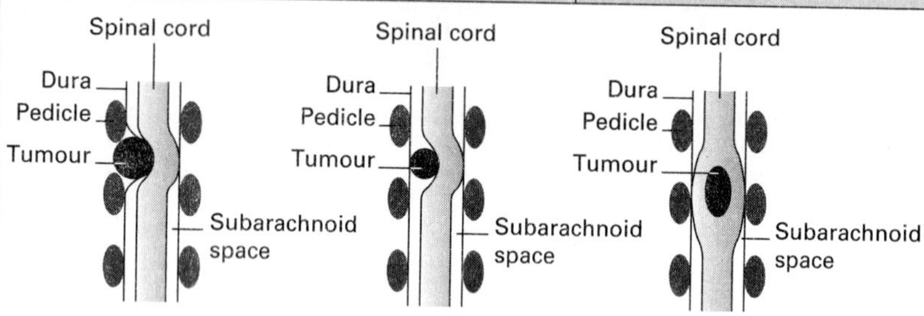

EXTRADURAL MASS

1. **Prolapsed or sequestrated intervertebral disc** — occurs at all levels. Usually extradural, but occasionally penetrates dura, especially in thoracic region. May calcify, especially thoracic disc prolapse.
2. **Metastases, myeloma and lymphoma deposits** — common; look for associated vertebral infiltration, destruction in body or neural arch, collapse, paravertebral mass, other bone lesions, evidence of primary tumour. Most common sites of primary tumours are prostate, breast and lung. Thoracic spine is the most common site affected, but there may be multiple sites.
3. **Neurofibroma** — solitary, or multiple in neurofibromatosis. Lateral indentation of theca at the level of the intervertebral foramen.
4. **Neuroblastoma and ganglioneuroma** — tumours of childhood arising in adrenal or sympathetic chain, close to spine: direct invasion of spinal canal may occur.

5. **Meningioma** — may be extradural, but most are largely intradural (see below). Commonest site is thoracic, middle-aged females predominate.
6. **Haematoma** — may be due to trauma, dural AVM, anticoagulant therapy, some spontaneous. Long-segment, extradural mass on MRI, which may show signal characteristics of blood.
7. **Abscess** — usually secondary to disc or vertebral sepsis. Long segment extradural mass, with marginal enhancement on CT and MRI.
8. **Arachnoid cyst** — secondary to developmental dural defect. Uncommon, most spinal arachnoid cysts are intradural.

INTRADURAL MASS

1. **Meningioma** — as above commonly thoracic, mainly in middle-aged females. Occasional calcification.
2. **Neurofibroma** — usually extradural, but intradural neurofibromas occur, especially in cauda equina.
3. **Metastases** — from remote primary tumours, or due to CSF seeding in CNS tumours, e.g. pineal tumours, ependymoma, medulloblastoma and primitive neuroectodermal tumour (PNET). Lymphoma may also occur intradurally, particularly in lumbosacral canal.
4. **Subdural empyema.**

INTRAMEDULLARY MASS

1. **Ependymoma** — can occur anywhere in spinal canal, but commonest at conus and in lumbar canal (from filum terminale). Very slow-growing, and bone remodelling is often seen with expansion of the spinal canal. Best shown on MRI: high signal mass on T_2W images, low on T_1W, but with enhancement. Associated cord cavitation may occur.
2. **Astrocytoma** — commonest intramedullary tumour. Appearances similar to ependymoma, but faster growing, and bone changes not a feature.
3. **Dermoid (including lipoma, teratoma)** — most commonly seen in conus medullaris. Different tissue elements include lipomatous tissue: low attenuation on CT, bright on T_1W MRI, cystic spaces (low attenuation on CT, low signal on T_1W, high on T_2W MRI), and soft tissue (intermediate density on CT, and intermediate signal on T_1W MRI, enhancing after gadolinium).

4. **Infarct** — expanding in acute phase.
5. **Haematoma** — cord swelling only on CT, but features of blood on MRI.

Further Reading

Koeler K.K., Rosenblum R.S. & Morrison A.L. (2000) Neoplasms of the spinal cord and filum terminale: radiologic-pathologic correlation. *RadioGraphics,* 20: 1721–49.

Loughrey G.J., Collins C.D., Todd S.M. *et al.* (2000) Magnetic resonance imaging in the management of suspected spinal canal disease in patients with known malignancy. *Clin. Radiol.,* 55: 849–55.

3 Joints

with contributions by Mark Davies

3.1 MONOARTHRITIS

1. **Trauma** — pointers to the diagnosis are: (a) the history, (b) the presence of a fracture, and (c) a joint effusion, especially a lipohaemarthrosis.
2. **Osteoarthritis** — including the late complication of avascular necrosis.
3. **Crystal-induced arthritis**
   (a) Gout*.
   (b) Calcium pyrophosphate dihydrate deposition disease*.
   (c) Calcium hydroxyapatite deposition disease.
4. **Rheumatoid arthritis*** — occasionally. Also juvenile idiopathic arthritis.
5. **Pyogenic arthritis** — commonest joints affected are the hip, knee and small joints of the hands and feet. 15% of those due to *Staphylococcus aureus* and 80% of those of gonococcal aetiology involve two or more joints. The joint may be radiographically normal at first presentation. Initially there is soft-tissue swelling due to effusion and synovial enlargement. Periarticular erosions progress to involve all of the articular cartilage and subchondral bone. Periosteal reaction. Osteoporosis follows the destructive changes.
6. **Tuberculous arthritis** — sometimes associated with pulmonary or renal tuberculosis. Similar sites of predilection to pyogenic arthritis. Insidious onset with radiological changes present at the time of first examination. Slowly developing osteoporosis precedes the destructive changes. Erosions first develop at peripheral non-contact points of the joint.
7. **Pigmented villonodular synovitis*** — most commonly at the knee.
8. **Sympathetic** — a joint effusion can occur as a response to a tumour in the adjacent bone.
9. **Neuropathic arthropathy*.**

Further Reading

Allman R.M., Brower A.C. & Kotlyarov E.B. (1988) Neuropathic bone and joint disease. *Radiol. Clin. North Am.*, 26: 1373–81.
Goldman A.B. & DiCarlo E.F. (1988) Pigmented villonodular synovitis. Diagnosis and differential diagnosis. *Radiol. Clin. North Am.*, 26(6): 1327–47.
Greenspan A. & Tehranzadeh J. (2001) Imaging of infectious arthritis. *Radiol. Clin. North Am.*, 39(2): 267–76.
Lin J., Jacobson J.A., Jamadar D.A.. *et al.* (1999) Pigmented villonodular synovitis and related lesions: the spectrum of imaging findings. *Am. J. Roentgenol.*, 172: 191–7.
Llauger J., Palmer J., Roson N. *et al.* (2000) Nonseptic monoarthritis: imaging features with clinical and histopathologic correlation. *RadioGraphics*, 20: S263–78.

3.2 NON-SEPTIC MONOARTHRITIS

1. **Gout*.**
2. **Synovial chondromatosis.**
3. **Amyloidosis.**
4. **Pigmented villonodular synovitis*.**
5. **Neuropathic arthropathy.**
6. **Milwaukee shoulder** — calcium hydroxyapatite and calcium pyrophosphate deposition.
7. **Rapid destructive arthritis of the hip.**

Further Reading

Gold R.H., Bassett L.W. & Seeger L.L. (1988) The other arthritides. *Radiol. Clin. North Am.*, 26: 1195–212.
Llauger J., Palmer J., Roson N. *et al.* (2000) Nonseptic monoarthritis: imaging features with clinical and histopathologic correlation. *RadioGraphics*, 20: S263–78.

3.3 THE MAJOR POLYARTHRITIDES

Inflammatory

Periarticular (synovial) erosions
Osteoporosis
Tendon-related erosions
Periosteal reaction
Syndesmophytes
Malalignment

Rheumatoid and its variants

Symmetrical
Small joints – esp. MCPJ and PIPJ
Osteoporosis

Rheumatoid arthritis
Systemic lupus erythematosus
Scleroderma
Dermatomyositis

Seronegative

Asymmetrical
Large joints – SIJs, spine and DIPJs of hand
Osteoporosis less marked
Periosteal reaction
Syndesmophytes

Ankylosing spondylitis
Reiter's syndrome
Psoriatic arthropathy
Enteropathic arthritis
Juvenile idiopathic arthritis

Chondropathic

Subchondral erosions
Subchondral sclerosis
Osteophytes
Chondroalcinosis
Normal bone density

Degenerative

Weight bearing joints, DIPJs and first CMCJs
Localized cartilage loss
Marginal calcification

Osteoarthritis
Neuropathic
Haemophilic

Metabolic

Atypical distribution
Uniform cartilage loss
Diffuse chondrocalcinosis
Large subchondral cysts
Greater destruction

Calcium pyrophosphate
Haemochromatosis
Alkaptonuria
Hyperparathyroidism
Wilson's disease

Depositional

Soft-tissue masses
Extra-articular erosions
– well defined
– roofed
– mass-related
Normal bone density

Gout
Hypercholesterolaemia
Reticulohistiocytosis
Amyloidosis

Further Reading

Gold R.H., Bassett L.W. & Seeger L.L. (1988) The other arthritides. Roentgenologic features of osteoarthritis, erosive osteoarthritis, ankylosing spondylitis, psoriatic arthritis, Reiter's disease, multicentric reticulohistiocytosis, and progressive systemic sclerosis. *Radiol. Clin. North Am.*, 26(6): 1195–212.

3.4 ARTHRITIS WITH OSTEOPOROSIS

1. **Rheumatoid arthritis*.**
2. **Juvenile idiopathic arthritis.**
3. **Systemic lupus erythematosus*.**
4. **Pyogenic arthritis.**
5. **Tuberculous arthritis.**
6. **Reiter's syndrome*** — in the acute phase.
7. **Scleroderma*.**
8. **Haemophilia*.**

3.5 ARTHRITIS WITH PRESERVATION OF BONE DENSITY

1. **Osteoarthritis.**
2. **Calcium pyrophosphate arthropathy** — see Calcium pyrophosphate dihydrate deposition disease*.
3. **Gout*.**
4. **Psoriatic arthropathy*.**
5. **Ankylosing spondylitis.**
6. **Reiter's syndrome*** — in chronic or recurrent disease.
7. **Neuropathic arthropathy*** — especially in the spine and lower extremities.
8. **Pigmented villonodular synovitis*.**

3.6 ARTHRITIS WITH A PERIOSTEAL REACTION

1. **Juvenile idiopathic arthritis*.**
2. **Reiter's syndrome*.**
3. **Pyogenic arthritis.**
4. **Psoriatic arthropathy*.**
5. **Rheumatoid arthritis*** — in less than 5% of patients.
6. **Hypertrophic osteoarthropathy.**
7. **Haemophilia*.**
8. **AIDS-associated arthritis.**

3.7 ARTHRITIS WITH PRESERVED OR WIDENED JOINT SPACE

1. **Early infective or inflammatory arthritis** — because of joint effusion.
2. **Psoriatic arthropathy*** — due to deposition of fibrous tissue.
3. **Acromegaly*** — due to cartilage overgrowth.
4. **Gout*.**
5. **Pigmented villonodular synovitis.**

3.8 ARTHRITIS WITH SOFT-TISSUE NODULES

1. **Gout*.**
2. **Rheumatoid arthritis*.**
3. **Pigmented villonodular synovitis*.**
4. **Multicentric reticulohistiocytosis.**
5. **Amyloidosis.**
6. **Sarcoidosis*.**

3.9 ARTHRITIS MUTILANS

A destructive arthritis of the hands and feet with resorption of bone ends and telescoping joints (main-en lorgnette).

1. **Rheumatoid arthritis***.
2. **Juvenile idiopathic arthritis***.
3. **Psoriatic arthropathy***.
4. **Diabetes.**
5. **Leprosy.**
6. **Neuropathic arthropathy***.
7. **Reiter's syndrome*** — in the feet.

3.10 DIFFUSE TERMINAL PHALANGEAL SCLEROSIS

1. **Normal variant** — in 10% of normal individuals.
2. **Rheumatoid arthritis*** — most commonly in association with erosive arthropathy but may occur in its absence.
3. **Scleroderma***.
4. **Systemic lupus erythematosus***.
5. **Sarcoidosis***.

Further Reading

Goodman N. (1967) The significance of terminal phalangeal osteosclerosis. *Radiology,* 89: 709–12.

Williams M. & Barton E. (1984) Terminal phalangeal sclerosis in rheumatoid arthritis. *Clin. Radiol.,* 35: 237–8.

3.11 CALCIFIED LOOSE BODY (SINGLE OR MULTIPLE) IN A JOINT

1. **Detached osteophyte** — larger and more variable in size than synovial osteochondromata. Other signs of degenerative arthritis.
2. **Osteochondral fracture.**
3. **Osteochondritis dissecans** — most commonly the knee, talus and elbow. A corresponding defect in the parent bone may be visible.
4. **Neuropathic arthropathy*** — joint disorganization.
5. **Synovial osteochondromatosis** — knee most commonly; hip, ankle, wrist and shoulder less commonly. Multiple small nodules of fairly uniform size. Faintly calcified initially; later ossified. Secondary erosion of intracapsular bone, joint-space narrowing and osteophyte formation may occur later in the disease.

3.12 CALCIFICATION OF ARTICULAR (HYALINE) CARTILAGE (CHONDROCALCINOSIS)

1. **Calcium pyrophosphate dihydrate deposition disease*.**
2. **Hyperparathyroidism*.**
3. **Haemochromatosis*.**
4. **Alkaptonuria.**
5. **Acromegaly*.**
6. **Gout*.**
7. **Wilson's disease.**

Further Reading

Jensen P. (1988) Chondrocalcinosis and other calcifications. *Radiol. Clin. North Am.*, 26: 1315–25.

3.13 SACROILIITIS

1. Changes initially in the lower and middle thirds of the joint and the iliac side is more severely affected than the sacral side.
2. Periarticular osteoporosis, superficial erosions and sclerosis of subchondral bone.
3. Further erosion leads to widening of the joint space.
4. Subchondral sclerosis progresses to bony ankylosis.
5. Eventual return of the bones to normal density.

The most typical patterns of distribution are:

BILATERAL SYMMETRICAL

1. **Ankylosing spondylitis*** — may be asymmetrical early in the disease. Radiological signs as above.
2. **Inflammatory bowel disease** — ulcerative colitis, Crohn's disease and Whipple's disease. Identical appearances to ankylosing spondylitis.
3. **Psoriatic arthropathy*** — ankylosis is less frequent than in ankylosing spondylitis. Occurs in 30–50% of patients with arthropathy. Less commonly is asymmetrical or unilateral.
4. **Osteitis condensans ilii** — predominantly in young, multiparous women. A triangular segment of bone sclerosis on the inferior aspect of the iliac side of the joint is associated with a well-defined joint margin and a normal joint space.
5. **Hyperparathyroidism*** — subchondral bone resorption and joint-space widening only.
6. **Paraplegia** — joint-space narrowing and osteoporosis.

BILATERAL ASYMMETRICAL

1. **Reiter's syndrome*.**
2. **Psoriatic arthropathy*** — this pattern in 40% of cases.
3. **Rheumatoid arthritis*** — rare. Minimal sclerosis and no significant bony ankylosis.
4. **Gouty arthritis (see Gout*)** — large well-defined erosions with surrounding sclerosis.
5. **Osteoarthritis** — the articular margins are smooth and well defined. Joint-space narrowing, subchondral sclerosis and anterior osteophytes are observed.

UNILATERAL

1. **Infection.**

3.14 PROTRUSIO ACETABULI

1. **Rheumatoid arthritis*** — including juvenile idiopathic arthritis.
2. **Osteoporosis** (q.v.).
3. **Osteomalacia and rickets** (q.v.)*.
4. **Paget's disease*.**
5. **Ankylosing spondylitis*.**
6. **Osteoarthritis** — occasionally.
7. **Psoriatic arthropathy*.**
8. **Trauma** — acetabular fractures.
9. **Familial or idiopathic.**
10. **Marfan's syndrome*** — 45% show evidence of protrusio acetabuli. Of these, 50% are unilateral and 90% have an associated scoliosis.

Further Reading

Kuhlman J.E., Scott W.W., Fishman E.K. *et al.* (1987) Acetabular protrusion in the Marfan Syndrome. *Radiology,* 164: 415–7.

3.15 WIDENING OF THE SYMPHYSIS PUBIS

> 10 mm in the newborn.
> 9 mm at age 3 years.
> 8 mm at 7 years and over.

ACQUIRED

1. **Pregnancy** — resolves by the 3rd postpartum month.
2. **Trauma.**

3. **Osteitis pubis** — one or more months after parturition or pelvic surgery, especially prostatic surgery. It may also be observed as a chronic stress reaction in athletes. Symmetrical bone resorption with subchondral bony irregularity and sclerosis. Ankylosis may be a late finding.
4. **Osteolytic metastases.**
5. **Infection** — low-grade osteomyelitis shows similar radiological features to osteitis pubis.
6. **Ankylosing spondylitis* and rheumatoid arthritis*** — early in the disease.
7. **Hyperparathyroidism*** — due to subperiosteal bone resorption.

CONGENITAL

With normal ossification

1. **Exstrophy of the bladder.**
2. **Epispadias** — the degree of widening correlates well with the severity of the epispadias.
3. **Hypospadias.**
4. **Imperforate anus with rectovaginal fistula.**
5. **Urethral duplication.**
6. **Prune belly syndrome.**
7. **Sjögren–Larsson syndrome.**
8. **Goltz syndrome.**

Poorly ossified cartilage

1. **Achondrogenesis.**
2. **Campomelic dysplasia.**
3. **Chondrodysplasia punctata (Conradi–Hünermann syndrome).**
4. **Chromosome 4p– syndrome (Wolf's syndrome).**
5. **Chromosome 9(p+) trisomy syndrome.**
6. **Cleidocranial dysplasia*.**
7. **Hypochondrogenesis.**
8. **Hypophosphatasia.**
9. **Hypothyroidism*.**
10. **Larsen syndrome.**
11. **Pycnodysostosis.**
12. **Spondyloepimetaphyseal dysplasia.**
13. **Spondyloepiphyseal dysplasia congenita.**

Further Reading

Abramson D., Roberts S.M. & Wilson P.D. (1934) Relaxation of pelvic joints in pregnancy. *Surg. Gynecol. Obstet.*, 58: 595–613.

Cortina H., Vallcanera A., Andres V. *et al.* (1979) The non-ossified pubis. *Pediatr. Radiol.*, 8: 87–92.

Muecke E.C. & Currarino G. (1968) Congenital widening of the symphysis pubis. Associated clinical disorders and roentgen anatomy of affected bony pelves. *Am. J. Roentgenol.*, 103: 179–85.

Patel K. & Chapman S. (1993) Normal symphysis pubis width in children. *Clin. Radiol.*, 47: 56–7.

Taybi H. & Lachman R.S. (1996) *Radiology of Syndromes, Metabolic Disorders, and Skeletal Dysplasias*, 4th edn. St Louis: Mosby, p. 1045.

Vix V.A. & Ryu C.Y. (1971) The adult symphysis pubis: normal and abnormal. *Am. J. Roentgenol.*, 112: 517–25.

3.16 FUSION OR BRIDGING OF THE SYMPHYSIS PUBIS

1. **Post-traumatic.**
2. **Postinfective.**
3. **Osteitis pubis** — see 3.16.
4. **Osteoarthritis.**
5. **Ankylosing spondylitis*.**
6. **Alkaptonuria*.**
7. **Fluorosis.**

3.17 FEMORAL HEAD AND NECK ABNORMALITIES

COXA MAGNA

The remodelled femoral head becomes wider and flatter.

1. **Developmental dysplasia of the hip.**
2. **Perthes' disease.**
3. **Septic arthritis.**

COXA PLANA

Flattened femoral head.

1. **Avascular necrosis**
   (a) Primary
      (i) Children — Perthes' disease.
      (ii) Adult — Chandler disease.
   (b) Secondary
      (i) Vascular.
         - Disruption — fracture, dislocation.
         - Vasculitis — collagen vascular disease, radiation.
         - Embolic — nitrogen (Caisson's disease).
         - Fat (pancreatitis, alcoholism).
         - Red blood cells (haemoglobinopathies).
         - Infiltration — Gaucher's disease.
      (ii) Hormonal — steroids, Cushing's syndrome.
      (iii) Pregnancy.

MRI is 95–100% sensitive in the acute stage when bone marrow oedema is seen. There are no early plain film signs. The earliest changes seen (after several weeks) are trabecular mottling, then focal sclerosis and osteopenia. After a few months, a radiolucent crescent is seen at the anterosuperior femoral head, parallel to the articular surface (best seen with a 'frog' lateral), that indicates subchondral collapse. The joint space is preserved. Later there is articular surface flattening and femoral head sclerosis, followed by femoral head collapse, acetabular involvement, joint-space narrowing and degenerative changes.

COXA VALGA

In coxa valga the femoral angle is increased, so the femoral neck becomes more vertical. This angle is normally about 150° at birth but reduces to 120–130° by adulthood.

IDIOPATHIC

Developmental

1. **Neuromuscular disorders.**
2. **Abductor muscle weakness.**
3. **Cleidocranial dysplasia*.**
4. **Diaphyseal aclasis** — multiple metaphyseal exostoses. Point away from the joint. May be associated with Madelung's deformity and supernumerary digits. The cartilaginous cap may show punctate calcification.
5. **Hunter's syndrome** — underdeveloped superior acetabular region, wide femoral neck, wide ribs with posterior tapering.
6. **Multiple enchondromatosis.**
7. **Diastrophic dwarfism.**

Inflammatory

1. **Juvenile idiopathic arthritis.**
2. **Poliomyelitis.**

Traumatic

1. **Femoral neck fracture.**

COXA VARA

In coxa vara the femoral angle is reduced so the femoral neck becomes more horizontal.

Developmental

1. **Neuromuscular disorders.**
2. **Developmental dysplasia of the hip.**
3. **Fibrous dysplasia*.**
4. **Cleidocranial dysplasia*.**
5. **Multiple epiphyseal dysplasia.**
6. **Osteogenesis imperfecta*.**
7. **Infantile (developmental) coxa vara** — M = F. 60–75% unilateral. Presents in the first few years of life. Painless lurching gait. Growth plate is widened and more vertically orientated than normal. A triangular piece of bone is seen in the femoral neck adjacent to the head that is bounded by two radiolucent bands traversing the neck and forming an inverted 'V'. Later a prominent greater trochanter is seen with thickened cortex along the medial aspect of the femoral neck due to remodelling.

8. **Proximal femoral focal deficiency** — a disease spectrum relating to partial absence and shortening of the proximal portion of the femur. Congenital but not inherited.

Inflammatory

1. **Rheumatoid arthritis*.**

Traumatic

1. **Slipped capital femoral epiphysis*.**
2. **Femoral neck fracture.**

Vascular

1. **Perthes' disease.**
2. **Avascular necrosis.**

Metabolic

1. **Renal osteodystrophy*.**
2. **Rickets*.**
3. **Paget's disease*.**

3.18 EROSION (ENLARGEMENT) OF THE INTERCONDYLAR NOTCH OF THE DISTAL FEMUR

1. **Juvenile idiopathic arthritis*.**
2. **Haemophilia*.**
3. **Psoriatic arthropathy*.**
4. **Tuberculous arthritis.**
5. **Rheumatoid arthritis*.**

3.19 PLANTAR CALCANEAL SPUR

1. **Idiopathic.**
2. **Diffuse idiopathic skeletal hyperostosis (DISH).**
3. **Ankylosing spondylitis*.**
4. **Psoriatic arthropathy*.**
5. **Reiter's syndrome*.**
6. **Rheumatoid arthritis*.**

3.20 MRI SIGNAL INTENSITIES IN MUSCULOSKELETAL IMAGING

Tissue	T_1W	*Proton density*	T_2W	T_2*
Cortical bone	↓	↓	↓	↓
Bone marrow	↑	↑	Intermediate	↓
Articular cartilage	Intermediate	Intermediate	↓	↑
Fibrocartilage	↓	↓	↓	↓
Ligament/tendon	↓	↓	↓	↓
Fat	↑	↑	Intermediate	↓
Nerve	↓	↓	↓	↓
Muscle	Intermediate	Intermediate	↓	↓
CSF	↓	Intermediate	↑	↑
Annulus fibrosus	↓	↓	↓	↓
Nucleus pulposus	Intermediate	Intermediate	↑	↑

3.21 INTRAMENISCAL SIGNAL CHANGES ON KNEE MRI

1. **Myxoid degeneration.**
2. **Meniscal tear.**
3. **Postoperative scar tissue.**

PITFALLS

1. **Popliteus tendon sheath.**
2. **Posterior ligaments of Humphry and Wrisberg.**
3. **Transverse ligaments.**
4. **Truncation artefact.**

Further Reading

Rubin D.A. (1997) MR imaging of the knee menisci. *Radiol. Clin. North Am.*, 35(1): 21–44.

4 Respiratory tract

4.1 ACUTE UPPER AIRWAY OBSTRUCTION

Most commonly in infants, because of the small calibre of the airways. Small or normal volume lungs with distension of the upper airway proximal to the obstruction during inspiration.

1. **Choanal atresia** — bilateral (33%) or unilateral, bony (90%) or membranous, complete or incomplete. When bilateral and complete, presentation is with severe respiratory distress at birth. Incomplete obstruction is associated with respiratory difficulty during feeding. Diagnosis is by failure to pass a catheter through the nose, and nasopharyngography or CT.
2. **Laryngo-tracheobronchitis** — narrowing of the glottic and subglottic regions. Indistinct tracheal margin because of oedema.
3. **Acute epiglottitis** — the epiglottis is swollen and may be shortened. Other components of the supraglottic region — aryepiglottic folds, arytenoids, uvula and prevertebral soft tissues — are also swollen. The hypopharynx and pyriform sinuses are distended with air.
4. **Retropharyngeal abscess** — enlargement of the prevertebral soft tissues which may contain gas or an air fluid level.
5. **Oedema** — caused by angio-oedema (allergic, anaphylactic or hereditary), inhalation of noxious gases or trauma. Predominantly laryngeal oedema.
6. **Foreign body** — more commonly produces a major bronchial occlusion rather than upper airway obstruction.
7. **Retropharyngeal haemorrhage** — due to trauma, neck surgery, direct carotid arteriography and bleeding disorders. Widening of the retropharyngeal soft-tissue space.

4.2 CHRONIC UPPER AIRWAY OBSTRUCTION IN A CHILD

May be associated with overinflation of the lungs.

NASAL

1. **Choanal atresia** — See 4.1.
2. **Nasal angiofibroma** — adolescent males. Symptoms of nasal obstruction and/or epistaxis. Plain films may show: (a) anterior bowing of the posterior wall of the maxillary antrum; (b) deviation of the nasal septum; and (c) a nasopharyngeal soft-tissue mass with erosion of contiguous bony structures.
3. **Antrochoanal polyp.**

SUPRAGLOTTIC

1. **Grossly enlarged tonsils and adenoids.**
2. **Laryngomalacia** — presents at or shortly after birth, persists for several months and usually resolves by 2 years. Diagnosis is confirmed by direct laryngoscopy, but fluoroscopy reveals anterior motion of the aryepiglottic folds and distension of the hypopharynx.
3. **Micrognathia** — in the Pierre Robin syndrome.
4. **Cysts** — of the epiglottis or aryepiglottic folds. The degree of obstruction depends on the size and location.

GLOTTIC

1. **Laryngeal polyp, papilloma or cyst.**

SUBGLOTTIC AND TRACHEAL

1. **Tracheomalacia** — weakness of tracheal wall which may be primary or secondary:

PRIMARY	Premature infants — probably related to intubation. Normal infants.
SECONDARY	With innominate artery compression — persistent narrowing of the anterior tracheal wall at the level of the thoracic inlet. With tracheo-oesophageal fistula/oesophageal atresia.

With vascular ring — most commonly a double aortic arch.
With external compression by tumour, etc.

2. **Subglottic haemangioma** — the most common subglottic soft-tissue mass in infancy. Occurs before 6 months. 50% have associated cutaneous haemangiomas. Characteristically it produces an asymmetrical narrowing of the subglottic airway.
3. **Following prolonged tracheal intubation** — see 4.3.
4. **External compression from other mediastinal structures** — e.g. lymphadenopathy or thymic enlargement.
5. **Respiratory papillomatosis** — occurs anywhere from the nose to the lungs. Irregular soft-tissue masses around the glottis or in the trachea mostly. (Papillomata in adults are usually single.)

Further Reading

Kushner, D.C. & Clifton Harris, G.B. (1978) Obstructing lesions of the larynx and trachea in infants and children. *Radiol. Clin. North Am.*, 16: 181–94.
Strife, J.L. (1988) Upper airway and tracheal obstruction in infants and children. *Radiol. Clin. North Am.*, 26: 309–22.

4.3 CHRONIC UPPER AIRWAY OBSTRUCTION IN AN ADULT

May be associated with overinflation of the lungs.

SUPRAGLOTTIC

1. **Supraglottic carcinoma of the larynx** — involving the posterior surface of the epiglottis, the ventricle or the superolateral part of the vestibule. Dyspnoea is a late feature.

GLOTTIC

1. **Vocal cord paralysis** — airway obstruction is most likely with bilateral recurrent nerve paresis and this most commonly occurs as a result of a thyroidectomy or malignant disease in the neck.
2. **Carcinoma of the glottis** — accounts for more than two-thirds of laryngeal carcinomas. Occurs mostly in the anterior two-thirds of the cords. Morphologically it can be proliferative or infiltrative.

SUBGLOTTIC AND TRACHEAL

1. **Extrinsic compression** — due to lymph nodes or local invasion from carcinomas of the bronchus, thyroid or oesophagus.
2. **Following prolonged tracheal intubation** — occurs in 5% of cases. The stenosis occurs most commonly at the level of the stoma. Less common sites are at the level of the inflatable cuff and where the tip impinges on the mucosa.
3. **Infraglottic carcinoma of the larynx** — either arising *de novo* at this site or as an extension from a glottic growth.
4. **Tracheal malignancy** — squamous cell carcinoma is the commonest tracheal primary.

Further Reading

Weber A.L. (ed.) (1978) The larynx and trachea. *Radiol. Clin. North Am.*, 16 (2).

4.4 UNEQUAL LUNG SIZE, LUCENCY AND VASCULARITY. WHICH IS THE ABNORMAL SIDE?

IF VASCULARITY IS DECREASED, THE LUNG IS ABNORMAL

IF VASCULARITY IS NORMAL OR INCREASED, THE LUNG IS PROBABLY NORMAL

A SMALL COMPLETELY OPAQUE HEMITHORAX IS ABNORMAL

When the small hemithorax is *completely* opaque the diagnosis is total collapse or agenesis. Furthermore, the atelectasis can be presumed to be resorptive (i.e. secondary to obstruction) rather than compressive (i.e. from an overdistended contralateral lung). This is because, *on the fully inspired film*, an overexpanded lung will never compress the other lung to the extent of obliterating the costophrenic angle.

WITH INSPIRATION – EXPIRATION, THE LUNG CHANGING LEAST OR NOT AT ALL, IS ABNORMAL

Further Reading

Swischuk L.E. & John S.D. (1995) *Differential Diagnosis in Paediatric Radiology*, 2nd edn. Baltimore: Williams & Wilkins, pp. 7–11.

4.5 UNILATERAL HYPERTRANSRADIANT HEMITHORAX

Exclude *contralateral* increased density, e.g. pleural effusion in a supine patient or pleural thickening.

ROTATION

1. **Poor technique**
2. **Scoliosis**

} the hypertransradiant hemithorax is the side to which the patient is turned.

CHEST WALL

1. **Mastectomy** — absent breast ± absent pectoral muscle shadows.
2. **Poliomyelitis** — atrophy of pectoral muscles ± atrophic changes in the shoulder girdle and humerus.
3. **Poland's syndrome** — unilateral congenital absence of pectoral muscles ± rib defects. Occurs in 10% of patients with syndactyly.

PLEURA

1. **Pneumothorax** — note the lung edge and absent vessels peripherally.

LUNG

1. **Compensatory emphysema** — following lobectomy (rib defects and opaque bronchial sutures indicate previous surgery) or lobar collapse.
2. **Obstructive emphysema** — due to bronchial stenosis or occlusion (q.v.). Air trapping on expiration results in increased lung volume and shift of the mediastinum to the contralateral side.
3. **Unilateral bullae** — vessels are absent rather than attenuated. May mimic pneumothorax.
4. **Macleod's syndrome** — the late sequela of childhood bronchiolitis. Small lung with small main and peripheral arteries. Air trapping occurs on expiration. Decreased number of bronchial divisions (5–10).
5. **Congenital lobar emphysema** — one-third present at birth. Marked overinflation of a lobe, most commonly the left upper lobe, right upper lobe or right middle lobe. The ipsilateral lobes

are compressed and there is mediastinal displacement to the contralateral side.

PULMONARY VESSELS

1. **Pulmonary embolus** (see Pulmonary embolic disease*) — to a major pulmonary artery (at least lobar in size). The pulmonary artery is dilated proximally and the affected lung shows moderate loss of volume.

4.6 BILATERAL HYPERTRANSRADIANT HEMITHORACES

WITH OVEREXPANSION OF THE LUNGS

1. **Chronic obstructive emphysema** — with large central pulmonary arteries and peripheral arterial pruning. ± Bullae.
2. **Asthma** — overinflation is secondary to bronchial constriction and mucus plugs.
3. **Acute bronchiolitis** — particularly affects children in the first year of life. Overexpansion is due to bronchial obstruction secondary to mucosal swelling, and this produces bronchial wall thickening on the radiograph. Collapse or consolidation is not a primary feature of the condition but is a frequent complication of it.
4. **Tracheal, laryngeal or bilateral bronchial stenoses** (see 4.7).

WITH NORMAL OR SMALL LUNGS

1. **Congenital heart disease producing oligaemia** — includes those conditions with right heart obstruction and right-to-left shunts. The hila are usually small except when there is post-stenotic dilatation of the pulmonary artery.
2. **Pulmonary artery stenosis** — if due to valvar stenosis, there is post-stenotic dilatation. 60% of congenital lesions have other associated cardiovascular abnormalities.

3. **Multiple pulmonary emboli** 4. **Primary pulmonary hypertension (PPH)** 5. **Schistosomiasis** 6. **Metastatic trophoblastic tumour**	identical radiological picture of big hilar vessels with peripheral pruning. History is most important. PP occurs predominantly in young females and may be familial. Schistosomiasis more usually presents as a diffuse reticulonodular pattern.

Further Reading

Frazier A.A., Galvin J.R., Franks T.J. *et al.* (2000) Pulmonary vasculature: hypertension and infarction. *RadioGraphics*, 20: 491–524.

Takasugi J.E. & Godwin J.D. (1998) Radiology of chronic obstructive pulmonary disease. *Radiol. Clin. North Am.*, 36(1): 29–55.

4.7 BRONCHIAL STENOSIS OR OCCLUSION

IN THE LUMEN

1. **Foreign body** — air trapping is more common than atelectasis. The lower lobe is most frequently affected. The foreign body may be opaque. The column of air within the bronchus may be discontinuous: the 'interrupted bronchus sign'.
2. **Mucus plug** — in asthma or cystic fibrosis.
3. **Misplaced endotracheal tube.**
4. **Aspergillosis** — with thickened bronchial walls.

IN THE WALL

1. **Carcinoma of the bronchus** — tapered narrowing ± irregularity.
2. **Bronchial adenoma** — usually a smooth, rounded filling defect, convex toward the hilum.
3. **Sarcoid granuloma.**
4. **Fibrosis** — e.g. tuberculosis and fungi. Can mimic carcinoma but usually produces a longer constriction.
5. **Bronchial atresia** — most commonly the apico-posterior segment of the left upper lobe.
6. **Fractured bronchus.**

OUTSIDE THE WALL

1. **Lymph nodes**
2. **Mediastinal tumour**
3. **Enlarged left atrium**

(1–3: smooth, eccentric narrowing.)

4. **Aortic aneurysm**
5. **Anomalous origin of left pulmonary artery from right pulmonary artery** — producing compression of the right main bronchus as it passes over it, between the trachea and oesophagus to reach the left hilum. PA chest X-ray shows the right side of the trachea to be indented and the vessel is seen end-on between the trachea and oesophagus on the lateral view.

Further Reading

Franquet T., Muller N.L., Gimenez A. *et al.* (2001) Spectrum of pulmonary aspergillosis: histologic, clinical, and radiologic findings. *RadioGraphics,* 21: 825–37.

Lim-Dunham J.E. & Yousefzadeh D.K. (1999) The interrupted bronchus: a fluoroscopic sign of bronchial foreign body in infants and children. *Am. J. Roentgenol.,* 173: 969–72.

Ward S. & Morcos S.K. (1999) Congenital bronchial atresia – presentation of three cases and a pictorial review. *Clin. Radiol.,* 54: 144–48.

4.8 INCREASED DENSITY OF A HEMITHORAX

WITH CENTRAL MEDIASTINUM

1. **Consolidation** — ± air bronchogram. Includes pneumonia, unilateral oedema (see 4.18), aspiration pneumonia and radiation pneumonitis.
2. **Pleural effusion** — when the patient is supine a small or moderate effusion gravitates posteriorly, producing a generalized increased density with an apical cap of fluid. Erect or decubitus films confirm the diagnosis.
3. **Mesothelioma** — often associated with a pleural effusion which obscures the tumour. Encasement of the lung limits mediastinal shift. ± Pleural calcification.

WITH MEDIASTINAL DISPLACEMENT AWAY FROM THE DENSE HEMITHORAX

1. **Pleural effusion** (q.v.) — NB. A large effusion with no mediastinal shift implies underlying collapse which, in an older person, is often secondary to a bronchial carcinoma.
2. **Diaphragmatic hernia** — on the right side with herniated liver; on the left side the hemithorax is not usually opaque because of air within the herniated bowel. The left hemithorax may be opaque in the early neonatal period when air has not yet had time to reach the herniated bowel.

WITH MEDIASTINAL DISPLACEMENT TOWARDS THE DENSE HEMITHORAX

1. **Collapse.**
2. **Post-pneumonectomy** — rib resection ± opaque bronchial sutures.
3. **Lymphangitis carcinomatosa** — unilateral disease is uncommon. Linear and nodular opacities ± ipsilateral hilar and mediastinal lymphadenopathy. Septal lines.
4. **Pulmonary agenesis and hypoplasia** — usually asymptomatic. Absent or hypoplastic pulmonary artery.

NB. 70% of unilateral diffuse lung opacities involve the right lung. Pneumonia, aspiration, pulmonary oedema, lymphangitis carcinomatosa and radiotherapy account for 90% (Youngberg, 1977).

Further Reading

Youngberg A.S. (1977) Unilateral diffuse lung opacity. *Radiology*, 123: 277–82.

4.9 PNEUMATOCELES

One or more air-filled, thin-walled 'cysts'. They are usually infective in origin and are thought to result from a check valve obstruction of a communication between a cavity and a bronchus. They appear during the first 2 weeks of the pneumonia and resolve within several months. They may contain fluid levels.

INFECTIONS

1. ***Staphylococcus aureus*** — a characteristic feature of childhood staphylococcal pneumonia, developing in 40–60% of cases.
2. ***Streptococcus pneumoniae.***
3. ***Escherichia coli.***
4. ***Klebsiella pneumoniae.***
5. ***Haemophilus influenzae.***
6. ***Pneumocystis carinii*** — usually multiple and in the upper parts of the lungs. Patients with cysts are more likely to suffer pneumothorax.
7. ***Legionella pneumophila* (Legionnaire's disease).**

TRAUMATIC

1. **Interstitial emphysema** — may be followed by thin-walled, air-containing cysts.

NEOPLASTIC

1. **Following treatment of pulmonary metastases** — bladder cancer and germ cell tumours. May be visible only on CT.

Further Reading

Charig M.J. & Williams M.P. (1990) Pulmonary lacunae: sequelae of metastases following chemotherapy. *Clin. Radiol.*, 42: 93–6.

Chow C., Templeton P.A. & White C.S. (1993) Lung cysts associated with *Pneumocystis carinii* pneumonia. *Am. J. Roentgenol.*, 161: 527–31.

4.10 SLOWLY RESOLVING OR RECURRENT PNEUMONIA

1. **Bronchial obstruction** — especially neoplasm or foreign body.
2. **Inappropriate chemotherapy** — especially for tuberculosis, *Klebsiella* and mycoses.
3. **Repeated aspiration**
   (a) Pharyngeal pouch.
   (b) Achalasia.
   (c) Scleroderma*.
   (d) Hiatus hernia.
   (e) 'H'-type tracheo-oesophageal fistula.
   (f) Paralytic or neuromuscular disorders.
   (g) Chronic sinusitis.
4. **Underlying lung pathology**
   (a) Abscess.
   (b) Bronchiectasis — see 4.14.
   (c) Cystic fibrosis*.
5. **Immunological incompetence**
   (a) Cachexia.
   (b) Steroids and immunosuppressives.
   (c) Diabetes.
   (d) White-cell and immunoglobulin deficiency states.
6. **Pneumonias that resolve by fibrosis**
   (a) Tuberculosis.
   (b) Fungi.

Further Reading

Franquet T., Gimenez A., Roson N. *et al.* (2000) Aspiration diseases: findings, pitfalls and differential diagnosis. *RadioGraphics*, 20: 673–85.
Hansell D.M. (1998) Bronchiectasis. *Radiol. Clin. North Am.*, 36(1): 107–28.
Harisinghani M.G., McLoud T.C., Shepard J.-A.O. *et al.* (2000) Tuberculosis from head to toe. *RadioGraphics*, 20: 449–70.

4.11 PNEUMONIA WITH AN ENLARGED HILUM

Hilar lymph node enlargement may be secondary to the pneumonia or pneumonia may be secondary to bronchial obstruction by a hilar mass. Signs suggestive of a secondary pneumonia are:

(a) Segmental or lobar consolidation which is better defined than a primary pneumonia.
(b) Slow resolution.
(c) Recurrent consolidation in the same part of the lung.
(d) Associated collapse.

SECONDARY PNEUMONIAS

See 4.7, but note particularly 'Carcinoma of the bronchus'.

PRIMARY PNEUMONIAS

1. **Primary tuberculosis** — lymph node enlargement is unilateral in 80% and involves the hilar (60%), or combined hilar and paratracheal (40%) nodes.
2. **Viral pneumonias.**
3. **Mycoplasma** — lymph node enlargement is common in children but rare in adults. May be unilateral or bilateral.
4. **Primary histoplasmosis** — in endemic areas. Hilar lymphadenopathy is common, particularly in children. During healing the lymph nodes calcify and may cause bronchial obstruction, thereby initiating distal infection.
5. **Coccidioidomycosis** — in endemic areas. The pneumonic type consists of predominantly lower lobe consolidation which is frequently associated with hilar lymph node enlargement.

See also 4.31.

4.12 LOBAR PNEUMONIA

Consolidation involving the air spaces of an anatomically recognizable lobe. The entire lobe may not be involved and there may be a degree of associated collapse.

1. ***Streptococcus pneumoniae*** — the commonest cause. Usually unilobar. Cavitation rare. Pleural effusion is uncommon. Little or no collapse.
2. ***Klebsiella pneumoniae*** — often multilobar involvement. Great propensity for cavitation and lobar enlargement.
3. ***Staphylococcus aureus*** — especially in children. 40–60% of children develop pneumatocoeles. Effusion (empyema) and pneumothorax are also common. Bronchopleural fistula may develop. No lobar predilection.
4. **Tuberculosis** — in primary or post-primary tuberculosis, but more common in the former. Associated collapse is common. The right lung is affected twice as often as the left, and primary tuberculosis predilects the anterior segment of the upper lobe or the medial segment of the middle lobe.
5. ***Streptococcus pyogenes*** — affects the lower lobes predominantly. Often associated with pleural effusion.

4.13 CONSOLIDATION WITH BULGING OF FISSURES

Homogeneous or inhomogeneous air-space opacification with bulging of the bounding fissures.

1. **Infection with abundant exudates** — *Klebsiella pneumoniae* (Friedländer's pneumonia), *Streptococcus pneumoniae*, *Mycobacterium tuberculosis* and *Yersinia pestis* (plague pneumonia).
2. **Abscess** — when an area of consolidation breaks down. Organisms which commonly produce abscesses are *Staphylococcus aureus*, *Klebsiella* spp. and other Gram-negative organisms.
3. **Carcinoma of the bronchus** — this can fill and expand a lobe.

4.14 BRONCHIECTASIS

1. Peribronchial thickening and retained secretions.
2. Crowded vessels, i.e. loss of volume.
3. Compensatory emphysema.
4. Cystic spaces ± air fluid levels.
5. Coarse honeycomb pattern in very severe disease.
6. Normal radiograph in 7%.

1. **Secondary to childhood infections** — especially measles and pertussis.
2. **Secondary to bronchial obstruction** — foreign body, neoplasm, mucus plugs (cystic fibrosis and asthma) and aspergillosis.
3. **Chronic aspiration.**
4. **Congenital structural defects**
   (a) Kartagener's syndrome — bronchiectasis with immobile cilia, dextrocardia and absent frontal sinuses. 5% of patients with dextrocardia will eventually develop bronchiectasis.
   (b) Williams–Campbell syndrome — bronchial cartilage deficiency.
5. **Immune deficiency states** — e.g. hypogammaglobulinaemia, chronic granulomatous disease, AIDS and Chédiak–Higashi syndrome.
6. **Collagen vascular diseases.**

Further Reading

McGuinness G. & Naidich D.P. (2002) CT of airways disease and bronchiectasis. *Radiol. Clin. North Am.*, 40(1): 1–19.

4.15 WIDESPREAD AIR-SPACE (ACINAR) DISEASE

This is commonly referred to as alveolar shadowing but the term is incorrect because the lung densities are due to the anatomically larger acinus. The general term 'air-space' shadow, nodule or disease is recommended. The signs of air-space disease are:

1. Acinar nodules, 4–10 mm in diameter.
2. Ill-defined margins.
3. Coalescence.
4. Mostly non-segmental.
5. Air bronchogram. NB. This sign may also be a feature of relaxation atelectasis (e.g. collapsed lung behind a large pneumothorax), cicatrization atelectasis (e.g. bronchiectasis and radiation fibrosis) and adhesive atelectasis (e.g. acute radiation pneumonitis and hyaline membrane disease).
6. Air bronchiologram and alveologram — lucencies due to residual air in bronchioles and alveoli.

1. **Oedema** (see 4.17).
2. **Pneumonia** — most often the unusual types
   (a) Tuberculosis.
   (b) Histoplasmosis.
   (c) *Pneumocystis carinii.*
   (d) Influenza — particularly in patients with mitral stenosis or who are pregnant.
   (e) Chicken pox — may be confluent in the central areas of the lungs. ± Hilar lymph node enlargement.
   (f) Other viral pneumonias.
3. **Haemorrhage**
   (a) Trauma (contusion).
   (b) Anticoagulants, haemophilia, leukaemia and disseminated intravascular coagulopathy.
   (c) Goodpasture's syndrome.
   (d) Idiopathic pulmonary haemosiderosis — in the acute stage.
4. **Fat emboli** — 1–2 days post-trauma. Predominantly peripheral. Resolves in 1–4 weeks. Normal heart size. Pleural effusions uncommon. Neurological symptoms in up to 85% and skin abnormalities in 20–50%.

5. **Alveolar cell carcinoma** — effusions are common. Mediastinal lymph nodes are uncommon. Diagnosis by sputum cytology or lung biopsy.
6. **Haematogenous metastases** — especially choriocarcinoma. Others are rare.
7. **Lymphoma*** — usually with hilar or mediastinal lymphadenopathy.
8. **Sarcoidosis*** — often associated with a reticulonodular pattern elsewhere.
9. **Löffler's** — peripheral ('reversed bat's wing'), often in the upper zones.

Further Reading

Fraser R.S., Müller N.L., Colman N & Paré P.D. (1999) *Fraser & Paré's Diagnosis of Diseases of the Chest,* 4th edn. Philadelphia. Saunders.

4.16 LOCALIZED AIR-SPACE DISEASE

See 4.15.

1. **Pneumonia.**
2. **Infarction** (see Pulmonary embolic disease*) — usually in the lower lobes. Often indistinguishable from pneumonia.
3. **Contusion** — ± rib fractures or other signs of trauma.
4. **Oedema** (see 4.17).
5. **Radiation** — several weeks following radiotherapy. May have a straight margin, corresponding to the field of treatment.
6. **Alveolar cell carcinoma.**
7. **Lymphoma*.**

4.17 PULMONARY OEDEMA

1. **Heart failure.**
2. **Fluid overload** — excess i.v. fluids, renal failure and excess hypertonic fluids, e.g. contrast media.
3. **Cerebral disease** — cerebrovascular accident, head injury or raised intracranial pressure.
4. **Near drowning** — radiologically no significant differences between fresh-water and sea-water drowning.
5. **Aspiration (Mendelson's syndrome).**
6. **Radiotherapy** — several weeks following treatment. May have a characteristic straight edge.
7. **Rapid re-expansion of lung following thoracentesis.**
8. **Liver disease and other causes of hypoproteinaemia.**
9. **Transfusion reaction.**
10. **Drugs**
    (a) Those which induce cardiac arrhythmias or depress myocardial contractility.
    (b) Those which alter pulmonary capillary wall permeability, e.g. overdoses of heroin, morphine, methadone, cocaine, 'crack', dextropropoxyphene and aspirin. Hydrochlorothiazide, phenylbutazone, aspirin and nitrofurantoin can cause oedema as an idiosyncratic response. Interleukin-2 and tumour necrosis factor may cause increased permeability by an unknown pathophysiological process.

NB. Contrast media can induce arrhythmias, alter capillary wall permeability and produce a hyperosmolar load.

11. **Poisons**
    (a) Inhaled — NO_2, SO_2, CO, phosgene, hydrocarbons and smoke.
    (b) Circulating — paraquat and snake venom.
12. **Mediastinal tumours** — producing venous or lymphatic obstruction.
13. **Shock lung (adult respiratory distress syndrome)** — 24–72 hours after insult.
14. **High altitude (acute mountain sickness)** — following rapid ascent to > 3000 metres.

Further Reading

Gluecker T., Capasso P., Schnider P. *et al.* (1999) Clinical and radiologic features of pulmonary edema. *RadioGraphics,* 19: 1507–31.

Milne E.N., Pistolesi M., Miniati M. *et al.* (1985) The radiological distinction of cardiogenic and noncardiogenic edema. *Am. J. Roentgenol.,* 144: 879–94.

4.18 UNILATERAL PULMONARY OEDEMA

PULMONARY OEDEMA ON THE SAME SIDE AS A PRE-EXISTING ABNORMALITY

1. **Prolonged lateral decubitus position.**
2. **Unilateral aspiration.**
3. **Pulmonary contusion.**
4. **Rapid thoracentesis of air or fluid.**
5. **Bronchial obstruction.**
6. **Systemic artery to pulmonary artery shunts** — e.g. Waterston (on the right side). Blalock–Taussig (left or right side) and Pott's procedure (on the left side).

PULMONARY OEDEMA ON THE OPPOSITE SIDE TO A PRE-EXISTING ABNORMALITY

Oedema on the side opposite a lung with a perfusion defect.

1. **Congenital absence or hypoplasia of a pulmonary artery.**
2. **Macleod's syndrome.**
3. **Thromboembolism.**
4. **Unilateral emphysema.**
5. **Lobectomy.**
6. **Pleural disease.**

Further Reading

Calenoff L., Kruglik G.D. & Woodruff A. (1978) Unilateral pulmonary oedema. *Radiology,* 126: 19–24.

4.19 SEPTAL LINES (KERLEY B LINES)

1. Due to visible interlobular lymphatics and their surrounding connective tissue.
2. 1–3 cm long, less than 1 mm thick, extending from and perpendicular to the pleural surface.
3. Best seen in the costophrenic angles.

PULMONARY VENOUS HYPERTENSION

1. **Left ventricular failure.**
2. **Mitral stenosis.**

LYMPHATIC OBSTRUCTION

1. **Pneumoconioses** — surrounding tissues may contain a heavy metal, e.g. tin, which contributes to the density.
2. **Lymphangitis carcinomatosa.**
3. **Sarcoidosis*** — septal lines are uncommon.

4.20 'HONEYCOMB LUNG'

1. A generalized reticular pattern or miliary mottling which, when summated, produces the appearance of air containing 'cysts' 0.5–2.0 cm in diameter.
2. Obscured pulmonary vasculature.
3. Late appearance of radiological signs after the onset of symptoms.
4. Complications
   (a) pneumothorax is frequent.
   (b) cor pulmonale later in the course of the disease.

1. **Collagen disorders**
   (a) Rheumatoid lung — most pronounced at the bases and may be preceded by basal infiltrates. ± Small effusions.
   (b) Scleroderma* — predominantly basal. Less regular 'honeycomb' pattern, which is preceded by fine, linear, basal streaks. Cor pulmonale is unusual.
2. **Extrinsic allergic alveolitis*** — predominantly in the upper zones.
3. **Sarcoidosis*** — sparing of extreme apices. Hilar lymphadenopathy usually resolved by this stage but, if present, it is a useful sign.
4. **Pneumoconiosis** — particularly frequent in asbestosis*, but also in other reactive dusts.
5. **Cystic bronchiectasis** (see 4.14) — in lower and middle lobes especially. Bronchial wall thickening. + Localized areas of consolidation.
6. **Cystic fibrosis*.**
7. **Drugs** — nitrofurantoin, busulphan, cyclophosphamide, bleomycin and melphalan.
8. **Langerhans cell histiocytosis*** — 'honeycomb' pattern probably always preceded by disseminated nodules. May be predominantly in the mid and upper zones. Cor pulmonale is uncommon.
9. **Lymphangioleiomyomatosis.**
10. **Tuberous sclerosis*** — lung involvement in 5% of patients. Symptoms first in adult life. Differentiated clinically.
11. **Idiopathic interstitial fibrosis (cryptogenic fibrosing alveolitis)** — no specific differentiating features. More marked in the lower half of the lungs initially and progresses to involve the whole of the lungs.
12. **Neurofibromatosis*** — ± rib notching, 'ribbon' ribs and/or scoliosis. In 10%, but not before adulthood.

4.21 PNEUMOCONIOSES

INORGANIC DUSTS

Without fibrosis

1. **Ferric oxide** — siderosis.
2. **Ferric oxide + silver** — argyrosiderosis.
3. **Tin oxide** — stannosis.
4. **Barium** — barytosis.
5. **Calcium.**

With fibrosis

1. **Free silica** — silicosis*.
2. **Coal dust** — coal miner's pneumoconiosis*.
3. **Silicates** — asbestosis*, china clay, talc and mica.

With chemical pneumonitis

1. **Beryllium.**
2. **Manganese.**
3. **Vanadium.**
4. **Osmium.**
5. **Cadmium.**
6. **Paraquat.**
7. **Hydrogen sulphide.**
8. **Ammonia.**
9. **Hydrocarbons.**

Carcinogenic dusts

1. **Radioactive dusts** — e.g. uranium.
2. **Asbestos** — see Asbestos inhalation*.
3. **Arsenic.**

ORGANIC DUSTS (EXTRINSIC ALLERGIC ALVEOLITIS*)

1. **Mouldy hay** — farmer's lung.
2. **Bagasse (sugar cane dust)** — bagassosis.
3. **Cotton or linen dust** — byssinosis.
4. **Mouldy vegetable compost** — mushroom worker's lung.
5. **Pigeon and budgerigar excreta** — pigeon breeder's and budgerigar fancier's lung.

Further Reading

Akira M. (2002) High-resolution CT in the evaluation of occupational and environmental disease. *Radiol. Clin. North Am.*, 40(1): 43–60.

Kim K.-I., Kim C.W., Lee M.K. *et al.* (2001) Imaging of occupational lung disease. *RadioGraphics*, 21: 1371–91.

McLoud T.C. (ed.) (1992) Occupational lung disease. *Radiol. Clin. North Am.*, 30 (6).

4.22 MULTIPLE PIN-POINT OPACITIES

Must be of very high atomic number to be rendered visible.

1. **Post lymphangiography** — iodized oil emboli. Contrast medium may be visible at the site of termination of the thoracic duct.
2. **Silicosis*** — usually larger than pin-point but can be very dense, especially in gold miners.
3. **Stannosis** — inhalation of tin oxide. Even distribution throughout the lungs. With Kerley A and B lines.
4. **Barytosis** — inhalation of barytes. Very dense, discrete opacities. Generalized distribution but bases and apices usually spared.
5. **Limestone and marble workers** — inhalation of calcium.
6. **Alveolar microlithiasis** — familial. Lung detail obscured by miliary calcifications. Few symptoms but may progress to cor pulmonale eventually. Pleura, heart and diaphragm may be seen as negative shadows.

4.23 MULTIPLE OPACITIES (0.5–2 mm)

SOFT-TISSUE DENSITY

1. **Miliary tuberculosis** — widespread. Uniform size. Indistinct margins but discrete. No septal lines. Normal hila unless superimposed on primary tuberculosis.
2. **Fungal diseases** — miliary histoplasmosis, coccidioidomycosis, blastomycosis and *Cryptococcus* (torulosis). Similar appearance to miliary tuberculosis.
3. **Coal miner's pneumoconiosis*** — predominantly mid zones with sparing of the extreme bases and apices. Ill-defined and may be arranged in a circle or rosette. Septal lines.
4. **Sarcoidosis*** — predominantly mid zones. Ill-defined. Often with enlarged hila.
5. **Acute extrinsic allergic alveolitis*** — micronodulation in all zones, but predominantly basal.
6. **Fibrosing alveolitis** — initially most prominent in the lower halves of the lungs and later spreads upwards. Poorly defined. Obliteration of vascular markings.

GREATER THAN SOFT-TISSUE DENSITY

1. **Haemosiderosis** — secondary to chronic raised venous pressure (seen in 10–15% of patients with mitral stenosis), repeated pulmonary haemorrhage (e.g. Goodpasture's disease) or idiopathic. Septal lines. Smaller than miliary TB.
2. **Silicosis*** — relative sparing of bases and apices. Very well-defined and dense when due to pure silica: ill-defined and of lower density when due to mixed dusts. Septal lines.
3. **Siderosis** — lower density than silica. Widely disseminated. Asymptomatic.
4. **Stannosis** } see 4.22.
5. **Barytosis** }

Further Reading

Hatipoglu O.N. (1996) High resolution computed tomographic findings in pulmonary tuberculosis. *Thorax,* 51: 397–402.

Leung A.N. (1999) Pulmonary tuberculosis: the essentials. *Radiology,* 210: 307–22.

Miller W.T. (ed.) (1996) Fungus disease of the chest. *Semin. Roentgenol.,* 31(1).

4.24 MULTIPLE OPACITIES (2–5 mm)

REMAINING DISCRETE

1. **Carcinomatosis** — breast, thyroid, sarcoma, melanoma, prostate, pancreas or bronchus (eroding a pulmonary artery). Variable sizes and progressive increase in size. ± Lymphatic obstruction.
2. **Lymphoma*** — nearly always with hilar or mediastinal lymphadenopathy.
3. **Sarcoidosis*** — predominantly mid zones. Often with enlarged hila.

TENDING TO CONFLUENCE AND VARYING RAPIDLY

1. **Multifocal pneumonia** — including aspiration pneumonia and tuberculosis.
2. **Pulmonary oedema** (see 4.17).
3. **Extrinsic allergic alveolitis*** — predominantly basal.
4. **Fat emboli** — predominantly peripheral.

4.25 SOLITARY PULMONARY NODULE

GRANULOMAS

1. **Tuberculoma** — more common in the upper lobes and on the right side. Well defined. 0.5–4 cm. 25% are lobulated. Calcification frequent. 80% have satellite lesions. Cavitation is uncommon and when present is small and eccentric. Usually persist unchanged for years.
2. **Histoplasmoma** — in endemic areas (Mississippi and the Atlantic coast of USA). More frequent in the lower lobes. Well-defined. Seldom larger than 3 cm. Calcification is common and may be central, producing a target appearance. Cavitation is rare. Satellite lesions are common.

MALIGNANT NEOPLASMS

1. **Carcinoma of the bronchus** — usually greater than 2 cm. Accounts for less than 15% of all solitary nodules at 40 years: almost 100% at 80 years. However, up to 38% of small (< 1 cm) nodules identified by CT may be primary carcinoma of the bronchus. CXR appearances suggesting malignancy are:
   (a) Recent appearance or rapid growth (previous CXRs are very helpful here).
   (b) Size greater than 4 cm.
   (c) The lesion crosses a fissure (although some fungus diseases also do so).
   (d) Ill-defined margins.
   (e) Umbilicated or notched margin (if present it indicates malignancy in 80%).
   (f) Corona radiata (spiculation). (But also seen in PMF and granulomas).
   (g) Peripheral line shadows.
   (h) Calcification is very rare, except in scar carcinomas.
2. **Metastasis** — accounts for 3–5% of asymptomatic nodules. 25% of pulmonary metastases are solitary. Most likely primaries are breast, sarcoma, seminoma and renal cell carcinoma. Predilection for the lung periphery. Calcification is rare but occurs with metastatic osteosarcoma, chondrosarcoma and some other rarer metastases. When considering the diagnosis of pulmonary metastases in children the following points must be borne in mind:
   (a) Unlike adults, it is highly unlikely that there will be an incidental finding of pulmonary metastatic disease.
   (b) The majority of single lung nodules are benign and even in a child with known malignancy one-third of new lung nodules may be benign.
   (c) Multiple lung nodules are more likely to be malignant than a single nodule.
   (d) Therapy usually results in complete resolution of a metastatic nodule but occasionally there may be a residual scar.
3. **Alveolar cell carcinoma** — when localized, a mass is the most common presentation. More commonly ill-defined. Air bronchogram is common. No calcification. Pleural effusion in 5%. Mediastinal lymphadenopathy is much less common than with carcinoma of the bronchus.

BENIGN NEOPLASMS

1. **Adenoma** — 90% occur around the hilum: 10% are peripheral. Round or oval and well-defined. 25% present as a solitary nodule, 75% present with the effects of bronchial stenosis. Calcification and cavitation are rare. Histologically, 80–90% are carcinoids and 10–20% are cylindromas. The former may metastasize to bone (sclerotic secondaries) or to liver and may produce the carcinoid syndrome.
2. **Hamartoma** — 96% occur over 40 years. 90% are intrapulmonary and usually within 2 cm of the pleura. 10% produce bronchial stenosis. Usually less than 4 cm diameter. Well-defined. Lobulated rather than smooth. Calcification in 30%, although the incidence increases with the size of the lesion (in 75% when greater than 5 cm). Calcification is 'pop-corn', craggy or punctate.

INFECTIONS

1. **Pneumonia** — simple consolidation, especially pneumococcal. Air bronchogram.
2. **Hydatid** — in endemic areas. Most common in the lower lobes and more frequent on the right side. Well-defined. 1–10 cm. Solitary in 70%. May have a bizarre shape. Rupture results in the 'water lily' sign.

CONGENITAL

1. **Sequestration** — usually more than 6 cm. Two-thirds occur in the left lower lobe, one-third in the right lower lobe and contiguous to the diaphragm. Well-defined, round or oval. Diagnosis confirmed by aortography and venous drainage is via the pulmonary veins (intralobar type) or bronchial veins (extralobar type). Identification of the mass and its blood supply is possible by US, CT and MRI.
2. **Bronchogenic cyst** — peak incidence in the second and third decades. Two-thirds are intrapulmonary and occur in the medial one-third of the lower lobes. Round or oval. Smooth-walled and well-defined.

VASCULAR

1. **Pulmonary infarction** (see Pulmonary embolic disease*) — most frequent in the lower lobes. With a pleural effusion and elevation of the hemidiaphragm.
2. **Haematoma** — peripheral, smooth and well-defined. 2–6 cm. Slow resolution over several weeks.
3. **Arteriovenous malformation** — 66% are single. Well-defined, lobulated ('bag of worms'). Feeding or draining vessels may be demonstrable. Calcification is rare.

Further Reading

Coley S.C. & Jackson J.E. (1998) Pulmonary arteriovenous malformations. *Clin. Radiol.,* 53: 396–404.

Erasmus J.J., Connolly J.E., McAdams H.P. *et al.* (2000) Solitary pulmonary nodules: Part I. Morphologic evaluation for differentiation of benign and malignant lesions. *RadioGraphics,* 20: 43–58.

Erasmus J.J., McAdams H.P. & Connolly J.E. (2000) Solitary pulmonary nodules: Part II. Evaluation of the indeterminate nodule. *RadioGraphics,* 20: 59–66.

Franco J., Aliaga R., Domingo M.L. *et al.* (1998) Diagnosis of pulmonary sequestration by spiral CT angiography. *Thorax,* 53: 1089–92.

Hatipoglu O.N. (1996) High resolution computed tomographic findings in pulmonary tuberculosis. *Thorax,* 51: 397–402.

Ko S.-F., Ng S.-H., Lee T.-Y. *et al.* (2000) Non-invasive imaging of bronchopulmonary sequestration. *Am. J. Roentgenol.,* 175: 1005–12.

Leef III J.L. & Klein J.S. (2002) The solitary pulmonary nodule. *Radiol. Clin. North Am.,* 40(1): 123–44.

Leung A.N. (1999) Pulmonary tuberculosis: the essentials. *Radiology,* 210: 307–22.

Morcos S.K. (1999) Radiology of the solitary pulmonary nodule. *J. Bronchol.,* 6: 72–3.

Yankelevitz D.F. (ed.) (2000) The solitary pulmonary nodule. *Sem. Ultrasound CT MRI,* 21(2).

Yankelevitz D.F. & Henschke C.I. (2000) Small solitary pulmonary nodules. *Radiol. Clin. North Am.,* 38(3): 471–8.

4.26 MULTIPLE PULMONARY NODULES
(> 5 mm)

NEOPLASTIC

1. **Metastases** — most commonly from breast, thyroid, kidney, gastrointestinal tract and testes. In children, Wilms' tumour, Ewing's sarcoma, neuroblastoma and osteosarcoma. Predilection for lower lobes and more common peripherally. Range of sizes. Well-defined. Ill-definition suggests prostate, breast or stomach. Hilar lymphadenopathy and effusions are uncommon.

INFECTIONS

1. **Abscesses** — widespread distribution but asymmetrical. Commonly *Staphylococcus aureus*. Cavitation common. No calcification.
2. **Coccidioidomycosis** — in endemic areas. Well-defined with a predilection for the upper lobes. 0.5–3 cm. Calcification and cavitation may be present.
3. **Histoplasmosis** — in endemic areas. Round, well-defined and few in number. Sometimes calcify. Usually unchanged for many years.
4. **Hydatid** — more common on the right side and in the lower zones. Well-defined unless there is surrounding pneumonia. Often 10 cm or more. May rupture and show the 'water lily' sign.

IMMUNOLOGICAL

1. **Wegener's granulomatosis** — widespread distribution. 0.5–10 cm. Round and well-defined. No calcification. Cavitation in 30–50% of cases. ± Focal pneumonitis.
2. **Rheumatoid nodules** — peripheral and more common in the lower zones. Round and well-defined. No calcification. Cavitation common.
3. **Caplan's syndrome** — well-defined. Develop rapidly in crops. Calcification and cavitation occur. Background stippling of pneumoconiosis.

INHALATIONAL

1. **Progressive massive fibrosis** — mid and upper zones. Begin peripherally and move centrally. Peripheral emphysema. Oval in shape. Calcification and cavitation occur. Background nodularity of pneumoconiosis.

VASCULAR

1. **Arteriovenous malformations** — 33% are multiple. Well-defined. Lobulated. Tomography may show feeding or draining vessels. Calcification is rare.

4.27 LUNG CAVITIES

INFECTIVE, i.e. ABSCESSES

1. ***Staphylococcus aureus*** — thick-walled with a ragged inner lining. No lobar predilection. Associated with effusion and empyema ± pyopneumothorax — almost invariable in children, not so common in adults. Pneumatocoeles (see 4.9.). Multiple.
2. ***Klebsiella pneumoniae*** — thick-walled with a ragged inner lining. More common in the upper lobes. Usually single but may be multilocular ± effusion.
3. **Tuberculosis** — thick-walled and smooth. Upper lobes and apical segment of lower lobes mainly. Usually surrounded by consolidation. ± Fibrosis.
4. **Aspiration** — look for foreign body, e.g. tooth.
5. **Others** — Gram-negative organisms, actinomycosis, nocardiosis, histoplasmosis, coccidioidomycosis, aspergillosis, hydatid and amoebiasis.

NEOPLASTIC

1. **Carcinoma of the bronchus** — thick-walled with an eccentric cavity. Predilection for the upper lobes. Found in 2–10% of carcinomas and especially if peripheral. More common in squamous cell carcinomas and may then be thin-walled.
2. **Metastases** — thin- or thick-walled. May only involve a few of the nodules. Seen especially in squamous cell, colon and sarcoma metastases.
3. **Hodgkin's disease** — thin- or thick-walled and typically in an area of infiltration. With hilar or mediastinal lymphadenopathy.

VASCULAR

1. **Infarction** — three situations may be encountered. Primary infection due to a septic embolus almost invariably results in cavitation. There may be secondary infection of an initially sterile infarct. An aseptic cavitating infarct may subsequently become infected: tertiary infection. Aseptic cavitation is usually solitary and arises in a large area of consolidation after about 2 weeks. If localized to a segment the commonest sites are apical or the posterior segment of an upper lobe or apical segment of lower lobe (cf. lower lobe predominance with non-cavitating infarction). Majority have scalloped inner margins and cross cavity band shadows. ± Effusion.

ABNORMAL LUNG

1. **Cystic bronchiectasis** (see 4.14) — thin-walled. More common in the lower lobes.
2. **Infected emphysematous bulla** — thin-walled. ± Air fluid level.
3. **Sequestrated segment** — thick- or thin-walled. 66% in the left lower lobe, 33% in the right lower lobe. ± Air fluid level. ± Surrounding pneumonia.
4. **Bronchogenic cyst** — in medial third of lower lobes. Thin-walled. ± Air fluid level. ± Surrounding pneumonia.

GRANULOMAS

1. **Wegener's granulomatosis** — widespread. Cavitation in some of the nodules. Thick-walled, becoming thinner with time. Can be transient.
2. **Rheumatoid nodules** — thick-walled with a smooth inner lining. Especially in the lower lobes and peripherally. Well-defined. Become thin-walled with time.

3. **Progressive massive fibrosis** — predominantly in the mid and upper zones. Thick-walled and irregular. Background nodularity.
4. **Sarcoidosis*** — thin-walled. In early disease due to a combination of central necrosis of areas of coalescent granulomas and a check-valve mechanism beyond partial obstruction of airways by endobronchial sarcoidosis.

TRAUMATIC

1. **Haematoma** — peripheral. Air fluid level if it communicates with a bronchus.
2. **Traumatic lung cyst** — thin-walled and peripheral. Single or multiple. Unilocular or multilocular. Distinguished from cavitating haematomas as they present early, within hours of the injury.

Further Reading

John P.R., Beasley S.W. & Mayne V. (1989). Pulmonary sequestration and related congenital disorders. A clinico-radiological review of 41 cases. *Pediatr. Radiol.*, 20: 4–9.

Vourtsi A., Gouliamos A., Moulopoulos L. *et al.* (2001) CT appearance of solitary and multiple cystic and cavitary lung lesions. *Eur. Radiol.*, 11: 612–22.

Wilson A.G., Joseph A.E. & Butland R.J. (1986) The radiology of aseptic cavitation in pulmonary infarction. *Clin. Radiol.*, 37: 327–33.

4.28 MULTIPLE THIN-WALLED CYSTIC SPACES

CONGENITAL

1. **Cystic adenomatoid malformation** — an area of lung that does not contain cartilage leading to a mass that may be solid or cystic. The cysts may be small or large, single or multiple, thin- or thick-walled and air- or fluid-filled. The mass may compress local structures. It usually presents neonatally with respiratory distress.
2. **Bronchogenic cyst** — usually solitary.
3. **Klippel–Trenaunay–Weber syndrome.**

INFECTIVE

1. **Hydatid.**
2. **Tuberculoma.**
3. **Septic emboli.**

INFLAMMATORY

1. **Sarcoidosis*.**
2. **Wegener's granulomatosis** — initially thick-walled.

NEOPLASTIC

1. **Metastases** — particularly squamous cell carcinoma, colon and sarcoma.
2. **Lymphoma*.**

ABNORMAL LUNG

1. **Bullous emphysema.**
2. **Cystic bronchiectasis.**
3. **Honeycombing** — see 4.20.
4. **Pneumatocoeles** — local obstructive hyperinflation of lung parenchyma.
   (a) Infective — occur during healing phase and usually resolve. Gram-positive and -negative bacterial infections. *Pneumocystis carinii.*
   (b) Traumatic — usually resolve. May be due to:
      (i) pulmonary laceration
      (ii) inflammatory response to hydrocarbon inhalation
      (iii) haematoma.
5. **Langerhans cell histiocytosis*** — early in the disease there are centrilobular nodules which, as the disease progresses, cavitate to thick- and then thin-walled cysts. Spares the costophrenic angles and predominates in the upper lung. Intervening lung is normal. Lung volumes are normal or increased.
6. **Lymphangioleiomyomatosis** — Only females. Presents with dyspnoea due to spontaneous pneumothorax or chylous pleural effusion. Diffuse distribution of rounded lung cysts surrounded by normal lung. The bronchovascular bundle lies at the edge of the cyst. The lung volumes are normal or increased. An identical abnormality may occur in tuberous sclerosis.

4.29 OPACITY WITH AN AIR BRONCHOGRAM

INFECTIVE

1. **Pneumonia.**

INFLAMMATORY

1. **Radiation pneumonitis.**
2. **Progressive massive fibrosis.**

NEOPLASTIC

1. **Alveolar cell carcinoma.**
2. **Lymphoma*.**
3. **Lymphosarcoma.**

4.30 NON-THROMBOTIC PULMONARY EMBOLI

1. **Septic embolism** — associated with indwelling venous catheters, tricuspid valve endocarditis and peripheral septic thrombophlebitis. Variable size, poorly marginated nodules, predominantly in the lower lobes, and which tend to form cavities.
2. **Catheter embolism** — catheter fragments are most common in the basilica vein and pulmonary arteries.
3. **Fat embolism** — 1–2 days post-trauma. Predominantly peripheral. Resolves in 1–4 weeks. Normal heart size. Pleural effusions uncommon. Neurological symptoms in up to 85% and skin abnormalities in 20–50%.

4. **Venous air embolism** — when iatrogenic, prognosis is affected by volume of air and speed of injection. Clinical effects are the result of right ventricular outflow obstruction or obstruction of pulmonary arterioles. CXR may be normal or show air in the main pulmonary artery, heart or hepatic veins, focal pulmonary oligaemia or pulmonary oedema.
5. **Amniotic fluid embolism** — rare. The majority of patients suffer cardiopulmonary arrest and the CXR shows pulmonary oedema.
6. **Tumour embolism** — common sources are liver, breast, stomach, kidney, prostate and chorioncarcinoma. CXR is usually normal.
7. **Talc embolism** — in i.v. drug abusers.
8. **Iodinated oil embolism** — following contrast lymphangiography.
9. **Cotton embolism** — when cotton fibres adhere to angiographic catheters or guidewires and in i.v. drug abusers.
10. **Hydatid embolism.**

Further Reading

Rossi S.F., Goodman P.C. & Franquet I. (2000) Nonthrombic pulmonary emboli *Am. J. Roentgenol.*, 174: 1499–1508.

4.31 PULMONARY CALCIFICATION OR OSSIFICATION

LOCALIZED CALCIFICATION

1. **Tuberculosis** — demonstrable in 10% of those with a positive tuberculin test. Small central nidus of calcification. Calcification ≠ healed.
2. **Histoplasmosis** — in endemic areas, calcification due to histoplasmosis is demonstrable in 30% of those with a positive histoplasmin test. Calcification may be laminated, producing a target lesion. ± Multiple punctate calcifications in the spleen.
3. **Coccidioidomycosis.**
4. **Blastomycosis** — rare.

CALCIFICATION WITHIN A SOLITARY NODULE

Calcification within a nodule equates with a benign lesion. The exceptions are:

(a) Carcinoma engulfing a pre-existing calcified granuloma (eccentric calcification).
(b) Solitary calcifying/ossifying metastasis — osteosarcoma, chondrosarcoma, mucinous adenocarcinoma of the colon or breast, papillary carcinoma of the thyroid, cystadenocarcinoma of the ovary and carcinoid.
(c) 1° peripheral squamous cell or papillary adenocarcinoma.

DIFFUSE OR MULTIPLE CALCIFICATIONS

1. **Infections**
   (a) Tuberculosis — healed miliary.
   (b) Histoplasmosis.
   (c) Varicella — following chicken pox pneumonia in adulthood. 1–3 mm. Numbered in 10s.
2. **Chronic pulmonary venous hypertension** — especially mitral stenosis. Up to 8 mm. Most prominent in mid and lower zones. ± Ossification.
3. **Silicosis** — in up to 20% of those showing nodular opacities.
4. **Metastases** — as above.
5. **Alveolar microlithiasis** — often familial. Myriad minute calcifications in alveoli which obscure all lung detail. Because of the lung's increased density, the heart, pleura and diaphragm may be evident as negative shadows.

6. **Metastatic due to hypercalcaemia** — chronic renal failure, 2° hyperparathyroidism and multiple myeloma*. Predominantly in the upper zones.
7. **Lymphoma following radiotherapy.**

INTERSTITIAL OSSIFICATION

Branching calcific densities extending along the bronchovascular distribution of the interstitial space.

1. **Fibrosing alveolitis.**
2. **Long-term busulphan therapy.**
3. **Chronic pulmonary venous hypertension.**
4. **Idiopathic.**

Further Reading

Jacobs A.N., Neitzschman H.R. & Nice C.M. Jr (1973) Metaplastic bone formation in the lung. *Am. J. Roentgenol.*, 118: 344–6.

Kuplic J.B., Higley C.S. & Niewoehner D.E. (1972) Pulmonary ossification associated with long-term busulfan therapy in chronic myeloid leukaemia. Case report. *Am. Rev. Resp. Dis.*, 106: 759.

Maile C.W., Rodan B.A., Godwin J.D. *et al.* (1982) Calcification in pulmonary metastases. *Br. J. Radiol.*, 55: 108–13.

Mendeloff J. (1971) Disseminated nodular pulmonary ossification in the Hamman–Rich lung. *Am. Rev. Resp. Dis.*, 103: 269.

4.32 UNILATERAL HILAR ENLARGEMENT

LYMPH NODES

1. **Carcinoma of the bronchus** — the hilar enlargement may be due to the tumour itself or involved lymph nodes.
2. **Lymphoma*** — unilateral is very unusual; involvement is usually bilateral and asymmetrical.
3. **Infective**
   (a) Primary tuberculosis.
   (b) Histoplasmosis.
   (c) Coccidioidomycosis.
   (d) Mycoplasma.
   (e) Pertussis.
4. **Sarcoidosis*** — unilateral disease in only 1–5%.

PULMONARY ARTERY

1. **Post-stenotic dilatation** — on the left side.
2. **Pulmonary embolus** (see Pulmonary embolic disease*) — massive to one lung. Peripheral oligaemia.
3. **Aneurysm** — in chronic pulmonary arterial hypertension. ± Egg-shell calcification.

OTHERS

1. **Mediastinal mass** — superimposed on a hilum.
2. **Perihilar pneumonia** — ill-defined, ± air bronchogram.

See also 4.11.

Further Reading

Ko J.P., Drucker E.A., Shepard J.-O. *et al.* (2000) CT depiction of regional nodal stations for lung cancer staging. *Am. J. Roentgenol.*, 174: 775–82.

4.33 BILATERAL HILAR ENLARGEMENT

Due to lymph node enlargement or pulmonary artery enlargement.

IDIOPATHIC

1. **Sarcoidosis*** — symmetrical and lobulated. Bronchopulmonary ± unilateral or bilateral paratracheal lymphadenopathy.

NEOPLASTIC

1. **Lymphoma*** — asymmetrical.
2. **Lymphangitis carcinomatosa.**

INFECTIVE

1. **Viruses** — most common in children.
2. **Primary tuberculosis** — rarely bilateral and symmetrical.
3. **Histoplasmosis.**
4. **Coccidioidomycosis.**

VASCULAR

1. **Pulmonary arterial hypertension** — see section 5.16.

IMMUNOLOGICAL

1. **Extrinsic allergic alveolitis*** — in mushroom workers.

INHALATIONAL

1. **Silicosis*** — symmetrical.
2. **Chronic berylliosis** — only in a minority of cases. Symmetrical.

Further Reading

Baldwin D.R., Lambert L., Pantin C.F. *et al.* (1996) Silicosis presenting as bilateral hilar lymphadenopathy. *Thorax*, 51: 1165–7.

4.34 'EGG-SHELL' CALCIFICATION OF LYMPH NODES

The criteria for diagnosis were listed by Gross *et al.* and Jacobsen *et al.* as:

1. Shell-like calcifications up to 2 mm thick in the periphery of at least two lymph nodes.
2. Calcifications may be solid or broken.
3. In at least one of the lymph nodes the ring of calcification must be complete.
4. The central part of the lymph node may show additional calcifications.
5. One of the affected lymph nodes must be at least 1 cm in its greatest diameter.

1. **Silicosis*** — seen in approximately 5% of silicotics. Predominantly hilar lymph nodes but may also be observed in the anterior and posterior mediastinal lymph nodes, cervical lymph nodes and intraperitoneal lymph nodes. More frequently seen in complicated pneumoconiosis. Lungs show multiple small nodular shadows or areas of massive fibrosis.
2. **Coal miner's pneumoconiosis*** — occurs in only 1% of cases. Associated pulmonary changes include miliary shadowing or massive shadows.
3. **Sarcoidosis*** — calcification of lymph nodes occurs in approximately 5% of patients and is occasionally 'egg-shell' in appearance. There may be extensive lymph node involvement throughout the mediastinum. Calcification appears about 6 years after the onset of the disease and is almost invariably associated with advanced pulmonary disease and in some cases with steroid therapy. The pulmonary manifestations include reticulonodular, acinar or fibrotic changes in the mid to upper zones.
4. **Lymphoma following radiotherapy** — appears 1–9 years after radiotherapy.

DIFFERENTIAL DIAGNOSIS

1. **Pulmonary artery calcification** — a rare feature of pulmonary arterial hypertension.
2. **Aortic calcification** — especially in the wall of a saccular aneurysm.
3. **Anterior mediastinal tumours** — teratodermoids and thymomas may occasionally exhibit rim calcification.

Further Reading

Gross B.H., Schneider H.J. & Proto A.V. (1980) Eggshell calcification of lymph nodes: an update. *Am. J. Roentgenol.*, 135: 1265.
Jacobsen G., Felson B., Pendergrass E.P. *et al.* (1967) Eggshell calcification in coal and metal miners. *Semin. Roentgenol.*, 2: 276–82.

4.35 RETICULONODULAR OPACITY

Definition — combination of interlacing lines and nodules.

PULMONARY FIBROSIS

Any cause. See 4.20.

INFLAMMATORY

1. **Infective** — atypical and opportunist.
2. **Hypersensitivity pneumonia.**
3. **Lipoid pneumonia.**
4. **Bronchiolitis obliterans organizing pneumonia.**
5. **Cystic fibrosis*.**
6. **Collagen vascular disease** — lower lobe predominance.
7. **Sarcoidosis*.**
8. **Amyloid.**

NEOPLASTIC

1. **Lymphangitis carcinomatosa.**
2. **Lymphoma*.**

OTHER

1. **Pulmonary oedema — chronic.**
2. **Langerhans cell histiocytosis*.**
3. **Alveolar microlithiasis.**
4. **Gaucher's disease.**
5. **Alveolar proteinosis.**

4.36 BASAL INTERSTITIAL OPACITY

PULMONARY FIBROSIS

See 4.21.

INFLAMMATORY

1. **Aspiration.**
2. **Collagen vascular disease** — particularly rheumatoid arthritis and systemic sclerosis. Usually produces fine reticulation.
3. **Drugs** — e.g. amiodarone (and see 4.20).

NEOPLASTIC

1. **Lymphangitis carcinomatosa** — typically coarse and may be nodular.
2. **Lymphoma*.**

OTHER

1. **Pulmonary oedema.**
2. **Neurofibromatosis*** — rare.
3. **Tuberous sclerosis*** — rare.

4.37 INTERSTITIAL LUNG DISEASE WITH INCREASED LUNG VOLUMES

1. **Emphysema.**
2. **Lymphangioleiomyomatosis.**
3. **Langerhans cell histiocytosis*.**
4. **Cystic fibrosis*.**
5. **Sarcoidosis*.**

4.38 UPPER ZONE FIBROSIS

1. **Tuberculosis** — calcification frequent.
2. **Radiotherapy** — no calcification. ± Evidence of the cause, e.g. mastectomy for carcinoma, or radiation osteonecrosis of ribs or clavicle.
3. **Sarcoidosis*** — no calcification. ± 'Egg-shell' calcification of lymph nodes.
4. **Chronic extrinsic allergic alveolitis*.**
5. **Histoplasmosis** — similar to tuberculosis.
6. **Progressive massive fibrosis** — conglomerate infiltrates with peripheral emphysema. Background nodularity. ± 'Egg-shell' calcification of lymph nodes.
7. **Ankylosing spondylitis*** — resembles tuberculosis. Cavitation frequent with mycetoma. Disease is almost invariably bilateral and associated with severe spondylitis.

Further Reading

Howarth F.H., Kendall M.J., Lawrence D.S. *et al.* (1975) Chest radiograph in ankylosing spondylitis. *Clin. Radiol.*, 26: 455–60.

Mesurolle B., Qanadli S.D., Merad M. *et al.* (2000) Unusual radiologic findings in the thorax after radiation therapy. *RadioGraphics*, 20: 67–81.

Park K.J., Chung J.Y., Chun M.S. *et al.* (2000) Radiation-induced lung disease and the impact of radiation methods on imaging features. *RadioGraphics*, 20: 83–98.

4.39 PLEURAL EFFUSION

TRANSUDATE (protein < 30 g l^{-1})

1. **Cardiac failure.**
2. **Hepatic failure.**
3. **Nephrotic syndrome.**
4. **Meigs syndrome.**

EXUDATE (protein >30 g l^{-1})

1. **Infection.**
2. **Malignancy.**
3. **Pulmonary infarction** — see Pulmonary embolic disease*.
4. **Collagen vascular diseases.**
5. **Subphrenic abscess.**
6. **Pancreatitis.**

HAEMORRHAGIC

1. **Carcinoma of the bronchus.**
2. **Trauma.**
3. **Pulmonary infarction** — see Pulmonary embolic disease*.
4. **Bleeding disorders.**

CHYLOUS

1. **Obstructed thoracic duct** — due to trauma, malignant invasion or filariasis.

4.40 PLEURAL EFFUSION DUE TO EXTRATHORACIC DISEASE

1. **Pancreatitis** — acute, chronic or relapsing. Effusions are predominantly left-sided. Elevated amylase content.
2. **Subphrenic abscess** — with elevation and restriction of movement of the ipsilateral diaphragm and basal atelectasis or consolidation.
3. **Following abdominal surgery** — most often seen on the side of the surgery and larger after upper abdominal surgery. Disappears after 2 weeks.
4. **Meigs syndrome** — pleural effusion + ascites + benign pelvic tumour (most commonly an ovarian fibroma, thecoma, granulosa cell tumour or cystadenoma).
5. **Nephrotic syndrome.**
6. **Fluid overload** — e.g. due to renal disease.
7. **Cirrhosis.**

4.41 PLEURAL EFFUSION WITH AN OTHERWISE NORMAL CHEST X-RAY

Effusion may be the only abnormality or other signs may be obscured by the effusion.

INFECTIVE

1. **Primary tuberculosis** — more common in adults (40%) than children (10%). Rarely bilateral.
2. **Viruses and mycoplasma** — effusions occur in 10–20% of cases but are usually small.

NEOPLASTIC

1. **Carcinoma of the bronchus** — effusion occurs in 10% of patients and a peripheral carcinoma may be hidden by the effusion.
2. **Metastases** — most commonly from breast; less commonly pancreas, stomach, ovary and kidney.
3. **Mesothelioma** — effusion in 90%; often massive and obscures the underlying pleural disease.
4. **Lymphoma*** — effusion occurs in 30% but is usually associated with lymphadenopathy or pulmonary infiltrates.

IMMUNOLOGICAL

1. **Systemic lupus erythematosus*** — effusion is the sole manifestation in 10% of cases. Usually small but may be massive. Bilateral in 50%. 35–50% of those with an effusion have associated cardiomegaly.
2. **Rheumatoid disease** (see Rheumatoid arthritis*) — observed in 3% of patients. Almost exclusively males. Usually unilateral and may predate joint disease. Tendency to remain unchanged for a long time.

EXTRATHORACIC DISEASES

See 4.40.

OTHERS

1. **Pulmonary embolus** (see Pulmonary embolic disease*) — effusion is a common sign and it may obscure an underlying area of infarction.
2. **Closed chest trauma** — effusion may contain blood, chyle or food (due to oesophageal rupture). The latter is almost always left-sided.
3. **Asbestosis*** — mesothelioma and carcinoma of the bronchus should be excluded but an effusion may be present without these complications. Effusion is frequently recurrent and usually bilateral. Usually associated with pulmonary disease.

Further Reading

Ng C.S., Munden R.F. & Libshitz H.I. (1999) Malignant pleural mesothelioma: the spectrum of manifestations on CT in 70 cases. Clin Radiol., 54: 415–21.

4.42 PNEUMOTHORAX

1. **Spontaneous** — M:F, 8:1. Especially those of tall thin stature. ? due to ruptured blebs or bullae. 20% are associated with a small pleural effusion.
2. **Iatrogenic** — e.g. postoperative, after chest aspiration, during artificial ventilation, after lung biopsy or following attempted insertion of a subclavian venous line.
3. **Traumatic** — ± rib fractures, haemothorax, surgical emphysema or mediastinal emphysema.
4. **Secondary to mediastinal emphysema** (see 4.43).
5. **Secondary to lung disease**
   (a) Emphysema.
   (b) 'Honeycomb lung' (q.v.).
   (c) Cystic fibrosis*.
   (d) Pneumonia.
   (e) Bronchopleural fistula, e.g. due to lung abscess or carcinoma.
   (f) Lung neoplasms — especially metastases from osteogenic sarcomas and other sarcomas.
6. **Pneumoperitoneum** — air passes through a pleuroperitoneal foramen.

4.43 PNEUMOMEDIASTINUM

Radiographic signs depend on air outlining normal anatomical structures.

1. Thymic sail sign.
2. Air anterior to the pericardium.
3. Air around the pulmonary artery or its major branches.
4. Air around the aorta or its major branches.
5. Double bronchial wall sign.
6. Subcutaneous emphysema.

May be associated with a pneumothorax.

1. **Lung tear** — a sudden rise in intra-alveolar pressure, often with airway narrowing, causes air to dissect through the interstitium to the hilum and then to the mediastinum.
   (a) Spontaneous — the most common cause and may follow coughing or strenuous exercise.
   (b) Asthma — but usually not < 2 years of age.
   (c) Diabetic ketoacidosis related to severe and protracted vomiting.
   (d) Childbirth — because of repeated Valsalva manoeuvres.
   (e) Artificial ventilation.
   (f) Chest trauma.
   (g) Foreign body aspiration — especially if < 2 years.
2. **Perforation of oesophagus, trachea or bronchus** — ruptured oesophagus is often associated with a hydrothorax or hydropneumothorax, usually on the left side.
3. **Perforation of a hollow abdominal viscus** — with extension of gas via the retroperitoneal space.

Further Reading

Burton E.M., Riggs Jr W., Kaufman R.A. *et al.* (1989) Pneumomediastinum caused by foreign body aspiration in children. *Pediatr. Radiol.*, 20: 45–7.

Fraser R.G., Paré J.A.P., Paré P.D. *et al.* (1991) Pneumomediastinum. In: *Diagnosis of Diseases of the Chest,* 3rd edn, Vol. 4, Ch. 19. Philadelphia: Saunders, pp. 2801–13.

Zylak C.M., Standen J.R., Barnes G.R. *et al.* (2000) Pneumomediastinum. *RadioGraphics,* 20: 1043–57.

4.44 RIGHT-SIDED DIAPHRAGMATIC HUMPS

AT ANY SITE

1. **Collapse/consolidation of adjacent lung.**
2. **Localized eventration.**
3. **Loculated effusion.**
4. **Subphrenic abscess.**
5. **Hepatic abscess.**
6. **Hydatid cyst.**
7. **Hepatic metastasis.**

MEDIALLY

1. **Pericardial fat pad.**
2. **Aortic aneurysm.**
3. **Pleuro-pericardial (spring water cyst).**
4. **Sequestrated segment.**

ANTERIORLY

1. **Morgagni hernia.**

POSTERIORLY

1. **Bochdalek hernia.**

Further Reading

Baron R.L., Lee J.K.T. & Melson G.L. (1980) Sonographic evaluation of right juxtadiaphragmatic masses in children using transhepatic approach. *J. Clin. Ultrasound,* 8: 156–8.

Kangerloo H., Sukov R., Sample F. *et al.* (1977) Ultrasonic evaluation of juxtadiaphragmatic masses in children. *Radiology,* 125: 785–7.

Khan A.N. & Gould D.A. (1984) The primary role of ultrasound in evaluating right sided diaphragmatic humps and juxtadiaphragmatic masses: a review of 22 cases. *Clin. Radiol.,* 35: 413–8.

4.45 UNILATERAL ELEVATED HEMIDIAPHRAGM

CAUSES ABOVE THE DIAPHRAGM

1. **Phrenic nerve palsy** — smooth hemidiaphragm. No movement on respiration. Paradoxical movement on sniffing. The mediastinum is usually central. The cause, e.g. bronchial carcinoma or mediastinal nodes, may be evident on the X-ray.
2. **Pulmonary collapse.**
3. **Pulmonary infarction** — see Pulmonary embolic disease*.
4. **Pleural disease** — especially old pleural disease, e.g. haemothorax, empyema or thoracotomy.
5. **Splinting of the diaphragm** — associated with rib fractures or pleurisy.
6. **Hemiplegia** — an upper motor neuron lesion.

DIAPHRAGMATIC CAUSES

1. **Eventration** — more common on the left side. The heart is frequently displaced to the contralateral side. Limited movement on normal respiration and paradoxical movement on sniffing. Stomach may show a partial volvulus.

CAUSES BELOW THE DIAPHRAGM

1. **Gaseous distension of the stomach or splenic flexure** — left hemidiaphragm only.
2. **Subphrenic inflammatory disease** — subphrenic abscess, hepatic or splenic abscess and pancreatitis.

SCOLIOSIS

The raised hemidiaphragm is on the side of the concavity.

DECUBITUS FILM

The raised hemidiaphragm is on the dependent side.

DIFFERENTIAL DIAGNOSIS

1. **Subpulmonary effusion** — movement of fluid is demonstrable on a decubitus film. On the left side there is increased distance between the lung and stomach fundal gas.
2. **Ruptured diaphragm** — more common on the left. Barium meal confirms the diagnosis.

4.46 BILATERAL ELEVATED HEMIDIAPHRAGMS

POOR INSPIRATORY EFFORT

OBESITY

CAUSES ABOVE THE DIAPHRAGMS

1. **Bilateral basal pulmonary collapse** — which may be secondary to infarction of subphrenic abscesses.
2. **Small lungs** — fibrotic lung disease, e.g. fibrosing alveolitis.

CAUSES BELOW THE DIAPHRAGMS

1. **Ascites.**
2. **Pregnancy.**
3. **Pneumoperitoneum.**
4. **Hepatosplenomegaly.**
5. **Large intra-abdominal tumour.**
6. **Bilateral subphrenic abscesses.**

DIFFERENTIAL DIAGNOSIS

1. **Bilateral subpulmonary effusions.**

4.47 PLEURAL CALCIFICATION

1. **Old empyema**
2. **Old haemothorax**

} amorphous bizarre plaques, often with a vacuolated appearance near the inner surface of greatly thickened pleura. Usually unilateral.

3. **Asbestos inhalation*** — small curvilinear plaques in the parietal pleura. More delicate than (1) and (2). Often multiple and bilateral and found over the domes of the diaphragms and immediately deep to the ribs. Observed in 10–15% of people exposed to asbestos but not before 20 years have elapsed. Not necessarily associated with asbestosis, i.e. pulmonary disease.
4. **Silicosis***
5. **Talc exposure**

} similar appearances to asbestos exposure.

Further Reading

Peacock C., Copley S.J. & Hansell D.M. (2000) Asbestos-related benign pleural disease. *Clin. Radiol.*, 55: 422–32.

4.48 LOCAL PLEURAL MASSES

1. **Loculated pleural effusion.**
2. **Metastases** — from bronchus or breast. Often multiple.
3. **Malignant mesothelioma** — nearly always due to asbestos exposure. Extensive thickening of the pleura which may be partly obscured by an effusion. Little mediastinal shift. Adjacent bone destruction in 12%.
4. **Pleural fibroma (local benign mesothelioma)** — a smooth lobular mass, 2–15 cm diameter, arising more frequently from the visceral pleura than the parietal pleura. Tendency to change position with respiration as 30–50% are pedunculated. They form an obtuse angle with the chest wall which indicates their extrapulmonary location. Usually found in patients over 40 years of age and usually asymptomatic. However, it causes hypertrophic osteoarthropathy in a greater proportion of cases than any other disease.
5. **Fibrin balls** — develop in a serofibrinous pleural effusion and become visible following absorption of the fluid. They are small and tend to be situated near the lung base. They may disappear spontaneously or remain unchanged for many years.

DIFFERENTIAL DIAGNOSIS

1. **Extrapleural masses** — see 4.49.
2. **Plombage** — the insertion of foreign material into the extrapleural space as a treatment for tuberculosis. The commonest materials used were solid Lucite spheres, hollow ‘ping-pong’ balls (which may have fluid levels in them) or crumpled cellophane. They produce a well-defined, smooth pleural surface, convex inferiorly and medially and displacing the lung apex. The pleura makes an acute angle with the chest wall.

Further Reading

Ng C.S., Munden R.F. & Libshitz H.I. (1999) Malignant pleural mesothelioma: the spectrum of manifestations on CT in 70 cases. *Clin. Radiol.*, 54: 415–21.

4.49 RIB LESION WITH AN ADJACENT SOFT-TISSUE MASS

NEOPLASTIC

1. **Bronchogenic carcinoma** — solitary site unless metastatic.
2. **Metastases** — solitary or multiple.
3. **Multiple myeloma*** — classically multiple sites and bilateral.
4. **Mesothelioma** — rib destruction occurs in 12%.
5. **Lymphoma*.**
6. **Fibrosarcoma** — similar appearances to mesothelioma.
7. **Neurofibroma** — rib notching.

INFECTIVE

1. **Tuberculosis osteitis** — commonest inflammatory lesion of a rib. Second only to malignancy as a cause of rib destruction. Clearly defined margins ± abscess.
2. **Actinomycosis** } usually a single rib. Adjacent consolidation.
3. **Nocardiosis** }
4. **Blastomycosis** — adjacent patchy or massive consolidation ± hilar lymphadenopathy.

INFLAMMATORY

1. **Radiation osteitis.**

METABOLIC

1. **Renal osteodystrophy** } rib fractures and osteopenia associated with a subpleural haematoma.
2. **Cushing's syndrome** }

Further Reading

Guttentag A. & Salwen J.K. (1999) Keep your eyes on the ribs: the spectrum of normal variants and diseases that involve ribs. *RadioGraphics*, 19: 1125–42.

Steiner R.M., Cooper M.W. & Brodovsky H. (1982) Rib destruction: a neglected finding in malignant mesothelioma. *Clin. Radiol.*, 33: 61–5.

4.50 THE CHEST RADIOGRAPH FOLLOWING CHEST TRAUMA

SOFT TISSUES

1. **Foreign bodies.**
2. **Surgical emphysema.**

RIBS

1. **Simple fracture**
2. **Flail chest**

} may be associated with surgical emphysema, pneumothorax, extrapleural haematoma or haemothorax. First rib fractures have a high incidence of other associated injuries.

STERNUM

1. **Fracture** — may be associated with a clinically unsuspected dorsal spine fracture.
2. **Sternoclavicular dislocation.**

CLAVICLES AND SCAPULAE

1. **Fracture** — scapular fractures are usually associated with other bony or intrathoracic injuries.

SPINE

1. **Fracture** — when present, are multiple in 10% and non-contiguous in 80% of these. Thoracic spine injuries have a much higher incidence of neurological deficit than cervical or lumbar spine injuries.
2. **Cord trauma.**
3. **Nerve root trauma** — especially to the brachial plexus.

PLEURA

1. **Pneumothorax** — simple (in 20–40% of patients with blunt chest trauma and 20% of patients with penetrating injuries) or tension. Signs of a small pneumothorax on a supine chest radiograph include a deep costophrenic sulcus, basal hyperlucency, a 'double'

diaphragm, unusually clear definition of the right cardiophrenic angle or left cardiac apex and visualization of apical pericardial fat tags. CT is more sensitive than plain film radiography.

2. **Haemothorax** — in 25–50% of patients with blunt chest trauma and 60–80% of patients with penetrating wounds.

LUNG

1. **Contusion** — non-segmental alveolar opacities which resolve in a few days.
2. **Haematoma** — usually appears following resolution of contusion. Round, well-defined nodule. Resolution in several weeks.
3. **Aspiration pneumonia.**
4. **Foreign body.**
5. **Pulmonary oedema** — following blast injuries or head injury (neurogenic oedema).
6. **Adult respiratory distress syndrome** — widespread air-space shadowing appearing 24–72 hours after injury.
7. **Fat embolism** — 1–2 days post-trauma. Resembles pulmonary oedema, but normal heart size and pleural effusions are uncommon. Resolves in 1–4 weeks. Neurological symptoms in up to 85% and skin abnormalities in 20–50%.

TRACHEA AND BRONCHI

1. **Laceration or fracture** — initially surgical emphysema and pneumomediastinum followed by collapse of the affected lung or lobe.

DIAPHRAGM

1. **Rupture** — in 3–7% of patients with blunt and 6–46% of patients with penetrating thoraco-abdominal trauma. Diagnosis may be delayed months or years. Plain film findings include herniated stomach or bowel above the diaphragm, pleural effusion, a supradiaphragmatic mass or a poorly visualized or abnormally contoured diaphragm. Probable equal incidence on both sides but rupture of the right hemidiaphragm is not so easily diagnosed.

MEDIASTINUM

1. **Aortic injury** — 90% of aortic ruptures occur just distal to the origin of the left subclavian artery. The majority of patients with

this complication die before radiological evaluation, especially when rupture involves the ascending aorta. Plain film radiographic abnormalities of aortic rupture are:

(a) Widening of the mediastinum (sensitivity 53–100%; specificity 1–60%).
(b) Abnormal aortic contour (sensitivity 53–100%; specificity 21–42%).
(c) Tracheal displacement to the right (sensitivity 12–100%; specificity 80–95%).
(d) Nasogastric tube displacement to the right of the T4 spinous process (sensitivity 9–71%; specificity 90–96%).
(e) Thickening of the right paraspinal stripe (sensitivity 12–83%; specificity 89–97%).
(f) Depression of the left mainstem bronchus > 40° below the horizontal (sensitivity 3–80%; specificity 80–100%).
(g) Loss of definition of the aortopulmonary window (sensitivity 0–100%; specificity 56–83%).

A normal chest radiograph has a 98% negative predictive value for traumatic aortic rupture.

2. **Mediastinal haematoma** - blurring of the mediastinal outline.
3. **Mediastinal emphysema** (see 4.43).
4. **Haemopericardium.**
5. **Oesophageal rupture.**

Further Reading

Desai S.R. (2002) Acute respiratory distress syndrome: imaging of the injured lung. *Clin. Radiol.*, 57: 8–17.

Groskin S.A. (1992) Selected topics in chest trauma. *Radiology*, 183: 605–17.

Patel N.H., Stephens K.E., Mirvis S.E. *et al.* (1998) Imaging of acute thoracic aortic injury due to blunt trauma: a review. *Radiology*, 209: 335–48.

Reynolds J. & Davis J.T. (1966) Thoracic injuries. The radiology of trauma. *Radiol. Clin. North Am.*, 4: 383–402.

Tack D., Defrance P., Delcour C. *et al.* (2000) The CT fallen lung-sign. *Eur. Radiol.*, 10: 719–21.

Wintermark M., Wicky S. & Schnyder P. (2002) Imaging of acute traumatic injuries of the thoracic aorta. *Eur. Radiol.*, 12: 431–42.

4.51 NEONATAL RESPIRATORY DISTRESS

PULMONARY CAUSES

A. With no mediastinal shift

1. **Hyaline membrane disease (surfactant deficiency disease)** — in premature infants. Infants are symptomatic soon after birth but maximum radiographic findings develop at 12–14 hours. Fine granular pattern throughout both lungs, air bronchograms and, later, obscured heart and diaphragmatic outlines. Often cardiomegaly. May progress to a complete 'white-out'. Interstitial emphysema, pneumomediastinum and pneumothorax are frequent complications of ventilator therapy. As oxygenation improves, bidirectional or left-to-right shunting through the ductus arteriosus may lead to pulmonary oedema and cardiomegaly.
2. **Transient tachypnoea of the newborn** — prominent interstitial markings and vessels, thickened septa, small effusions and mild cardiomegaly. May resemble hyaline membrane disease, meconium aspiration or neonatal pneumonia. Resolves within 2–3 days.
3. **Meconium aspiration syndrome** — predominantly postmature infants. Coarse linear and irregular opacities of uneven size, generalized hyperinflation and focal areas of collapse and emphysema. Spontaneous pneumothorax and effusions in 20%. Pleural effusion in up to two-thirds; never in hyaline membrane disease. No air bronchograms.
4. **Pneumonia** — in < 1% of newborns. Risk factor – prolonged rupture of membranes. Most commonly Group B *Streptococcus*. Segmental or lobal consolidation. May resemble hyaline membrane disease or meconium aspiration syndrome, but should be suspected if unevenly distributed.
5. **Pulmonary haemorrhage** — 75% are less than 2.5 kg. Onset at birth or delayed several days. Resembles meconium aspiration syndrome or hyaline membrane disease.
6. **Upper airway obstruction** — e.g. choanal atresia and micrognathia.
7. **Mikity–Wilson syndrome (pulmonary dysmaturity)** — always premature infants and usually less than 1.5 kg. Initially well but there is an insidious onset of respiratory distress between 1 and 6 weeks. Streaky opacities radiating from both hila with small bubbly areas of focal hyperaeration throughout both lungs.

Moderate hyperinflation. Severe disease leads to death but infants may recover fully. Resolution over a period of 12 months. Bases clear before apices and hyperinflation is the last feature to disappear.

8. **Abnormal thoracic cage**
   (a) neuromuscular abnormalities — often with thin ribs and clavicles.
   (b) skeletal dysplasias — e.g. Jeune's asphyxiating thoracic dysplasia, thanatophoric dwarfism, osteogenesis imperfecta and metatropic dwarfism.

B. With mediastinal shift away from the abnormal side

1. **Diaphragmatic hernia** — six times more common on the left side. Multiple lucencies due to gas containing bowel in the chest. Herniated bowel may appear solid if X-rayed too early but there will still be a paucity of gas in the abdomen.
2. **Congenital lobar emphysema** — involves the left upper, right upper and right middle lobes (in decreasing order of frequency) with compression of the lung base (cf. pneumothorax which produces symmetrical lung compression). CT is useful, particularly to exclude external compression of a bronchus by an aberrant vessel.
3. **Cystic adenomatoid malformation** — translucencies of various shapes and sizes scattered throughout an area of opaque lung with well-defined margins.
4. **Pneumothorax** — may complicate resuscitation or positive pressure ventilation, or may be spontaneous. Spontaneous pneumothorax is associated with renal anomalies. In the supine neonate, pleural air collects anteriorly and may not collapse the lung medially. In the absence of a lung edge, other signs which suggest the presence of a pneumothorax are:
   (a) sharp ipsilateral heart border.
   (b) depression or inversion of the ipsilateral hemidiaphragm.
   (c) sharp ipsilateral parietal pleura in the upper medial part of the hemithorax. If there is tension this may herniate across the superior mediastinum.
   (d) medial deviation of the ipsilateral compressed thymic lobe.
   (e) mediastinal shift to the contralateral side.
5. **Pleural effusion (empyema, chylothorax)** — rare.

C. With mediastinal shift towards the abnormal side

1. **Atelectasis** — most commonly due to incorrect placement of an endotracheal tube down a major bronchus. Much less commonly, primary atelectasis may occur without any other abnormality.
2. **Agenesis** — rare. May be difficult to differentiate from collapse but other congenital defects, especially hemivertebrae, are commonly associated.

CARDIAC CAUSES (Q.V.)

CEREBRAL CAUSES

Haemorrhage, oedema and drugs. After cardiopulmonary causes these account for 50% of the remainder.

METABOLIC CAUSES

Metabolic acidosis, hypoglycaemia and hypothermia.

ABDOMINAL CAUSES

Massive organomegaly, e.g. polycystic kidneys, elevating the diaphragms.

Further Reading

Agrons G.A. & Harty M.P. (1998) Lung disease in premature neonates: impact of new treatments and technologies. *Semin. Roentgenol.*, 33(2): 101–16.

Alford B.A. & McIlhenny J. (1999) An approach to the asymmetric neonatal chest radiograph. *Radiol. Clin. North Am.*, 37(6) 1079–92.

Cleveland R.H. (1995) A radiologic update on medical diseases of the newborn chest. *Pediatr. Radiol.*, 25: 631–7.

Donnelly L.F. & Frush D.P. (1999) Localized radiolucent chest lesions in neonates. *Am. J. Roentgenol.*, 172: 1651–8.

Markowitz R.I. & Fellows K.E. (1998) The effects of congenital heart disease on the lungs. *Semin. Roentgenol.*, 33(2): 126–35.

Newman B. (1999) Imaging of medical disease of the newborn lung. *Radiol. Clin. North Am.*, 37(6): 1049–65.

Schwartz D.S., Reyes-Mugica M. & Keller M.S. (1999) Imaging of surgical diseases of the newborn chest. *Radiol. Clin. North Am.*, 37(6): 1067–78.

4.52 RING SHADOWS IN A CHILD

NEONATE

1. **Diaphragmatic hernia** — unilateral.
2. **Interstitial emphysema** — secondary to ventilator therapy. Bilateral.
3. **Cystic adenomatoid malformation** — unilateral.
4. **Mikity–Wilson syndrome** — bilateral.

OLDER CHILD

1. **Cystic bronchiectasis** (q.v.).
2. **Cystic fibrosis*.**
3. **Pneumatocoeles** (q.v.).
4. **Langerhans cell histiocytosis*** } see 4.20.
5. **Neurofibromatosis*** }

See also 4.51.

4.53 DRUG-INDUCED LUNG DISEASE

DIFFUSE ALVEOLAR OPACITIES

1. **Pulmonary oedema** — cocaine, cytosine arabinoside (Ara-C), heroin overdose, interleukin 2, morphine overdose, OKT3 (in association with fluid overload), sympathomimetics (ritodrine and terbutaline), salicylate overdose and tricyclic antidepressant overdose.
2. **Pulmonary haemorrhage** — anticoagulants and those drugs which produce an idiosyncratic thrombocytopenia, crack cocaine, penicillamine and quinidine.
3. **Allergic alveolitis** — pituitary snuff.

FOCAL ALVEOLAR OPACITIES

1. **Phospholipidosis** — amiodarone.
2. **Pulmonary eosinophilia** — sulphonamides (sulphasalazine), nitrofurantoin, para-aminosalicylic acid and penicillin.
3. **Vasculitis** — ampicillin, penicillin and sulphonamides.

DIFFUSE INTERSTITIAL OPACITIES

1. **Acute interstitial reactions** — all-trans retinoic acid, methotrexate, nitrofurantoin, procarbazine and drugs causing pulmonary oedema.
2. **Chronic interstitial reactions** — cytotoxic agents (BCNU, bleomycin, busulphan, cyclophosphamide, methotrexate and mitomycin-C).
3. **Non-cytotoxic agents** — amiodarone, gold salts and nitrofurantoin.

BRONCHOSPASM

1. **β-blockers.**
2. **Histamine liberators** — iodine containing contrast media and morphine.
3. **Drugs as antigens** — antisera, penicillins and cephalosporins.
4. **Others** — aspirin, anti-inflammatory agents, paracetamol.

HILAR ENLARGEMENT OR MEDIASTINAL WIDENING

1. **Phenytoin**
2. **Steroids**

INCREASED OPPORTUNISTIC INFECTIONS

1. **Antimitotics.**
2. **Steroids.**
3. **Actinomycin C.**
4. **Drug-induced neutropenia or aplastic anaemia** — idiosyncratic or dose-related.

Further Reading

Aronchik J.M. & Gefter W.B. (1995) Drug-induced pulmonary disorders. *Semin. Roentgenol.*, 30(1): 18–34.

Ellis S.J., Cleverley J.R. & Muller N.L. (2000) Drug-induced lung disease: high resolution CT findings. *Am. J. Roentgenol.*, 175: 1019–24.

Erasmus J.J., McAdams H.P. & Rossi S.E. (2002) High-resolution CT of drug-induced lung disease. *Radiol. Clin. North Am.*, 40(1): 61–72.

Gefter W.B., Aronchik J.M., Miller W.T. Jr. *et al.* (1990) Drug-induced chest disorders. In: *A Categorical Course in Diagnostic Radiology, RSNA Scientific Assembly.* Chicago: RSNA, pp. 167–80.

Rossi S.E., Erasmus J.J., McAdams P. *et al.* (2000) Pulmonary drug toxicity: radiologic and pathologic manifestations. *RadioGraphics,* 20: 1245–59.

4.54 HIGH RESOLUTION CT – NODULES

These may be centrilobular, perilymphatic or random.

CENTRILOBULAR

The most peripheral nodules are > 5 mm from the pleural surfaces. They are often seen close to small vessels and are related to endobronchial and small airway disease. A 'tree in bud' appearance suggests endobronchial disease.

1. **Tuberculosis.**
2. **Endobronchial spread of tumour** — e.g. bronchoalveolar carcinoma.
3. **Hypersensitivity pneumonitis.**
4. **Bronchiolitis** — bronchiolitis obliterans, bronchiolitis obliterans organizing pneumonia, respiratory bronchiolitis.
5. **Diseases associated with bronchiectasis.**

PERILYMPHATIC

Nodules will be seen closely related (i.e. < 5 mm) to the pleural surfaces, large vessels and bronchi, interlobular septa and centrilobular regions.

1. **Sarcoidosis*.**
2. **Lymphangitis carcinomatosa.**
3. **Silicosis*.**
4. **Coal miner's pneumoconiosis*.**
5. **Lymphoma*.**
6. **Lymphoid interstitial pneumonia.**
7. **Amyloidosis.**

RANDOM

Nodules are seen randomly distributed in relationship to the secondary pulmonary lobule and thus also involve the pleural surfaces.

1. **Miliary tuberculosis.**
2. **Haematogenous metastasis.**
3. **Fungi.**
4. **Silicosis*.**
5. **Coal miner's pneumoconiosis.**
6. **Langerhans cell histiocytosis*.**

4.55 HIGH RESOLUTION CT – LINES

INTERLOBULAR SEPTAL THICKENING

Outlines the secondary pulmonary lobule and thus contains a visible central arterial branch. If seen peripherally the lines may extend to the pleural surface.

1. **Lymphangitis carcinomatosa** — typically nodular but may be smooth.
2. **Sarcoidosis*** - typically nodular.
3. **Pulmonary oedema** — smooth.
4. **Alveolar proteinosis** — typically smooth with associated ground-glass opacity.
5. **Pulmonary fibrosis** — usually smooth.

INTRALOBULAR SEPTAL THICKENING

Occurs within the secondary pulmonary nodule.

1. **Early pulmonary fibrosis.**
2. **Lymphangitis carcinomatosa.**
3. **Sarcoidosis*.**
4. **Pulmonary oedema.**
5. **Alveolar proteinosis.**

PARENCHYMAL BANDS

Any cause of pulmonary fibrosis.

4.56 HIGH RESOLUTION CT – GROUND-GLASS OPACITY

This is a hazy increase in lung density without obscuring the pulmonary vessels. It is frequently patchy and is seen in early interstitial or air space disease. Although it is associated with active disease, in areas where there is coexistent fibrosis the appearances are likely to be due to the fibrosis rather than to reversible disease.

NB. Refer to its differentiation from mosaic attenuation (see 4.58).

1. **Interstitial pneumonitis.**
2. **Pneumonia** — *Pneumocystis carinii*, viral, eosinophilic, hypersensitivity (extrinsic allergic alveolitis).

3. **Pulmonary oedema.**
4. **Pulmonary haemorrhage.**
5. **Sarcoidosis*.**
6. **Bronchiolitis obliterans organizing pneumonia.**
7. **Alveolar proteinosis.**
8. **Any developing cause of consolidation** — see 4.15.

Further Reading

Ellis S.M. & Hansell D.M. (2002) Idiopathic interstitial pneumonias: imaging-pathology correlation. *Eur. Radiol.*, 12: 610–26.

Reynolds J.H. & Hansell D.M. (2000) The interstitial pneumonias: understanding the acronyms. *Clin. Radiol.*, 55: 249–60.

Webb W.R., Müller N.L. & Naidich D.P (2000) *High Resolution CT of the Lung.* Philadelphia: Lippincott Williams & Wilkins.

Webb W.R., Brant W.E. & Helms C.A. (1997) *Fundamentals of Body CT.* Philadelphia: Saunders.

4.57 HIGH RESOLUTION CT – CONSOLIDATION

Similar to ground-glass but the pulmonary vessels are now obscured. The pattern of consolidation may be helpful in determining aetiology.

PERIPHERAL

1. **Pneumonia** — eosinophilic, bronchiolitis obliterans organizing pneumonia.
2. **Neoplasia** — bronchoalveolar carcinoma, lymphoma.
3. **Pulmonary infarction.**

PERIBRONCHIAL

1. **Infection** — airway invasive aspergillosis.
2. **Neoplasia** — lymphoma, Kaposi's sarcoma.
3. **Bronchiolitis obliterans organizing pneumonia.**

4.58 HIGH RESOLUTION CT – MOSAIC ATTENUATION

Refers to areas of altered attenuation on HRCT. It reflects vascular obstruction or abnormal ventilation. However, ground-glass opacity can look similar and is more common. To differentiate an area of ground-glass opacity from mosaic attenuation, look at the inspiratory HRCT scan and compare the 'lucent' and 'opaque' areas. Try to determine which area has the bigger centrilobular vessels. This area is normal. (NB. This differentiation may be difficult as, in practice, with ground-glass opacity, the vessels are often the same size throughout the lung.) If the lucent area is judged to be normal then the opaque area represents ground-glass opacity. If the lucent area is judged to be abnormal then the lucent area represents mosaic attenuation. In cases judged to be mosaic attenuation further information can be obtained by an expiratory scan.

IF THERE IS AIR TRAPPING THE DIAGNOSIS IS AIRWAYS DISEASE

1. **Bronchiolitis obliterans.**
2. **Other causes of small airways obstruction** — e.g. bronchiectasis and cystic fibrosis.
3. **Large bronchial obstruction.**

IF THERE IS NO AIR TRAPPING THE DIAGNOSIS IS VASCULAR DISEASE

1. **Pulmonary emboli** — of any cause.

Further Reading

Webb W.R., Brant W.E. & Helms C.A. (1997) *Fundamentals of Body CT.* Philadelphia: Saunders.

Webb W.R., Müller N.L. & Naidich D.P (2000) *High Resolution CT of the Lung.* Philadelphia: Lippincott Williams & Wilkins.

4.59 HIGH RESOLUTION CT — PATTERNS OF PARENCHYMAL DISEASE PROCESSES

Normal vessels are only visualized up to a distance of 1 cm from the pleura. Any linear opacity distal to this is abnormal. Although HRCT is sensitive in detecting interstitial opacification, there is an overlap of appearances for different disease processes which can cause difficulty in making a specific diagnosis. Scans must be done prone to avoid the gravitational effect obscuring early interstitial fibrosis.

PERIPHERAL, BASE

1. **Cryptogenic fibrosing alveolitis**
   (a) Early — ground-glass opacities, subpleural reticulation at lung base.
   (b) Later — reticulation extends centrally.
   (c) Chronic — small cyst formation commencing at subpleural site.
2. **Asbestos-related lung disease**
   (a) Earliest changes are at the lung bases posteriorly.
   (b) Thickened curvilinear subpleural lines.

   (c) Thickened subpleural septal (interlobular) lines.

   (d) Coarse parenchymal lines extending centrally separate from pulmonary vessels.

   (e) 'Honeycombing'.

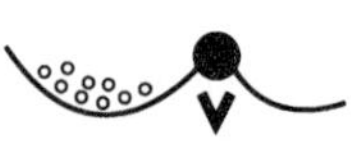

   (f) ± Rounded atelectasis — wedge-shaped contiguous with pleural, thickening 'comet tail' vessels.

CENTRAL, UPPER/MID ZONE

1. **Sarcoidosis** — thickened bronchovascular sheath ± 'beading' centrally. ± Patchy alveolar opacification. Nodules — subpleural and peribronchovascular.

PERIPHERAL AND CENTRAL

1. **Lymphangitis** — can mimic sarcoidosis, but rarely has alveolar opacification. Approx. 50% cases are focal — CT can be used to guide optimum biopsy site.

WIDESPREAD

1. **Lymphangioleiomyomatosis**

Further Reading

Hansell D.M. (2001) Computed tomography of diffuse lung disease: functional correlates. *Eur. Radiol.*, 11: 1666–80.
Kazerooni E.A. (2001) High-resolution CT of the lungs. *Am. J. Roentgenol.*, 177: 501–19.
Lynch D.A. (ed.) (2001) High resolution CT of the lung I. *Radiol. Clin. North Am.*, 39(6).
Lynch D.A. (ed.) (2002) High resolution CT of the lung II. *Radiol. Clin. North Am.*, 40(1).
Reynolds J.H. & Hansell D.M. (2000) The interstitial pneumonias: understanding the acronyms. *Clin. Radiol.*, 55: 249–60.
Schaefer-Prokop C., Prokop M., Fleischmann D. *et al.* (2001) High-resolution CT of diffuse interstitial lung disease: key findings in common disorders. *Eur. Radiol.*, 11: 373–92.
Takasugi J.E. & Godwin J.D. (1998) Radiology of chronic obstructive pulmonary disease. *Radiol. Clin. North Am.*, 36: 29–56.
Worthy S.A. & Muller N.L. (1998) Small airway diseases. *Radiol. Clin. North Am.*, 36: 163–73.

4.60 CT OF DIFFUSE INTERSTITIAL LUNG DISEASE IN CHILDREN

KNOWN AETIOLOGY

1. **Aspiration.**
2. **Chronic infection.**
3. **Hypersensitivity pneumonia.**
4. **Lipid storage diseases.**

UNKNOWN AETIOLOGY

1. **Desquamative interstitial pneumonitis (DIP)** — most cases less than 1 year of age. Widespread ground-glass attenuation.
2. **Lymphocytic interstitial pneumonitis (LIP)** — associated with immunodeficiency states and connective tissue disorders. Widespread ground-glass attenuation with small nodules.
3. **Follicular bronchiolitis** — widespread ground-glass attenuation with small nodules.
4. **Non-specific interstitial pneumonitis** — widespread ground-glass attenuation, but with upper zone predominance of a honeycomb pattern and parenchymal distortion.
5. **Idiopathic pulmonary haemosiderosis.**
6. **Obliterative bronchiolitis.**
7. **Cryptogenic organizing pneumonitis.**
8. **Alveolar proteinosis** — bilateral ground-glass appearance, consolidation and thickened interlobular septa giving a 'crazy paving' pattern.
9. **Pulmonary lymphangiomatosis** — thickened interlobular septa, peribronchial thickening, ground-glass attenuation, pleural effusions and pleural thickening, and increased attenuation of mediastinal fat.
10. **Pulmonary alveolar microlithiasis.**

SYSTEMIC DISORDERS WITH LUNG INVOLVEMENT

1. **Neurocutaneous disorders.**
2. **Connective tissue disorders** — particularly systemic sclerosis.
3. **Langerhan's cell histiocytosis*** — as part of multisystem involvement. Lung disease may regress in younger children. In older children there are multiple nodules which are the precursors of multiple thin-walled cysts, < 1 cm, predominantly in the upper and mid zones with relative sparing of the costophrenic angles.

UNIQUE TO CHILDHOOD

1. **Persistent tachypnoea of the newborn.**
2. **Bronchopulmonary dysplasia.**
3. **Cellular interstitial pneumonitis of infancy.**
4. **Infantile pulmonary haemosiderosis.**
5. **Chronic pneumonitis of infancy (CPI).**
6. **Surfactant protein B deficiency** — AR. Similar appearance to hyaline membrane disease but in a full-term newborn infant.
7. **Familial desquamative interstitial pneumonitis** — worse prognosis than DIP.

Further Reading

Copley S.J. & Padley S.P. (2001) High-resolution CT of paediatric lung disease. *Eur. Radiol.*, 11: 2564–75.

Koh D.M. & Hansell D.M. (2000) Computed tomography of diffuse interstitial lung disease in children. *Clin. Radiol.*, 55: 659–67.

Lynch D.A., Hay T., Newell J.D. *et al.* (1999) Pediatric diffuse lung disease: diagnosis and classification using high-resolution CT. *Am. J. Roentgenol.*, 173: 713–8.

Schaefer-Prokop C., Prokop M., Fleischmann D. *et al.* (2001) High-resolution CT of diffuse interstitial lung disease: key findings in common disorders. *Eur. Radiol.*, 11: 373–92.

4.61 THE THYMUS

The normal thymus is a bilobed anterosuperior mediastinal structure. It is only visible on plain films of infants and young children, and is inconstantly visible after 2–3 years of age. On plain films three radiological signs aid diagnosis — the 'sail' sign (a triangular projection to one or both sides of the mediastinum), the 'wave' sign (a rippled thymic contour due to indentations by the anterior rib ends) or the 'notch' sign (an indentation at the junction of thymus with heart). A large normal thymus may be seen in:

(a) Well nourished children.
(b) Following recovery from illness (rebound overgrowth in 25% following previous involution).
(c) Hyperthyroidism and euthyroid children following treatment for hypothyroidism.

It has the following CT characteristics:

1. **Incidence** — identifiable in 100% < 30 years of age, decreasing to 17% > 49 years. However, < 10 years of age the distinction from great vessels is very difficult without the use of contrast enhancement.
2. **Shape** — quadrilateral shape in childhood with, usually, convex, undulating margins. After puberty two separate lobes (ovoid, elliptical, triangular or semilunar) or an arrowhead (triangle). The normal thymus is never multilobular.
3. **Size** — progressive enlargement during childhood. Maximum absolute size is in the 12–19-year age group but relative to body size it is largest in infancy. Left lobe nearly always larger than right lobe. Becomes narrower with increasing age. Maximum thickness (the perpendicular to the long axis) of one lobe in those > 20 years is 1.3 cm. In those > 40 years there may be linear or oval soft-tissue densities but they are never > 7 mm in size and never alter the lateral contour of the mediastinal fat.
4. **Density** — homogeneous, isodense or hyperdense when related to chest wall musculature in childhood. After puberty becoming inhomogeneous and progressively lower in attenuation due to fatty infiltration. In those > 40 years the majority will have total fatty involution.

On MRI the normal thymus is:

1. Larger than is seen by CT (probably because the study is undertaken during quiet respiration rather than with suspended full inspiration).

2. Homogeneous in childhood (T_1W slightly greater than muscle, T_2W similar to fat).
3. Heterogeneous in adults (T_1W and T_2W similar to fat).

Further Reading

Baron R.L., Lee J.K., Sagel S.S. *et al.* (1982) Computed tomography of the normal thymus. *Radiology,* 142: 121–5.

Baron R.L., Lee J.K., Sagel S.S. *et al.* (1982) Computed tomography of the abnormal thymus. *Radiology,* 142: 127–34.

Francis I.R., Glazer G.M., Bookstein F.L. *et al.* (1985) The thymus: re-examination of age-related changes in size and shape. *Am. J. Roentgenol.,* 145: 249–54.

de Geer G., Webb W.R. & Gamsu G. (1986) Normal thymus: assessment with MR and CT. *Radiology,* 158: 313–7.

Han B., Babcock D. & Oestreich A. (1989) Normal thymus in infancy: sonographic characteristics. *Radiology,* 170: 471–4.

Leonidas J.C. (1998) The thymus: from past misconception to present recognition. *Pediatr. Radiol.,* 28: 275–82.

Siegal M.J., Glazer H.S., Wiener J.I. *et al.* (1989) Normal and abnormal thymus in childhood: MR imaging. *Radiology,* 172: 367–71.

Williams M.P. (1989) Problems in radiology: CT assessment of the thymus. *Clin. Radiol.,* 40: 113–4.

4.62 ANTERIOR MEDIASTINAL MASSES IN CHILDREN

The anterior mediastinum is bounded by the clavicles (superiorly), the diaphragm (inferiorly), the sternum (anteriorly) and the anterior surfaces of the heart and great vessels (posteriorly). 45% of paediatric mediastinal masses occur at this site.

CONGENITAL

1. **Normal thymus** — see 4.61.
2. **Cystic hygroma** — 5% of anterior mediastinal masses but the majority are extensions from the neck with only 1% being purely mediastinal.
3. **Morgagni hernia.**

NEOPLASTIC

1. **Hodgkin's disease (HD), non-Hodgkin's lymphoma (NHL) and leukaemia** — the majority of neoplastic anterior mediastinal masses are due to Hodgkin's disease. At presentation, mediastinal lymph nodes are seen in 23% of HD, 14% of NHL and 5–10% of leukaemics. Comparing mediastinal involvement in HD with NHL:

Hodgkin's disease	*Non-Hodgkin's lymphoma*
Usually > 10 yrs old	Any age in children
Mostly localized. Mediastinal lymphadenopathy (LN) in 85% of those with cervical LN	Disseminated disease in > 75% at presentation
Histology usually nodular sclerosing	Histology usually lymphoblastic
Displacement of other mediastinal structures rather than compression	Tracheal compression is more likely
Paratracheal > hilar > subcarinal LN. Hilar LN without mediastinal LN is rare	
Lung involvement in 10% at diagnosis – direct spread from LNs	Pulmonary involvement is higher
	Pleural effusion is more common but may be 2° to ascites or lymphatic obstruction.

After treatment for lymphoma a residual anterior mediastinal mass may present a diagnostic difficulty. If CT shows this to be homogeneous and there is no other lymphadenopathy then tumour is unlikely to be present but only the lack of deterioration on follow-up imaging studies will provide confirmation.

2. **Germ cell tumours** — 5–10% of germ cell tumours arise in the mediastinum. Two age peaks: at 2 years and during adolescence. Majority (80%) are teratomas and benign. Endodermal sinus (yolk sac) tumours are more aggressive. Seminomas are rare. All tumours are moderate to large in size and may contain calcification (including teeth), fat and cystic/necrotic areas. Radiological appearance does not accurately correlate with histology but large size, marked mass effect and local infiltration suggest an aggressive lesion.
3. **Thymoma** — 5–8% of mediastinal tumours in childhood. Most occur after 10 years of age. 50% discovered incidentally. Calcification in 10% — linear. Only rarely associated with myasthenia gravis.

INFLAMMATORY

1. **Lymphadenopathy** — inflammatory lymph node masses are less common than neoplasia. Most frequent causes are tuberculosis and histoplasmosis.

Further Reading

Cohen M.D. (1992) *Imaging of Children With Cancer,* Ch. 4. St Louis: Mosby Year Book, pp. 89–133.

Crisci K.L., Greenberg S.B. & Wolfson B.J. (1997) Cardiopulmonary and thoracic tumours of childhood. *Radiol. Clin. North Am.*, 35(6): 1341–66.

Meza M.P., Benson M. & Slovis T. (1993) Imaging of mediastinal masses in children. *Radiol. Clin. North Am.*, 31: 583–604.

4.63 MIDDLE MEDIASTINAL MASSES IN CHILDREN

The middle mediastinum is bordered by the anterior and posterior mediastinum. 20% of paediatric mediastinal masses occur at this site.

NEOPLASTIC

1. Most middle mediastinal tumours are extensions of those which arise primarily in the anterior mediastinum (see 4.62).

INFLAMMATORY

1. **Lymphadenopathy** — tuberculosis, histoplasmosis and sarcoidosis.

CONGENITAL

1. **Foregut duplication cysts** — account for 10–20% of paediatric mediastinal masses. The spectrum of abnormalities includes bronchogenic cysts, oesophageal duplication cysts and neurenteric cysts.
   Bronchogenic cyst — round or oval, unilocular, homogeneous, water-density mass (usually 0–20 HU, but up to 100 HU due to mucus or milk of calcium contents) with well-defined borders. There may be airway obstruction and secondary infection, both within the cyst and in the surrounding lung. Communication with the tracheobronchial tree, resulting in a cavity, is rare. Four groups may be defined according to location:
   (a) Paratracheal cysts are attached to the tracheal wall above the carina.
   (b) Carinal cysts are the most common and are attached to the carina ± anterior oesophageal wall.
   (c) Hilar cysts are attached to a lobar bronchus and appear to be intrapulmonary.
   (d) Para-oesophageal cysts may be attached or communicate with the oesophagus but have no communication with the bronchial tree.

   Oesophageal Duplication cyst — 10–15% of intestinal duplications. Less common than bronchogenic cysts, usually larger and usually situated to the right of the midline extending into the posterior mediastinum. May be an incidental finding or produce symptoms related to oesophageal or tracheobronchial tree compression. May contain ectopic gastric mucosa (positive ^{99m}Tc-pertechnetate scan) which causes ulceration, haemorrhage or perforation. Communication with the oesophageal lumen is rare.

Neurenteric cyst — located in the middle or posterior mediastinum, contains neural tissue and maintains a connection with the spinal canal. More commonly right-sided. Vertebral body anomalies (hemivertebra, butterfly vertebra and scoliosis) are usually superior to the cyst.

2. **Cystic hygroma** — 5% of cystic hygromas extend into the mediastinum from the neck. Most present at birth. Cystic with some solid components on all imaging modalities.
3. **Hiatus hernia.**
4. **Achalasia.**
5. **Cardiomegaly or vena caval enlargement** — see Chapter 5.

Further Reading

Berrocal T., Torres I., Gutierrez J. *et al.* (1999) Congenital anomalies of the upper gastrointestinal tract. *RadioGraphics,* 19: 855–72.

Merten D.F. (1992) Diagnostic imaging of mediastinal masses in children. *Am. J. Roentgenol.,* 158: 825–32.

Meza M.P., Benson M. & Slovis T. (1993) Imaging of mediastinal masses in children. *Radiol. Clin. North Am.,* 31: 583–604.

4.64 POSTERIOR MEDIASTINAL MASSES IN CHILDREN

The posterior mediastinum is bounded by the thoracic inlet (superiorly), the diaphragm (inferiorly), the bodies of the thoracic vertebrae and paravertebral gutters (posteriorly), and the pericardium (anteriorly). In children, 30–40% of mediastinal masses lie in the posterior mediastinum and 95% of these are of neurogenic origin.

Left-sided paravertebral soft tissues greater than the width of the adjacent pedicle (particularly on radiographs taken in the upright position) and any right-sided paravertebral soft-tissue shadows are abnormal.

NEOPLASTIC

1. **Ganglion cell tumours** — neuroblastoma (most malignant, usually < 5 years), ganglioneuroblastoma (age 5–10 years) and ganglioneuroma (benign, usually > 10 years). Imaging features of all three types are similar but metastases do not occur with ganglioneuroma. Plain films show a paravertebral soft-tissue mass with calcification in 30%. Thinning of posterior ribs, separation of ribs and enlargement of intervertebral foramina. CT shows calcification in 90%. Both CT and MRI may show extradural extension.

CONGENITAL

1. **Bochdalek hernia** — most present at, or shortly after, birth with respiratory distress, but 5% present after the neonatal period. Rarely it may complicate Group B streptococcal infection. Bochdalek hernias include:
   (a) Persistence of the pleuroperitoneal canal with a posterior lip of diaphragm.
   (b) Larger defects with no diaphragm.
   (c) Herniation through the costolumbar triangles.

The appearance of herniated liver may provoke thoracentesis and herniated bowel may mimic pneumothorax, pneumatocoeles or cystic adenomatoid malformation.

Further Reading

Berman L., Stringer D.A., Ein S. *et al.* (1988) Childhood diaphragmatic hernias presenting after the neonatal period. *Clin. Radiol.*, 39: 237–44.

Donnelly L.F., Frush D.P., Zheng J.-Y. *et al.* (2000) Differentiating normal from abnormal inferior thoracic paravertebral soft tissues on chest radiography in children. *Am. J. Roentgenol.*, 175: 477–83.

4.65 ANTERIOR MEDIASTINAL MASSES IN ADULTS

Anterior to the pericardium and trachea. Superiorly the retrosternal air space is obliterated. For ease of discussion it can be divided into three regions:

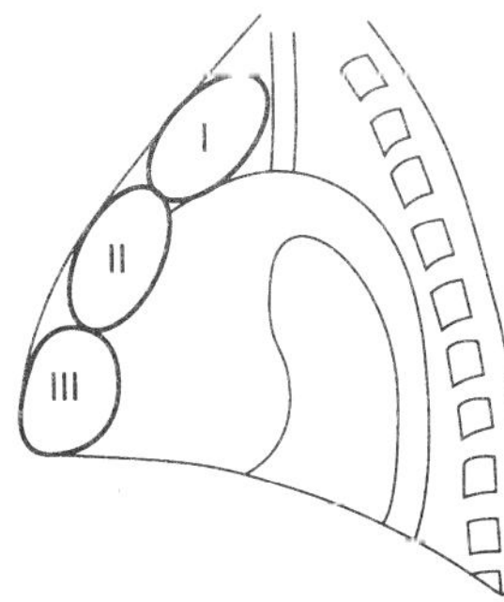

REGION I

1. **Retrosternal goitre** — goitre extends into the mediastinum in 3–17% of cases. On a PA chest X-ray it appears as an inverted truncated cone with its base uppermost. It is well-defined, smooth or lobulated. The trachea may be displaced posteriorly and laterally, and may be narrowed. Calcification is common. CT shows the connection with the cervical thyroid. Relatively high attenuation compared with other mediastinal structures and other tumours. Uptake by ^{123}I is diagnostic when positive but the thyroid may be non-functioning.
2. **Tortuous innominate artery** — a common finding in the elderly.
3. **Lymph nodes** — due to reticuloses, metastases or granulomas.
4. **Thymic tumours** — are uncommon but occur in 15% of adult patients with myasthenia gravis. They are round or oval and smooth or lobulated. They may contain nodular or rim calcification. If the tumour contains a large amount of fat (thymolipoma) then it may be very large and soft and reach the diaphragm, leaving the superior mediastinum clear.
5. **Aneurysm of the ascending aorta.**

REGION II

1. **Germinal cell neoplasms** — including dermoids, teratomas, seminomas, choriocarcinomas, embryonal carcinomas and endodermal sinus tumours. More than 80% are benign and they

occur with equal incidence to thymic tumours. Usually larger than thymomas (but not thymolipomas). Round or oval and smooth. They usually project to one or other side of the mediastinum on the PA view. Calcification, especially rim calcification, and fragments of bone or teeth may be demonstrable, the latter being diagnostic.

2. **Thymic tumours** — see above.
3. **Sternal tumours** — metastases (breast, bronchus, kidney and thyroid) are the most common. Of the primary tumours, malignant (chondrosarcoma, myeloma, reticulum cell sarcoma and lymphoma) are more common than benign (chondroma, aneurysmal bone cyst and giant cell tumour).

REGION III (ANTERIOR CARDIOPHRENIC ANGLE MASSES)

1. **Pericardiac fat pad** — especially in obese people. A triangular opacity in the cardiophrenic angle on the PA view. It appears less dense than expected because of the fat content. CT is diagnostic. Excessive mediastinal fat can be due to steroid therapy.
2. **Diaphragmatic hump** — or localized eventration. Commonest on the anteromedial portion of the right hemidiaphragm. A portion of liver extends into it and this can be confirmed by ultrasound or isotope examination of the liver.
3. **Morgagni hernia** — through the defect between the septum transversum and the costal portion of the diaphragm. It is almost invariably on the right side but is occasionally bilateral. It usually contains a knuckle of colon or, less commonly, colon and stomach. Appears solid if it contains omentum and/or liver. Ultrasound and/or barium studies will confirm the diagnosis.
4. **Pericardial cysts** — either a true pericardial cyst ('spring water' cyst) or a pericardial diverticulum. The cyst is usually situated in the right cardiophrenic angle and is oval or spherical. CT confirms the liquid nature of the mass.

Further Reading

Buckley J.A. & Stark P. (1999) Intrathoracic mediastinal thyroid goiter: imaging manifestations. *Am. J. Roentgenol.*, 173: 471–5.

Drevelegas A., Palladas P. & Scordalaki A. (2001) Mediastinal germ cell tumours: a radiologic-pathologic review. *Eur. Radiol.*, 11: 1925–32.

Landwehr P., Schulte O. & Lackner K. (1999) MR imaging of the chest: mediastinum and chest wall. *Eur. Radiol.*, 9: 1737–44.

4.66 MIDDLE MEDIASTINAL MASSES IN ADULTS

Between the anterior and posterior mediastinum and containing the heart, great vessels and pulmonary roots. Causes of cardiac enlargement are excluded.

1. **Lymph nodes** — the paratracheal, tracheobronchial, bronchopulmonary and/or subcarinal nodes may be enlarged. This may be due to neoplasm (most frequently metastatic bronchial carcinoma), reticuloses (most frequently Hodgkin's disease), infection (most commonly tuberculosis, histoplasmosis or coccidioidomycosis) or sarcoidosis.
2. **Carcinoma of the bronchus** — arising from a major bronchus.
3. **Aneurysm of the aorta** — CT scanning after i.v. contrast medium or, if this is not available, aortography is diagnostic. Peripheral rim calcification is a useful sign if present.
4. **Bronchogenic cyst** — see 4.63.

Further Reading

Landwehr P., Schulte O. & Lackner K. (1999) MR imaging of the chest: mediastinum and chest wall. *Eur. Radiol.*, 9: 1737–44.

4.67 POSTERIOR MEDIASTINAL MASSES IN ADULTS

For ease of discussion it can be divided into three regions:

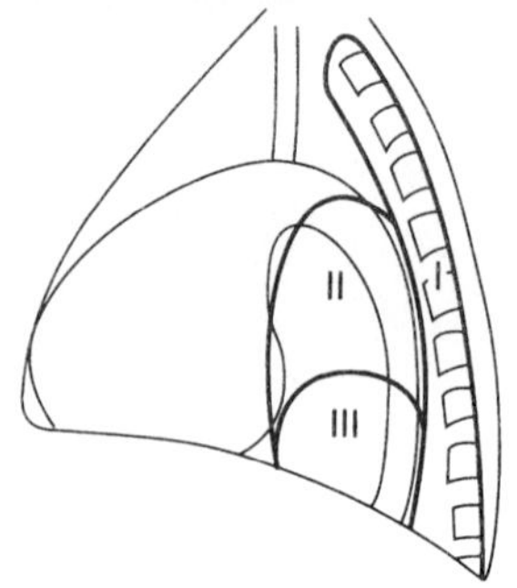

REGION I (PARAVERTEBRAL)

1. **Reticuloses, myeloma and metastases** — bone destruction with preserved discs.
2. **Extramedullary haemopoiesis** — with splenomegaly ± bone changes of specific disease entities, e.g. haemolytic anaemias.
3. **Abscess** — with disc space and vertebral body destruction.
4. **Ganglioneuroma** — see 4.64.

REGION II

1. **Dilated oesophagus** — especially achalasia. Contains mottled gas shadows ± an air fluid level. Diagnosis is confirmed by barium swallow.
2. **Aorta** — unfolded, dilated or ruptured.

REGION III

1. **Hiatus hernia** — often contains an air fluid level which is projected through the cardiac shadow on a penetrated PA view.

Further Reading

Landwehr P., Schulte O. & Lackner K. (1999) MR imaging of the chest: mediastinum and chest wall. *Eur. Radiol.*, 9: 1737–44.

4.68 CT MEDIASTINAL MASS CONTAINING FAT

1. **Teratodermoid** — well-defined soft-tissue mass containing fat and calcification.
2. **Diaphragmatic hernia** — bowel, liver, kidney or stomach may also be present. Anterior (Morgagni) hernias are usually on the right, and posterior (Bochdalek) hernias usually on the left. Linear soft-tissue densities representing omental vessels help to distinguish hernias which only contain omental fat from pericardial fat pads.
3. **Lipoma** — relatively rare. Can occur anywhere in the mediastinum.
4. **Liposarcoma** — can contain calcification, and may also appear as a soft-tissue mass with no visible fat, due to excess soft-tissue component of the sarcoma.
5. **Thymolipoma** — occurs in children and young adults. Accounts for 2–9% of thymic tumours. Usually asymptomatic.
6. **Mediastinal lipomatosis** — associated with Cushing's, steroid treatment and obesity.
7. **Hamartoma.**
8. **Chylolymphatic cyst** — fat/fluid level in cyst.
9. **Neurofibroma** — can have a negative CT attenuation due to myelin content.

Further Reading

Phillips G.W.L., Serapati A. & Young A.E. (1988) Chylolymphatic-mesenteric cyst: a diagnostic appearance on computed tomography. *Br. J. Radiol.*, 61: 413–4.

Reed D.H. (1988) The changing mediastinum. *Br. J. Radiol.*, 61: 695–6.

Shirkhoda A., Chasen M.H., Eftekhari F. *et al.* (1987) M.R. Imaging of mediastinal thymolipoma. *J. Comput. Assist. Tomogr.*, 11: 364–5.

4.69 CT MEDIASTINAL CYSTS

1. **Congenital**
   (a) Bronchogenic cyst — usually subcarinal or right paratracheal site. 50% homogeneous water density, 50% soft-tissue density due to mucus or milk of calcium content. Occasional calcification in cyst wall, and air in cyst if communicating with airway.
   (b) Enteric cyst — para-oesophageal site.
   (c) Neuroenteric cyst — associated anomaly of spine.
2. **Pericardial cyst** — usually cardiophrenic angle.
3. **Thymic cyst** — can develop following radiotherapy for Hodgkin's.
4. **Cystic tumours**
   (a) Lymphangioma.
   (b) Teratoma.
   (c) Teratodermoid.
5. **Pancreatic pseudocyst** — can track up into mediastinum.
6. **Meningocele** — 75% association with neurofibromatosis.
7. **Chronic abscess.**
8. **Old haematoma.**

Further Reading

Aviv R.I., McHugh K. & Hunt J. (2001) Angiomatosis of bone and soft tissue: a spectrum of disease from diffuse lymphangiomatosis to vanishing bone disease in young patients. *Clin. Radiol.*, 56; 184–90.

Charruau L., Parrens M., Jougon J. *et al.* (2000) Mediastinal lymphangioma in adults: CT and MR imaging features. *Eur. Radiol.*, 10: 1310–4.

DuMontier C., Graviss E.R., Silberstein M.J. *et al.* (1985) Bronchogenic cysts in children. *Clin. Radiol.*, 36: 431–6.

Nakata H, Sato Y., Nakayama T. *et al.* (1986) Bronchogenic cyst with high C.T. numbers: analysis of contents. *J. Comput. Assist. Tomogr.*, 10: 360–2.

4.70 CT THYMIC MASS

Normal shape of thymus is an arrowhead with maximum length < 2 cm and maximum width < 1.8 cm if age < 20 years, and 1.3 cm if age > 20 years. However, measurements are misleading, and a multilobular appearance or focal alteration in shape is abnormal at any age. Fatty involution occurs after the age of 30.

1. **Thymoma** — occurs in 15% of those with myasthenia gravis (usually occurring in the fourth decade) and 40% of these will be malignant. If malignant it is usually locally invasive and can extend along pleura to involve diaphragm and even spread into abdomen. Can contain calcification.
2. **Thymic hyperplasia**
   (a) Lymphoid — occurs in 65% of those with myasthenia gravis. Only medulla enlarges and this is not sufficient to be visible on CT.
   (b) True hyperplasia — occurs in myasthenia gravis, post-chemotherapy rebound, Graves thyrotoxicosis, Addison's and acromegaly. Thymus increases in size but is normal in shape.
3. **Germ cell tumour** — teratodermoid, benign and malignant teratomas.
4. **Lymphoma*** — thymus is infiltrated in 35% of Hodgkin's disease but there is always associated lymphadenopathy.
5. **Thymolipoma** — usually children or young adults. Asymptomatic.

Further Reading

Heron C.W., Husband, J.E. & Williams M.P. (1988) Hodgkin's disease: C.T. of the thymus. *Radiology*, 167: 647–51.
Moore N.R. (1989) Imaging in myasthenia gravis. *Clin. Radiol.*, 40: 115–6.
Williams M.P. (1989) Problems in radiology: C.T. assessment of the thymus. *Clin. Radiol.*, 40: 113–4.

4.71 VENTILATION PERFUSION MISMATCH

MISMATCHED PERFUSION DEFECTS

Perfusion defect greater than ventilation defect.

1. **Pulmonary embolus** — especially if multiple and segmental.
2. **Bronchial carcinoma** — but more commonly matched.
3. **Tuberculosis** — typically affecting an apical segment.
4. **Vasculitis** — polyarteritis nodosa, systemic lupus erythematosus, etc.
5. **Tumour embolus.**
6. **Fat embolus.**
7. **Post-radiotherapy.**
8. **Pulmonary hypertension.**

MISMATCHED VENTILATION DEFECTS

Bronchial obstruction with normal blood supply. Ventilation defect greater than perfusion defect.

1. **Chronic obstructive airways disease.**
2. **Pneumonia.**
3. **Carcinoma** — the rarest appearance with bronchial carcinoma.
4. **Lung collapse** — of any cause.
5. **Pleural effusion.**

Further Reading

Carvandho P. & Lavender J.P. (1988) Incidence and aetiology of the reverse (V/Q) mismatch defect. *Nucl. Med. Commun.*, 9: 167.

4.72 MULTIPLE MATCHED VENTILATION/PERFUSION DEFECTS

See 4.71.

1. **Chronic bronchitis.**
2. **Pulmonary infarct** (do not confuse with the mismatched perfusion defect of embolus).
3. **Asthma or acute bronchitis** — may also show mismatched ventilation or perfusion defects.
4. **Collagen vascular disease.**
5. **Lymphangitis carcinomatosa.**
6. **Pulmonary hypertension.**
7. **Sarcoidosis.***
8. **Intravenous drug abuse.**

Further Reading

Benson M.L. & Balseiro J. (1993) Multiple matched ventilation–perfusion defects in illicit drug use. *Semin. Nucl. Med.*, 23: 180–3.

5 Cardiovascular system

5.1 SITUS AND CARDIAC MALPOSITIONS

Assess the positions of the cardiac apex, aortic arch, left and right main bronchi, stomach bubble, liver and spleen. (Isolated right-sided aortic arch is not considered a malposition.)

1. **Situs solitus** — normal. All structures are concordant.
2. **Situs inversus** — cardiac apex, aortic arch and stomach are on the right; visceral organs are on the opposite side to normal. Slight increase in the incidence of congenital heart disease. Patients have sinusitis and bronchiectasis (Kartagener's syndrome).
3. **Situs solitus with dextrocardia** — cardiac apex on right with stomach bubble on left. Caused by failure of rotation of the embryonic cardiac loop and > 90% of cases are associated with congenital heart disease, usually cyanotic (corrected TGA, VSD and pulmonary stenosis). Scimitar syndrome is dextrocardia, hypoplastic right lung and partial anomalous pulmonary venous drainage into the inferior cava.
4. **Levoversion with abdominal situs inversus** — incidence of congenital heart disease 100%.
5. **Situs ambiguous with bilateral 'right-sidedness': asplenia syndrome** — absent spleen, bilateral trilobed lungs, right and left lobes of liver are similar size. Cardiac apex left, right or midline. Complex cardiac anomalies ± small bowel malrotation.
6. **Situs ambiguous with bilateral 'left-sidedness': polysplenia syndrome** — bilateral bilobed lungs, absent hepatic segment of IVC and enlarged azygos and hemiazygos veins. Intracardiac anomalies, but less complex than in bilateral 'right-sidedness'.

Further Reading

Applegate K.E. (1999) Situs revisited: imaging of the heterotaxy syndrome. *RadioGraphics*, 19: 837–52.

5.2 GROSS CARDIAC ENLARGEMENT

May be difficult to assess in the young infant because of a large thymus. If uncertainty persists, a lateral film is helpful. The normal size heart does not cross a line drawn from the trachea to the diaphragm.

1. **Multiple valvular disease** — aortic and mitral valve disease, particularly with regurgitation.
2. **Pericardial effusion** — no recognizable chamber enlargement. Flask-shaped heart on the erect film which becomes globular on the supine film. Acute angle between right heart border and right hemidiaphragm. The effusion masks ventricular wall movement; therefore, unusually sharp cardiac outline on chest radiography and poor pulsation on fluoroscopy. Rapid change in size on serial films. Diagnosis best made by echocardiography.
3. **ASD** — with pulmonary pleonaemia or an Eisenmenger situation.
4. **Cardiomyopathy** — including ischaemia.
5. **Ebstein's anomaly** — the posterior or septal cusp of the tricuspid valve arises distally from the wall of the right ventricle. Marked tricuspid incompetence. Marked right atrioventricular enlargement. Small aorta. Oligaemic lungs. Sharp cardiac outline.

Further Reading

Baron M.G. (1999) Plain film diagnosis of common cardiac anomalies in the adult. *Radiol. Clin. North Am.*, 37: 401–19.

5.3 SMALL HEART

1. **Normal variant.**
2. **Emphysema.**
3. **Addison's disease.**
4. **Dehydration/malnutrition.**
5. **Constrictive pericarditis.**

5.4 ENLARGED RIGHT ATRIUM

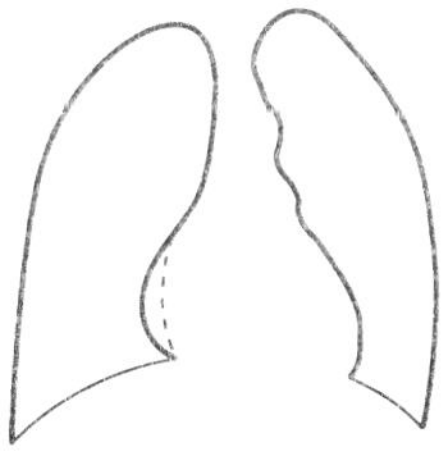

PA
Prominent right heart bordor

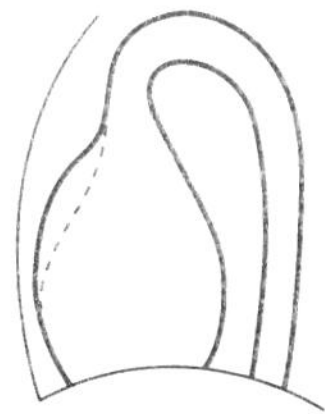

Lateral
Prominent anterosuperior part of cardiac shadow

VOLUME OVERLOAD

1. **ASD.**
2. **AV canal.**
3. **Tricuspid incompetence** — including Ebstein's anomaly, endocardial fibroelastosis and endomyocardial fibrosis. In 9% of patients following mitral valve replacement. In Uhl's disease there is a thin-walled, dilated right ventricle due to focal or complete absence of right ventricular myocardium.
4. **Anomalous pulmonary venous drainage.**

PRESSURE OVERLOAD

1. **Tricuspid stenosis** — NB. In tricuspid atresia a shunt must exist to preserve life. This decompresses the right atrium, so that it is not large (typically a straight right heart border).
2. **Myxoma of the right atrium** — may cause tricuspid obstruction.

SECONDARY TO RIGHT VENTRICULAR FAILURE

See 5.5.

Further Reading

Baron M.G. (1999) Plain film diagnosis of common cardiac anomalies in the adult. *Radiol. Clin. North Am.*, 37: 401–19.

Gross G.W. & Steiner R.M. (1991) Radiographic manifestations of congenital heart disease in the adult patient. *Radiol. Clin. North Am.*, 29: 293–318.

Rubin S.A., Hightower C.W. & Flicker S. (1987) Giant right atrium after mitral valve replacement: plain film findings in 15 patients. *Am. J. Roentgenol.*, 49: 257–60.

5.5 ENLARGED RIGHT VENTRICLE

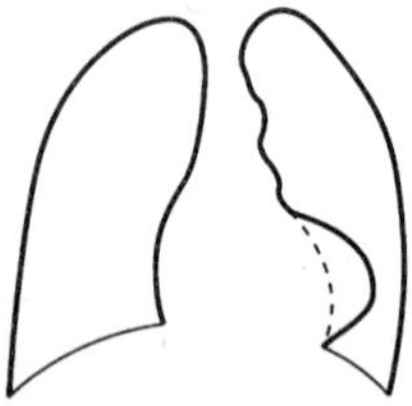

PA
Prominent left heart border
Elevated apex

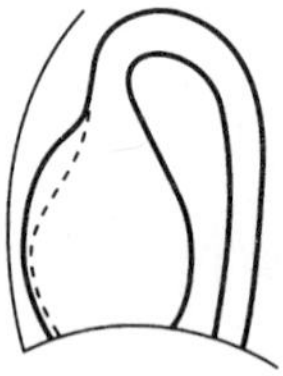

Lateral
Prominent anterior part of cardiac shadow

SECONDARY TO LEFT HEART FAILURE/MITRAL VALVE DISEASE

See 5.7.

PULMONARY ARTERIAL HYPERTENSION

1. **Diffuse lung disease** — e.g. chronic obstructive airways disease, interstitial fibrosis, cystic fibrosis etc.
2. **Pulmonary emboli** — see Pulmonary embolic disease*.
3. **Chronic left to right shunt** — with pulmonary hypertension and right ventricular failure.
4. **Vasculitis** — e.g. polyarteritis nodosa.
5. **Idiopathic** — mostly young females.

PRESSURE OVERLOAD

1. **Pulmonary stenosis.**

VOLUME OVERLOAD

1. **ASD.**
2. **VSD.**

Further Reading

Baron M.G. (1999) Plain film diagnosis of common cardiac anomalies in the adult. *Radiol. Clin. North Am.*, 37: 401–19.

Gross G.W. & Steiner R.M. (1991) Radiographic manifestations of congenital heart disease in the adult patient. *Radiol. Clin. North Am.*, 29: 293–318.

5.6 ENLARGED LEFT ATRIUM

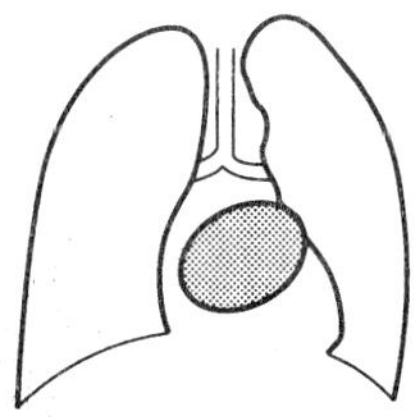

PA
1 Prominent left atrial appendage
2 'Double' right heart border
3 Increased density due to left atrium
4 Splaying of carina and elevated left main bronchus

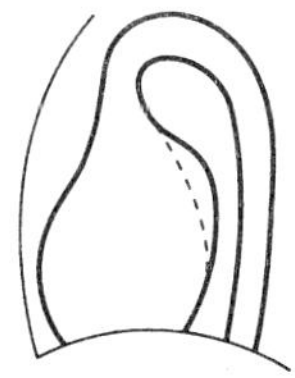

Lateral
1 Prominent posterosuperior part of cardiac shadow
2 Prominent left atrial impression on oesophagus during barium swallow

VOLUME OVERLOAD

1. **Mitral incompetence.**
2. **VSD.**
3. **PDA.**
4. **ASD with shunt reversal** — Eisenmenger complex or tricuspid atresia.

PRESSURE OVERLOAD

1. **Mitral stenosis.**
2. **Myxoma of the left atrium.**

SECONDARY TO LEFT VENTRICULAR FAILURE

Further Reading

Baron M.G. (1999) Plain film diagnosis of common cardiac anomalies in the adult. *Radiol. Clin. North Am.*, 37: 401–19.
Gross G.W. & Steiner R.M. (1991) Radiographic manifestations of congenital heart disease in the adult patient. *Radiol. Clin. North Am.*, 29: 293–318.

5.7 ENLARGED LEFT VENTRICLE

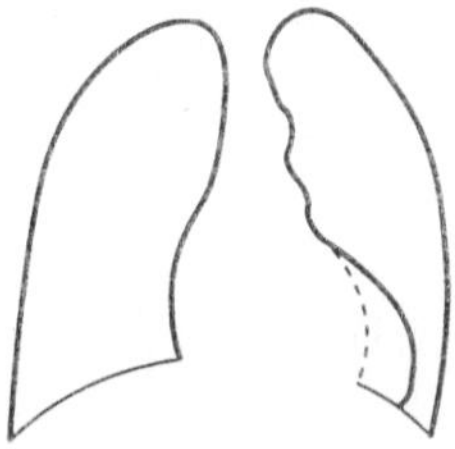

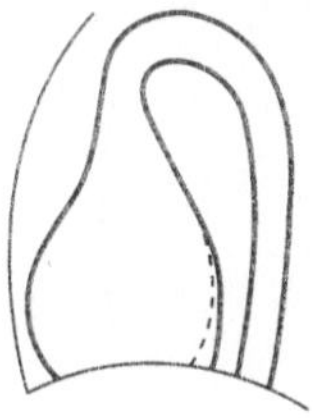

PA
1 Prominent left heart border
2 Rounding of left heart border
3 Apex displaced inferiorly

Lateral
Prominent posteroinferior part of cardiac shadow

MYOCARDIAL

1. **Ischaemia.**
2. **Cardiomyopathy/myocarditis.**

VOLUME OVERLOAD

1. **Aortic incompetence.**
2. **Mitral incompetence.**
3. **VSD.**
4. **PDA.**

HIGH OUTPUT STATES

1. **Anaemia.**
2. **Hyperthyroidism.**
3. **Paget's disease*.**
4. **AV fistula.**

PRESSURE OVERLOAD (DILATATION IS END STAGE)

1. **Aortic stenosis.**
2. **Hypertension.**
3. **Coarctation of the aorta.**

Further Reading

Baron M.G. (1999) Plain film diagnosis of common cardiac anomalies in the adult. *Radiol. Clin. North Am.*, 37: 401–19.

Gross G.W. & Steiner R.M. (1991) Radiographic manifestations of congenital heart disease in the adult patient. *Radiol. Clin. North Am.*, 29: 293–318.

5.8 BULGE ON THE LEFT HEART BORDER

1. **Enlarged left atrial appendage.**
2. **Ventricular aneurysm.**
3. **Pericardial cyst.**
4. **Pericardial sac defect.**
5. **Myocardial mass** — e.g. neoplasm, hydatid.
6. **Coronary artery aneurysm.**

Further Reading

Baron M.G. (1999) Plain film diagnosis of common cardiac anomalies in the adult. *Radiol. Clin. North Am.*, 37: 401–19.

Gross G.W. & Steiner R.M. (1991) Radiographic manifestations of congenital heart disease in the adult patient. *Radiol. Clin. North Am.*, 29: 293–318.

Konen E., Feinberg M.S., Morag B. *et al.* (2001) Giant right coronary aneurysm: CT, angiographic and echocardiographic findings. *Am. J. Roentgenol.*, 177: 689–91.

5.9 CARDIAC CALCIFICATION

PERICARDIAL

Primarily located over the right-sided chambers and in the atrioventricular grooves; less frequently over the base of the left ventricle and rarely over the apex of the left ventricle. When the left ventricle is involved there is always more extensive calcification elsewhere in the pericardium.

1. **Post-pericarditis** — TB, rheumatic fever, pyogenic, viral.
2. **Post-traumatic/postoperative.**
3. **Uraemia.**
4. **Asbestosis*** } may appear to be 'pericardial'.
5. **Coronary artery** }

MYOCARDIAL

Predominantly in the apex of the left ventricle or, uncommonly, in the posterior wall of the left ventricle.

1. **Calcified infarct.**
2. **Aneurysm.**
3. **Post-myocarditis** — especially rheumatic fever.
4. **Hydatid.**

INTRACARDIAC

1. **Calcified valve** — see 5.10.
2. **Calcified thrombus** — overlying an infarct or in an aneurysm.
3. **Atrial myxoma** — larger, more mobile and lobulated than a calcified thrombus.

Further Reading

MacGregor J.H., Chen J.T., Chiles C. *et al.* (1987) The radiographic distinction between pericardial and myocardial calcifications. *Am. J. Roentgenol.*, 148: 675–7.

Shawdon H.H. & Dinsmore R.E. (1967) Pericardial calcification: radiological features and clinical significance in twenty-six patients. *Clin. Radiol.*, 18: 205–14.

5.10 VALVE CALCIFICATION

AORTIC VALVE

1. **Bicuspid aortic valve.**
2. **Rheumatic heart disease.**
3. **Ageing.**
4. **Syphilis.**
5. **Ankylosing spondylitis*.**

MITRAL VALVE

1. **Rheumatic heart disease.**

PULMONARY VALVE

1. **Pulmonary valve stenosis** } in middle age.
2. **Fallot's tetralogy** } in middle age.
3. **Pulmonary hypertension**. } in middle age.
4. **Homograft** — for severe Fallot's tetralogy or pulmonary atresia.

TRICUSPID VALVE

1. **Pulmonary valve stenosis** (with high systolic pressures).
2. **ASD**.
3. **Isolated tricuspid regurgitation.**

5.11 LARGE AORTIC ARCH

1. **Unfolded (atherosclerotic) aorta** — parallel walls ± calcification.
2. **Hypertension** — on its own only leads to slight unfolding with left ventricular enlargement.
3. **Aortic incompetence** — prominent ascending aorta.
4. **Aortic stenosis** — post-stenotic dilatation. ± Aortic valve calcification.
5. **Aneurysm** — loss of parallelism of walls. Aetiologies include:
   (a) Atherosclerosis — calcification prominent.
   (b) Trauma.
   (c) Infection — e.g. syphilis, subacute bacterial endocarditis.
   (d) Intrinsic abnormality — e.g. Marfan's syndrome.
   Macroscopically the aneurysm may be:
   (a) Fusiform.
   (b) Saccular.
   (c) Dissecting — signs on the plain chest X-ray include:
      (i) Ill-defined aortic outline (because of mediastinal haematoma).
      (ii) Tracheal shift.
      (iii) Left pleural effusion (haemothorax).
      (iv) Left apical cap (also due to effusion).
      (v) Sudden increase in size of the aorta when compared with a previous film.
6. **PDA.**

Further Reading

Dow J., Roebuck E.J. & Cole F. (1970) Dissecting aneurysms of the aorta. *Br. J. Radiol.*, 39: 915–27.

Friedberg E.B. & Boxt L.M. (1999) Plain-film evaluation of the thoracic aorta. *Semin. Roentgenol.*, 34(3): 181–94.

5.12 SMALL AORTIC ARCH

1. **Decreased cardiac output** — e.g. mitral stenosis, HOCM.
2. **Intracardiac left to right shunt.**
3. **Coarctation** — long segment 'infantile' type.
4. **(Transposition of great arteries** — rotated but not small.)

5.13 RIGHT-SIDED AORTIC ARCH

1. Aortic knuckle on right side.
2. Absent left-sided aortic knuckle.
3. Trachea central or slightly to the left side.
4. In 0.1% of normal adults and 6% of neonates with significant congenital heart disease.

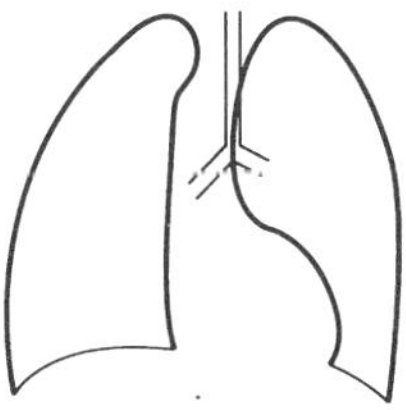

TYPE 1: MIRROR IMAGE BRANCHING

98% incidence of congenital heart disease — nearly all of which will be tetralogy of Fallot. However, because of the relative incidence of different cardiac defects the incidence of right-sided aortic arch in different congenital heart defects is:

1. **Dextrocardia with situs inversus** — a feature in 30% of cases.
2. **Fallot's tetralogy** — 25%.
3. **Pulmonary atresia + VSD** — 25%.
4. **Double outlet right ventricle** — 15%.
5. **Truncus arteriosus** — 15–50%.
6. **Corrected transposition of the great vessels** — 20%.
7. **Uncomplicated VSD** — 3%.

TYPE 2 (RARE)

TYPE 3: RIGHT-SIDED AORTIC ARCH WITH ABERRANT LEFT SUBCLAVIAN ARTERY

12% incidence of congenital heart disease — Fallot's tetralogy (70%), VSD (20%), coarctation (10%).

Further Reading

Glew D. & Hartnell G.G. (1991) The right aortic arch revisited. *Clin. Radiol.*, 43: 305–7.
Jaffe R.B. (1991) Radiographic manifestations of congenital anomalies of the aortic arch. *Radiol. Clin. North Am.*, 29: 319–34.
Knight L. & Edwards J.E. (1974) Right aortic arch. Types and associated anomalies. *Circulation*, 50: 1047–51.

5.14 ENLARGED SUPERIOR VENA CAVA

VOLUME OVERLOAD

1. **Tricuspid incompetence.**
2. **TAPVD** — if supracardiac. 'Cottage loaf' cardiac configuration, with pulmonary pleonaemia.

OBSTRUCTION

1. **Carcinoma of the bronchus.**
2. **Mediastinal mass.**
3. **Mediastinal fibrosis** — radiotherapy, idiopathic.
4. **Constrictive pericarditis.**

5.15 ENLARGED AZYGOS VEIN

If greater than 1 cm in diameter. (A normal or abnormal azygos vein will decrease in size in the erect position, on deep inspiration, and during a Valsalva manoeuvre.)

1. **Heart failure.**
2. **Portal hypertension.**
3. **Superior or inferior vena cava obstruction.**
4. **Pregnancy.**
5. **Constrictive pericarditis/pericardial effusion.**

DIFFERENTIAL DIAGNOSIS

1. **Sinus venosus defect** — right upper and middle lobe pulmonary veins drain into the superior vena cava (+ ASD).

5.16 ENLARGED PULMONARY ARTERIES

VOLUME OVERLOAD (enlarged central and peripheral vessels)

1. **Left-to-right shunt** — the sign is apparent when the shunt reaches 3:1.
2. **Hyperdynamic circulation** — e.g. thyrotoxicosis, severe anaemia, beri-beri and Paget's disease.

PERIPHERAL ARTERIAL VASOCONSTRICTION (enlarged central vessels only)

1. **Hypoxia** — e.g. due to chronic obstructive airways disease or cystic fibrosis.
2. **Secondary to pulmonary venous hypertension** — e.g. mitral stenosis or left ventricular failure.
3. **Secondary to left-to-right shunts.**

PERIPHERAL ARTERIAL OBLITERATION (enlarged central vessels only)

1. **Secondary to left-to-right shunts.**
2. **Thromboembolic disease** (see Pulmonary embolic disease*).
3. **Tumour emboli.**
4. **Schistosomiasis.**
5. **Vasculitides** — e.g. polyarteritis nodosa.
6. **Idiopathic pulmonary arterial hypertension** — typically in young females.

5.17 ENLARGED PULMONARY VEINS

LEFT VENTRICULAR FAILURE

OBSTRUCTION AT MITRAL OR ATRIAL LEVEL

1. **Mitral stenosis.**
2. **Left atrial myxoma.**
3. **Ball-valve thrombus.**
4. **Cor triatriatum.**

OBSTRUCTION PROXIMAL TO THE ATRIUM

1. **TAPVD.**
2. **Constrictive pericarditis** — rarely.
3. **Mediastinal fibrosis.**

5.18 NEONATAL PULMONARY VENOUS CONGESTION

1. **Prominent interstitial markings.**
2. **Indistinct vessels.**
3. **Perihilar haze.**
4. **Pleural effusions.**
5. **Cardiomegaly** – in all except the infradiaphragmatic type of TAPVD.

1ST WEEK

1. **Overhydration** — delayed clamping of the cord and twin–twin transfusion.
2. **Asphyxia** — the most common cause of cardiomegaly on the first day.
3. **Hypoplastic left heart** — heart size normal to mild cardiomegaly. Pulmonary vasculature normal or mild oedema. Often a marked discrepancy between the 'near normality' of the CXR and severity of clinical symptoms.
4. **Critical aortic stenosis.**
5. **TAPVD (obstructed).**

2ND–3RD WEEKS

1. **Coarctation of the aorta.**
2. **Interrupted aortic arch.**
3. **Critical aortic stenosis.**

4TH–6TH WEEKS

1. **Coarctation.**
2. **Critical aortic stenosis.**
3. **Endocardial fibroelastosis.**
4. **Anomalous left coronary artery.**

NB. Left-to-right shunts are usually asymptomatic during the neonatal period because of the high pulmonary vascular resistance. However, pulmonary vascular resistance in premature infants is lower, so shunts may present earlier in this particular group. PDA is the commonest shunt to cause heart failure in premature infants.

Further Reading

Strife J.L. & Sze R.W. (1999) Radiographic evaluation of the neonate with congenital heart disease. *Radiol. Clin. North Am.*, 37(6): 1093–107.

5.19 NEONATAL CYANOSIS

WITH PLEONAEMIA

Cyanosis and congestive cardiac failure — either may predominate.

1. **Transposition of the great arteries** — CXR may be normal and classic findings seen in only 50%:
   (a) narrow mediastinum because of the abnormal relationship of the great vessels and a small thymus.
   (b) poor visualization of the aorta and main pulmonary artery.
   (c) asymmetrical pulmonary flow, R > L. The lungs show only mild pleonaemia or may be normal.
2. **Truncus arteriosus.**
3. **TAPVD.**
4. **Single ventricle.**
5. **Hypoplastic left ventricle** } predominantly congestive cardiac
6. **Interrupted aortic arch** } failure, but may be cyanosed.

WITH OLIGAEMIA AND CARDIOMEGALY

1. **Pulmonary stenosis.**
2. **Ebstein's anomaly.**
3. **Pulmonary atresia with an intact ventricular septum.**
4. **Tricuspid atresia.**

WITH OLIGAEMIA BUT NO CARDIOMEGALY

Signs appear towards the end of the first week due to closure of the ductus arteriosus.

1. **Fallot's tetralogy** — small PA segment; large aorta; right-sided aortic arch in 25%.
2. **Pulmonary atresia** with a VSD.
3. **Tricuspid atresia.**

See also 'Neonatal respiratory distress' (4.50).

5.20 CARDIOVASCULAR INVOLVEMENT IN SYNDROMES

Cri-du-chat	Variable.
Down's*	AV canal, VSD, PDA, ASD, and aberrant right subclavian artery.
Ehlers–Danlos	Mitral valve prolapse, aortic root dilatation, dissecting aortic aneurysm and intracranial aneurysm.
Ellis–Van Creveld	ASD and common atrium.
Friedreich's ataxia	Hypertrophic cardiomyopathy.
Holt–Oram	ASD and VSD.
Homocystinuria*	Medial degeneration of the aorta and pulmonary artery causing dilatation. Arterial and venous thromboses.
Hurler's/Hunter's*	Intimal thickening of coronary arteries and valves.
Kartagener's	Situs inversus ± septal defects.
Marfan's	Cystic medial necrosis of the wall of the aorta, and less commonly the pulmonary artery, leading to dilatation and predisposing to dissection. Aortic and mitral regurgitation.
Morquio's*	Late onset of aortic regurgitation.
Noonan's	Pulmonary valve stenosis, and branch stenosis of pulmonary arteries, septal defects.
Osteogenesis imperfecta*	Aortic and mitral regurgitation. Ruptured chordae.
Rubella	Septal defects, PDA, pulmonary artery branch stenoses and myocardial disease.
Trisomy 13	VSD, ASD, PDA and dextroposition.
Trisomy 18	VSD, ASD and PDA.
Tuberous sclerosis*	Cardiomyopathy and rhabdomyoma of the heart.
Turner's	Coarctation, aortic and bicuspid aortic valve stenosis.

6 Abdomen and gastrointestinal tract

6.1 EXTRALUMINAL INTRA-ABDOMINAL GAS

1. **Pneumoperitoneum** — see 6.2.
2. **Gas in bowel wall**
   (a) Pneumatosis coli.
   (b) Linear pneumatosis intestinalis — infarction (e.g. due to vascular disease, volvulus, necrotizing enterocolitis).
3. **Biliary tree gas** (q.v.) — see 7.3.
4. **Portal vein gas** (q.v.) — see 7.4.
5. **Urinary tract gas** (q.v.) — see 8.7.
6. **Abscess** — mottled gas which may mimic gas within colonic faeces. A homogeneous gas distribution (less common) may mimic gas in normal bowel. Lack of mucosal pattern helps to differentiate it.
7. **Necrotic tumour** — especially following chemotherapy, radiotherapy and therapeutic embolization.
8. **Retroperitoneal gas** — small 'bubbles' or linear translucencies. Secondary to perforation or after nephrectomy.

Further Reading

Rice R.P., Thompson W.M. & Gedgandas R.K. (1982) The diagnosis and significance of extraluminal gas in the abdomen. *Radiol. Clin. North Am.*, 20: 819–37.

6.2 PNEUMOPERITONEUM

1. Erect — free gas under diaphragm or liver. Can detect 10 ml of air. Can take 10 min for all gas to rise.
2. Supine — gas outlines both sides of bowel wall, which then appears as a white line. In infants a large volume of gas will collect centrally, producing a rounded, relative translucency over the central abdomen. The falciform ligament may also be outlined by free gas. This is seen as a characteristic curvilinear white line in the right upper abdomen.

1. **Perforation**
   (a) Peptic ulcer — 30% do not have free air visible.
   (b) Inflammation — diverticulitis, appendicitis, toxic megacolon, necrotizing enterocolitis.
   (c) Infarction.
   (d) Malignant neoplasms.
   (e) Obstruction.
   (f) Pneumatosis coli — the cysts may rupture.
2. **Iatrogenic (surgery: peritoneal dialysis)** — may take 3 weeks to reabsorb (faster in obese and children), but serial views will show progressive diminution in volume of free air.
3. **Pneumomediastinum** — see 4.43.
4. **Introduction per vaginam** — e.g. douching.
5. **Pneumothorax** — due to a congenital pleuroperitoneal fistula.
6. **Idiopathic.**

6.3 GASLESS ABDOMEN

ADULT

1. **High obstruction.**
2. **Ascites** — see 6.4.
3. **Pancreatitis (acute)** — due to excess vomiting.
4. **Fluid-filled bowel** — closed-loop obstruction, total active colitis, mesenteric infarction (early), bowel wash-out.
5. **Large abdominal mass** — pushes bowel laterally.
6. **Normal.**

CHILD

1. **High obstruction**
   (a) Oesophageal atresia, without a fistula distally.
   (b) Duodenal atresia.
   (c) Annular pancreas.
   (d) Volvulus (secondary to malrotation).
   (e) Hypertrophic pyloric stenosis.
   (f) Choledochal cyst.
2. **Vomiting** — including excess nasogastric aspiration.
3. **Fluid-filled bowel** — see above.
4. **Congenital diaphragmatic hernia** — bowel in the chest.

6.4 ASCITES

1. Hazy appearance of entire abdomen.
2. Bowel gas 'floats' centrally on supine film.
3. Bulging flank lines.

1. **Cirrhosis.**
2. **Tumours**
   (a) Malignant — peritoneal metastases, primary carcinoma (particularly ovary and gastrointestinal tract).
   (b) Benign — fibroma of ovary (Meigs' syndrome).
3. **Hypoalbuminaemia** — e.g. nephrotic syndrome.
4. **Peritonitis** — particularly TB.
5. **Increased pressure in vascular system distal to liver** — congestive cardiac failure, constrictive pericarditis, thrombosis of inferior vena cava.
6. **Lymphatic obstruction** — chylous ascites, lymphoma, radiation, trauma or filariasis.

6.5 ABDOMINAL MASS IN A NEONATE

(After Kirks *et al.*, 1981.)

RENAL (55%) (q.v.)

1. **Hydronephrosis** (25%) — e.g. pelviureteric junction obstruction, posterior urethral valves, ectopic ureterocoele, prune-belly and ureterovesical junction obstruction.
2. **Multicystic kidney** (15%).
3. **Infantile polycystic kidneys** (see Polycystic disease*) — ± hepatic fibrosis.
4. **Mesoblastic nephroma** — benign hamartoma.
5. **Renal vein thrombosis** — complication of dehydration/sepsis.
6. **Renal ectopia.**
7. **Wilms' tumour.**

GENITAL (15%)

1. **Hydrometrocolpos** — dilated fluid-filled vagina and/or uterus, due to vaginal stenosis. ± Associated with imperforate anus or gastrointestinal fistula.
2. **Ovarian cyst** — uncomplicated or complicated by torsion or haemorrhage. A complicated cyst contains a fluid-debris level, septa or multiple echoes (mimicking a solid lesion). A small cyst along the wall of a cystic mass, the 'daughter cyst' sign, seems to be specific for ovarian cyst.

GASTROINTESTINAL (15%) — commonly associated with obstruction

1. **Duplication** — commonest bowel mass in neonates. Commonly in right lower quadrant.
2. **Mesenteric cyst.**

NON-RENAL RETROPERITONEAL (10%)

1. **Adrenal haemorrhage** — relatively common. Due to neonatal stress. ± Asymptomatic.
2. **Neuroblastoma.**
3. **Teratoma.**

HEPATO/SPLENO/BILARY (5%)

1. **Hepatoblastoma** — see 7.7.
2. **Hepatic cyst.**
3. **Splenic haematoma.**
4. **Choledochal cyst** — see 7.10.

Further Reading

Kirks D.R., Merten D.F., Grossman H. *et al.* (1981) Diagnostic imaging of paediatric abdominal masses: an overview. *Radiol. Clin. North Am.*, 19: 527–45.

Lee H.-J., Woo S.-K., Kim J.-S. *et al.* (2000) "Daughter cyst" sign: a sonographic finding of ovarian cyst in neonates, infants, and young children. *Am. J. Roentgenol.*, 174: 1013–15.

See also 8.22 — 'Renal mass in the newborn and young infant'.

6.6 ABDOMINAL MASS IN A CHILD

(After Kirks *et al.*, 1981.)

RENAL (55%)

1. **Wilms' tumour** — second commonest primary abdominal neoplasm in childhood (just behind neuroblastoma). See 8.17.
2. **Hydronephrosis** (20%) — see 8.23.
3. **Cysts** —see 8.20.

NON-RENAL RETROPERITONEAL (23%)

1. **Neuroblastoma (21%).**
   Age: 75% < 5 years; 15–30% < 1 year. Accounts for 50% of all neonatal tumours.
   Site: adrenal (40%), abdominal sympathetic chain (25%), posterior mediastinal sympathetic chain (15%), neck (5%), pelvis (5%), unknown (10%).

Staging: In addition to staging along conventional lines, stage IVS (or 4S) is defined as localized primary tumour not crossing the midline and with remote disease confined to liver, subcutaneous tissues and bone marrow but without evidence of cortical bone involvement. This group invariably presents in the first year of life and has an excellent prognosis.

Clinical presentation: 70% have metastases at presentation and a similar percentage have systemic symptoms. There may be local effects: pain, mass, spinal cord compression, dyspnoea or dysphagia, the effects of metastases (scalp masses, pain, weight loss, anaemia, fatigue etc.), or other effects due to hormone secretion (opsomyoclonus (cerebellar ataxia and jerky eye movements; 50% have neuroblastoma), hypertension, diarrhoea (due to vasoactive intestinal peptide, VIP), flushing and sweating).

Plain films: calcification in two-thirds, loss of psoas outline, bony metastases, enlargement of intervertebral foramina and, in the chest, abnormal posterior ends of ribs.

Ultrasound: heterogeneous, echogenic mass.

CT: soft-tissue mass with calcification in nearly all. Encasement rather than displacement of major vessels.

MRI: Prolonged T_1 and T_2 relaxation times. Calcification is not as readily recognized as on CT but MRI is superior for lymph node metastases, liver metastases and extradural spread of tumour.

Radionuclide scanning: bone scanning and meta-iodo-benzyl-guoniodine (MIBG) scanning are complementary techniques for the demonstration of skeletal metastases. MIBG is superior for follow-up of disease.

GASTROINTESTINAL (18%)

1. **Appendix abscess** (10%) — particularly spreads to pouch anterior to rectum.
2. **Hepatoblastoma** — more commonly in right lobe, but 40% in both lobes. 40% calcify. See 7.7.
3. **Haemangioma** — commonly multiple, involving entire liver. Rarely calcify. ± Associated with congestive heart failure and cutaneous haemangiomas.
4. **Choledochal cyst** — the classic triad of mass, pain and jaundice is only present in 10%. Dynamic radionuclide scintigraphy with ^{99}Tc-TBIDA is diagnostic. See 7.10.

GENITAL (4%)

1. **Ovarian cysts or teratoma.**

Further Reading

Abramson S.J. (1997) Adrenal neoplasms in children. *Radiol. Clin. North Am.*, 35(6): 1415–53.

Cohen M.D. (1992) *Imaging of Children with Cancer*, Ch. 6. St Louis: Mosby Year Book, pp. 134–76.

Haddad M.C., Birjawa G.A., Hemadeh M.S. *et al.* (2001) The gamut of abdominal and pelvic cystic masses in children. *Eur. Radiol.*, 11: 148–166.

Hiorns M.P. & Owens C.M. (2001) Radiology of neuroblastoma in children. *Eur. Radiol.*, 11: 2071–81.

Kirks D.R., Merten D.F., Grossman H. *et al.* (1981) Diagnostic imaging of paediatric abdominal masses: an overview. *Radiol. Clin. North Am.*, 19: 527–45.

6.7 INTESTINAL OBSTRUCTION IN A NEONATE

1. It is usually impossible to differentiate small from large bowel.
2. Not all gaseously distended bowel is obstructed. Resuscitation and infants on positive pressure ventilation may lead to significant abdominal distension. These bowel loops, unlike obstructed bowel, do not exhibit multiple fluid levels on the decubitus film.
3. Ileus is characterized by uniform dilatation of bowel. It is found in sepsis, NEC and electrolyte imbalance. Infants with sepsis and NEC are sick; those with uncomplicated bowel obstruction are usually otherwise well.
4. Bowel obstruction should be considered as 'high' (as far as the jejunum) or 'low' (for more distal obstructions). The former present with vomiting and are investigated by upper GI contrast study while the lower present with delayed passage of meconium and may require a contrast enema.

HIGH INTESTINAL OBSTRUCTION

1. **Pyloric atresia** — rare.
2. **Pyloric or prepyloric membrane/antral web** — gastric outlet obstruction in the presence of a normal pylorus and the appearance of two duodenal caps. The web may be identified by US.
3. **Duodenal stenosis/atresia** — marked dilatation of the proximal duodenum with the 'double bubble' sign, which may also be seen by ultrasound of the fetus (50% have a history of polyhydramnios). No gas distally when there is atresia, but a variable amount of gas in the distal bowel when there is stenosis. Bile-stained vomiting in the majority. Associated with annular pancreas (20%), Down's syndrome (30%), cardiac abnormalities (25%), oesophageal atresia (10%) and other abnormalities of gastrointestinal tract (60%).
4. **Preduodenal portal vein** — identified on US, CT or MRI. Associated with an intrinsic duodenal obstruction; the vein is not the direct cause of the obstruction.
5. **Malrotation and volvulus** — sudden onset of bile-stained vomiting. Few radiological signs if the obstruction is recent, intermittent or incomplete. Because of the acute nature of the condition, the duodenum is not dilated. If not recognized, obstruction progresses to bowel ischaemia, infarction and death. A contrast study should demonstrate the normal C-shaped duodenal loop which terminates to the left of the midline at the same level as the duodenal cap. In malrotation without volvulus the duodenojejunal flexure is to the right and below its normal position. Volvulus with incomplete obstruction is identified by a corkscrew pattern of the jejunum. When there is complete obstruction the distal duodenum terminates as a beak.
6. **Congenital fibrous band (of Ladd)** — connects caecum to posterolateral abdominal wall and commonly crosses the duodenum. May be complicated by malrotation and midgut volvulus.
7. **Jejunal atresia** — 50% of small bowel atresias and 50% are associated with other atretic sites distally (ileum > colon). AXR demonstrates a number of dilated, air-filled loops.

LOW INTESTINAL OBSTRUCTION

1. **Meconium ileus** — mottled lucencies due to gas trapped in meconium but only few fluid levels (since it is very viscous).

Bowel loops of variable calibre. Rapid appearance of fluid levels suggests volvulus. Peritoneal calcification due to perforation occurring *in utero* is seen in 30%. Secondary microcolon on contrast enema which also shows meconium pellets in the colon and distal ileum. Cystic fibrosis in the majority.

2. **Ileal atresia** — 50% of small bowel atresia, may be multiple and may coexist with jejunal atresia. Multiple dilated loops with fluid levels. Secondary microcolon.
3. **Inguinal hernia.**
4. **Meconium plug syndrome** — a long plug of meconium fills the rectosigmoid/descending colon. Infants should be followed up to exclude Hirschsprung's disease.
5. **Small left colon syndrome** — 50% associated with maternal diabetes. Infants should be followed up to exclude Hirschsprung's disease.
6. **Hirschsprung's disease** — multiple dilated loops of bowel. Diagnosis is made by contrast enema which demonstrates normal size, aganglionic distal bowel with a transition zone at the junction with proximal dilated ganglionic bowel.
7. **Inspissated milk** — presents from 3 days to 6 weeks of age. Dense, amorphous intraluminal masses frequently surrounded by a rim of air, ± mottled lucencies within them. Usually resolves spontaneously.
8. **Colonic atresia** — 5–15% of intestinal atresias. AXR may be similar to other distal bowel obstructions but some infants show a huge, disproportionately dilated loop (between the atretic segment and a competent ileocaecal valve).
9. **Imperforate anus**
   (a) High — ± sacral agenesis and gas in the bladder (due to a rectovesical fistula).
   (b) Low — ± perineal or urethral fistula.

Further Reading

Berrocal T., Torres I., Gutierrez J. *et al.* (1999) Congenital anomalies of the upper gastrointestinal tract. *RadioGraphics*, 19: 855–72.

Berrocal T., Lamas M., Gutierrez J. *et al.* (1999) Congenital anomalies of the small intestine, colon, and rectum. *RadioGraphics*, 19: 1219–36.

Buonomo C. (1997) Neonatal gastrointestinal emergencies. *Radiol. Clin. North Am.*, 35(4): 845–64.

Carty H. & Brereton R.J. (1983) The distended neonate. *Clin. Radiol.*, 34: 367–80.

Hernanz-Schulman M. (1999) Imaging of neonatal gastrointestinal obstruction. *Radiol. Clin. North Am.*, 37(6): 1163–86.

McAlister W.H., Kronemer K.A. (1996) Emergency gastrointestinal radiology of the newborn. *Radiol. Clin. North Am.*, 34(4): 819–44.

6.8 ABNORMALITIES OF BOWEL ROTATION

1. **Exomphalos** — total failure of the bowel to return to the abdomen from the umbilical cord. Bowel is contained within a sac. To be differentiated from gastroschisis, in which bowel protrudes through a defect in the abdominal wall.
2. **Non-rotation** — usually an asymptomatic condition with the small bowel on the right side of the abdomen and the colon on the left side. Small and large bowel lie on either side of the superior mesenteric artery (SMA) with a common mesentery. CT or transverse US scans show the superior mesenteric vein (SMV) lying to the left of the SMA, cf. the normal arrangement in which the SMV lies to the right of the SMA.
3. **Malrotation** — the duodenojejunal flexure lies to the right and caudad to its usual position which is to the left of the midline and approximately in the same axial plane as the first part of the duodenum. The caecum is usually more cephalad than normal but is normally sited in 5%. Malrotation nearly always complicates left-sided diaphragmatic hernia. US or CT shows the SMV immediately anterior to the SMA. *This sign is not reliable when the SMA lies to the left of the aorta, e.g. in association with hepatomegaly, aortic aneurysm or scoliosis, and a normal US does not exclude malrotation (3% false negative rate).*
4. **Reverse rotation** — rare. Colon lies dorsal to the SMA with jejunum and duodenum anterior to it.
5. **Paraduodenal hernia** — rare.
6. **Extroversion of the cloaca** — rare. No rotation of the bowel, and the ileum and colon open separately onto the extroverted area in the midline below the umbilical cord.

Further Reading

Dufour D., Delaet M.H., Dassonville M. *et al.* (1992) Midgut malrotation, the reliability of sonographic diagnosis. *Pediatr. Radiol.*, 22: 21–3.

Gaines P.A., Saunders A.J. & Drake D. (1987) Midgut malrotation diagnosed by ultrasound. *Clin. Radiol.*, 38: 51–3.

Houston C.S. & Wittenborg M.H. (1965) Roentgen evaluation of anomalies of rotation and fixation of the bowel in children. *Radiology*, 84: 1–17.

Long F.R., Kramer S.S., Markowitz R.I. *et al.* (1996) Intestinal malrotation in children: tutorial on radiological diagnosis in difficult cases. *Radiology*, 198: 775–80.

Nichols D.M. & Li D.K. (1983) Superior mesenteric vein rotation: a CT sign of midgut malrotation. *Am. J. Roentgenol.*, 141: 707–8.

6.9 INTRA-ABDOMINAL CALCIFICATIONS IN THE NEWBORN

EXTRALUMINAL

1. **Fetal perforation and meconium peritonitis.**

INTRAMURAL

1. **Bowel atresia.**
2. **Meconium ileus.**
3. **Intrauterine volvulus.**

INTRALUMINAL

1. **Non-hereditary intestinal obstructions** — imperforate anus, small bowel atresia and Hirschsprung's disease.
2. **Multiple gastrointestinal atresias with AR inheritance.**
3. **Without obstruction.**

See 7.9.

Further Reading

Beasley S.W. & de Campo M. (1986) Intraluminal calcification in the newborn: diagnostic and surgical implications. *Pediatr. Surg.*, 1: 249.

Berdon W.E., Baker D.H., Wigger H.J. *et al.* (1975) Calcified intraluminal meconium in newborn males with imperforate anus. *Am. J. Roentgenol.*, 125: 449–55.

Lang I., Daneman A., Cutz E. *et al.* (1997) Abdominal calcification in cystic fibrosis with meconium ileus: radiologic-pathologic correlation. *Pediatr. Radiol.*, 27: 523–7.

Miller J.P., Smith S.D. & Sukarochana K. (1988) Neonatal abdominal calcification: is it always meconium peritonitis? *J. Pediatr. Surg.*, 23: 555.

Yousefzadeh D.K., Jackson J.H. Jr, Smith W.L. *et al.* (1984) Intraluminal meconium calcification without distal obstruction. *Pediatr. Radiol.*, 14: 23–27.

6.10 HAEMATEMESIS

OESOPHAGUS

1. **Hiatus hernia.**
2. **Varices** — 20% of cases are bleeding from a coexisting peptic ulcer.
3. **Neoplasms.**
4. **Mallory–Weiss tears.**

STOMACH

1. **Ulcer.**
2. **Erosions** — may be associated with steroids, analgesics or alcohol.
3. **Carcinoma.**

DUODENUM

1. **Ulcer.**

OTHERS

1. **Blood dyscrasias.**
2. **Osler–Rendu–Weber (hereditary telangiectasia)** — AD. Telangiectases not prominent until age 20 years. Epistaxis is often the first symptom.
3. **Connective tissue disorders** — Ehlers–Danlos syndrome, pseudoxanthoma elasticum.

6.11 DYSPHAGIA – ADULT

INTRINSIC

1. **Reflux stricture.**
2. **Tumours** — carcinoma, lymphoma, leiomyoma.
3. **Ingestion** — corrosive, lye, foreign body.
4. **Iatrogenic** — radiotherapy, prolonged nasogastric intubation.
5. **Plummer–Vinson web** — narrow anterior indentation. Can occur from C4 to T1. Females with iron-deficiency anaemia; males after gastrectomy. Premalignant, but tumour can occur at different site.
6. **Schatzki ring** — marks the squamocolumnar junction lying above the diaphragm. Acute obstruction may occur if internal diameter is less than 6 mm.
7. ***Candida*** — painful dysphagia. Can involve entire oesophagus: 'shaggy', ulcerated. Immunosuppression, long-term antibiotics, hypoparathyroidism and debilitation all predispose. Herpes simplex and CMV may cause identical changes.
8. **Skin disorders** — epidermolysis bullosa and pemphigus can produce strictures.

EXTRINSIC

1. **Tumours** — lymph nodes, mediastinal tumours.
2. **Vascular** — aortic aneurysm; aberrant right subclavian artery (posterior indentation); aberrant left pulmonary artery (anterior indentation); right-sided aortic arch (right lateral and posterior indentation).
3. **Pharyngeal pouch** — ± air/fluid level in neck. Can cause superior mediastinal mass. Signs of aspiration on CXR.
4. **Goitre.**
5. **Enterogenous cyst** — adjacent to, but rarely communicates with, the oesophagus. Hemivertebra and anterior meningocoele may be associated (neurenteric cyst).
6. **Prevertebral abscess/haematoma.**

NEUROMUSCULAR

1. **Achalasia.**
2. **Scleroderma*.**

3. **Chagas' disease.**
4. **Myasthenia gravis*.**
5. **Bulbar/pseudobulbar palsy.**

PSYCHIATRIC

1. **Globus hystericus.**

Further Reading

Jones B. (1994) The pharynx. Disorders of function. *Radiol. Clin. North Am.*, 32(6): 1103–15.

Rubesin S.E. (1994) The pharynx. Structural disorders. *Radiol. Clin. North Am.*, 32(6): 1083–101.

Schima W., Ryan J.M., Harisisghani M. *et al.* (1998) Radiographic detection of achalasia: diagnostic accuracy of videofluoroscopy. *Clin. Radiol.*, 53: 372–5.

6.12 DYSPHAGIA – NEONATE

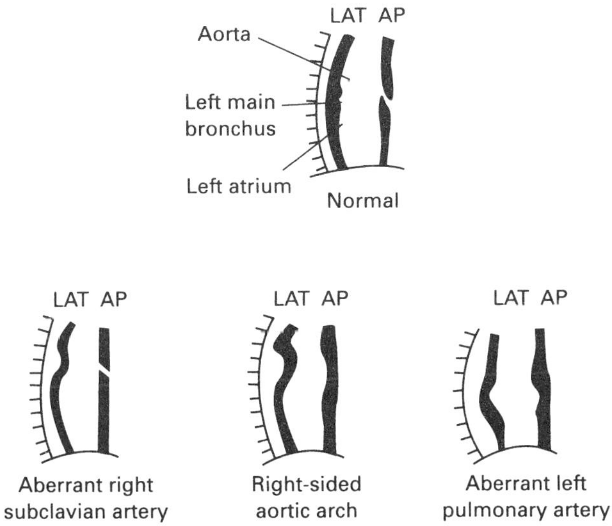

1. **Cleft palate.**
2. **Macroglossia/glossoptosis** — e.g. Beckwith–Wiedemann syndrome and Pierre Robin syndrome.
3. **Oesophageal atresia.**
4. **Vascular rings.**
5. **Choanal atresia.**
6. **Neuromuscular defects** — e.g. delayed maturation, prematurity and mental subnormality.

Further Reading

Berrocal T., Torres I., Gutierrez J. *et al.* (1999) Congenital anomalies of the upper gastrointestinal tract. *RadioGraphics*, 19: 855–72.

Mercado-Deane M.-G., Burton E.M. *et al.* (2001) Swallowing dysfunction in infants less than 1 year of age. *Pediatr. Radiol.*, 31: 423–8.

6.13 PHARYNGEAL/OESOPHAGEAL POUCHES AND DIVERTICULA

UPPER THIRD

1. **Zenker's diverticulum** — posteriorly, usually on left side, between the fibres of the inferior constrictor and cricopharyngeus. Can cause dysphagia, regurgitation, aspiration and hoarseness ± an air/fluid level. If large, can appear as a superior mediastinal mass. Food residue with it seen as 'mobile' filling defects.
2. **Lateral pharyngeal pouch and diverticulum** — through the unsupported thyrohyoid membrane in the anterolateral wall of the upper hypopharynx. Pouches are common and patients are asymptomatic. They fill with barium during a swallow and empty after the swallow has passed. Diverticula are uncommon and are seen in patients with chronically elevated intrapharyngeal pressure, e.g. glass blowers and trumpeters.
3. **Lateral cervical oesophageal pouch and diverticulum** — through the Killian–Jamieson space. Pouches are transient; diverticula are persistent. Patients are usually asymptomatic. The opening is below the level of cricopharyngeus.

MIDDLE THIRD

1. **Traction** — at level of carina. May be related to fibrosis after treatment for TB. Asymptomatic.
2. **Developmental** — failure to complete closure of tracheo-oesophageal communication.
3. **Intramural** — very rare. Multiple, tiny flask-shaped outpouchings. 90% have associated strictures, mainly in the upper third of the oesophagus.

LOWER THIRD

1. **Epiphrenic.**
2. **Ulcer** — peptic or related to steroids, immunosuppression and radiotherapy.
3. **Mucosal tears** — Mallory–Weiss syndrome, post-oesophagoscopy.
4. **After Heller's operation.**

Further Reading

Levine M.S., Moolten D.N., Herlinger H. *et al.* (1986) Esophageal intramural pseudodiverticulosis: a reevaluation. *Am. J. Roentgenol.*, 147: 1165–70.

Rubesin S.E. (1994) The pharynx. Structural disorders. *Radiol. Clin. North Am.*, 32(6): 1083–101.

Rubesin S.E. & Levine M.S. (2001) Killian–Jamieson diverticula: radiographic findings in 16 patients. *Am. J. Roentgenol*, 177: 85–9.

Schwartz E.E., Tucker J. & Holt G.P. (1981) Cervical dysphagia: pharyngeal protrusions and achalasia. *Clin. Radiol.*, 32: 643–50.

6.14 OESOPHAGEAL ULCERATION

In addition to ulceration there may be non-specific signs of oesophagitis:

1. Thickening of longitudinal folds (> 2 mm), which may be slightly scalloped.
2. Thickening of transverse folds resembling small bowel mucosal folds.
3. Reduced or absent peristalsis.

INFLAMMATORY

1. **Reflux oesophagitis** — ± hiatus hernia. Signs characteristic of reflux oesophagitis are:
   (a) a gastric fundal fold crossing the gastro-oesophageal junction and ending as a polypoid protuberance in the distal oesophagus
   (b) erosions — dots or linear streaks of barium in the distal oesophagus.
   (c) ulcers which may be round or, more commonly, linear or serpiginous.
2. **Barrett's oesophagus** — to be considered in any patient with oesophageal ulceration or stricture but especially if the abnormality is in the body of the oesophagus (although strictures are more common in the lower oesophagus). Hiatus hernia in 75–90%.

3. **Candida oesophagitis** — predominantly in immunosuppressed patients. Sudden onset of pain and dysphagia, not relieved by antacids. Early: small, plaque-like filling defects, often orientated in the long axis of the oesophagus. Advanced: cobblestone mucosal surface ± luminal narrowing. Ulceration is uncommon. Tiny bubbles along the top of the column of barium — the 'foamy' oesophagus.
   Patients with mucocutaneous candidiasis or oesophageal stasis due to achalasia, scleroderma etc. may develop chronic infection which is characterized by a lacy or reticular appearance of the mucosa ± nodular filling defects.
4. **Viral** — herpes and CMV occurring mostly in immunocompromised patients. May manifest as discrete ulcers, ulcerated plaques or mimic *Candida* oesophagitis. Discrete ulcers on an otherwise normal background mucosa are strongly suggestive of a viral aetiology.
5. **Caustic ingestion** — ulceration is most marked at the sites of anatomical hold-up and progresses to a long, smooth stricture.
6. **Radiotherapy** — ulceration is rare. Altered oesophageal motility is frequently the only abnormality.
7. **Crohn's disease*** — aphthoid ulcers and, in advanced cases, undermining ulcers, intramural tracking and fistulae.
8. **Drug-induced** — due to prolonged contact with tetracycline, quinidine and potassium supplements.
9. **Behçet's disease.**
10. **Intramural diverticulosis.**

NEOPLASTIC

1. **Carcinoma.**
2. **Leiomyosarcoma and leiomyoma.**
3. **Lymphoma*.**
4. **Melanoma.**

Further Reading

Chen M.Y. & Frederick M.G. (1994) Barrett esophagus and adenocarcinoma. *Radiol. Clin. North Am.*, 32(6): 1167–81

Cynn W.S., Chon H.K., Gureghian P.A. *et al.* (1975) Crohn's disease of the esophagus. *Am. J. Roentgenol.*, 125: 359–64.

Goldstein H.M., Rogers L.F. & Fletcher G.H. (1975) Radiological manifestations of radiation induced injury to the normal upper gastrointestinal tract. *Radiology,* 117: 135–40.

Ott D.J. (1994) Gastroesophageal reflux disease. *Radiol. Clin. North Am.*, 32(6): 1147–66.

Sam J.W., Levine M.S., Rubesin S.E. *et al.* (2000) The "foamy" esophagus: a radiographic sign of *Candida* esophagitis. *Am. J. Roentgenol.*, 174: 999–1002.

Yee J. & Wall S.D. (1994) Infectious esophagitis. *Radiol. Clin. North Am.*, 32(6): 1135–45.

6.15 OESOPHAGEAL STRICTURES – SMOOTH

INFLAMMATORY

1. **Peptic** — the stricture develops relatively late. Most frequently at the oesophagogastric junction and associated with reflux and a hiatus hernia. Less commonly, more proximal in the oesophagus and associated with heterotopic gastric mucosa (Barrett's oesophagus). ± Ulceration.
2. **Scleroderma*** — reflux through a wide open cardia may produce stricture. Oesophagus is the commonest internal organ to be affected. Peristalsis is poor, cardia wide open and the oesophagus dilated (contains air in the resting state).
3. **Corrosives** — acute: oedema, spasm, ulceration and loss of mucosal pattern at 'hold-up' points (aortic arch and oesophagogastric junction). Strictures are typically long and symmetrical, may take several years to develop and are more likely to be produced by alkalis than acid.
4. **Iatrogenic** — prolonged use of a nasogastric tube. Stricture in distal oesophagus probably secondary to reflux.

NEOPLASTIC

1. **Carcinoma** — squamous carcinoma may infiltrate submucosally. The absence of a hiatus hernia and the presence of an extrinsic soft-tissue mass should differentiate it from a peptic stricture but a carcinoma arising around the cardia may predispose to reflux.
2. **Mediastinal tumours** — carcinoma of the bronchus and lymph nodes. Localized obstruction ± ulceration and an extrinsic soft-tissue mass.
3. **Leiomyoma** — narrowing due to a smooth, eccentric, polypoid mass. ± Central ulceration.

OTHERS

1. **Achalasia** — 'rat-tail' tapering may mimic a stricture; this occurs below the diaphragm. Considerable oesophageal dilatation with food in the lumen.
2. **Skin disorders** — epidermolysis bullosa, pemphigus.

Further Reading

Sans N., Galy-Fourcade D., Bloom E. *et al.* (2000) Imaging of diffuse esophageal leiomyomatosis: two case reports and review of the literature. *Eur. Radiol.*, 10: 134–8.

6.16 OESOPHAGEAL STRICTURES – IRREGULAR

NEOPLASTIC

1. **Carcinoma** — increased incidence in achalasia, Plummer–Vinson syndrome, Barrett's oesophagus, coeliac disease, asbestosis, lye ingestion and tylosis. Mostly squamous carcinomas; adenocarcinoma is rare. Appearances include
   (a) Irregular filling defect — annular or eccentric.
   (b) Extraluminal soft-tissue mass.
   (c) Re-entrant angles at its margins (shouldering).
   (d) Ulceration.
   (e) Proximal dilatation.
2. **Leiomyosarcoma.**
3. **Carcinosarcoma** — big polypoid tumour ± pedunculated. Better prognosis than squamous carcinoma.
4. **Lymphoma*** — usually extension from gastric involvement.

INFLAMMATORY

1. **Reflux** — rarely irregular.
2. **Crohn's disease*** — rare.

IATROGENIC

1. **Radiotherapy** — rare, unless treating an oesophageal carcinoma. Dysphagia after radiotherapy is usually due to a motility disorder. Acute oesophagitis may occur with a dose of 50–60 Gy (5000–6000 rad).
2. **Fundoplication.**

Further Reading

Gore R.M. (1997) Esophageal cancer. Clinical and pathologic features. *Radiol. Clin. North Am.*, 35(2): 243–63.

Levine M.S. (1997) Esophageal cancer. Radiologic diagnosis. *Radiol. Clin. North Am.*, 35(2): 265–79.

Saunders H.S., Wolfman N.T. & Ott D.J. (1997) Esophageal cancer. Radiologic staging. *Radiol. Clin. North Am.*, 35(2): 281–94.

6.17 TERTIARY CONTRACTIONS IN THE OESOPHAGUS

Unco-ordinated, non-propulsive contractions.

1. **Reflux oesophagitis.**
2. **Presbyoesophagus** — impaired motor function due to muscle atrophy in the elderly. Occurs in 25% of people over 60 years.
3. **Obstruction at the cardia** — from any cause.
4. **Neuropathy**
   (a) Early achalasia — before dilatation occurs.
   (b) Diabetes.
   (c) Alcoholism.
   (d) Malignant infiltration.
   (e) Chagas' disease.

Further Reading

Ott D.J. (1994) Motility disorders of the esophagus. *Radiol. Clin. North Am.*, 32(6): 1117–32.

6.18 STOMACH MASSES AND FILLING DEFECTS

PRIMARY MALIGNANT NEOPLASMS

1. **Carcinoma** — most polypoidal carcinomas are 1–4 cm in diameter. (Any polyp greater than 2 cm in diameter must be considered to be malignant.) Granular/lobulated surface pattern is suggestive of carcinoma. Asbestosis, adenomatous polyps and Peutz–Jeghers syndrome predispose. Metastases may calcify and sclerotic or lytic bone metastases may occur.
2. **Lymphoma*** — primary gastric lymphoma is usually non-Hodgkin's. It can be ulcerative and infiltrative as well as polypoid. Often cannot be distinguished from carcinoma, but extension across the pylorus is suggestive of a lymphoma. Mucosa-associated lymphoid tissue (MALT) lymphoma is strongly associated with *Helicobacter pylori* infection.

POLYPS

1. **Hyperplastic** — accounts for 80–90% of gastric polyps. Usually multiple, small (< 1 cm in diameter) and occur randomly throughout stomach but predominantly affect body and fundus. Associated with chronic gastritis. Rarely can be very large (3–10 cm).
2. **Adenomatous** — usually solitary, 1–4 cm in diameter, sessile and occur in antrum. High incidence of malignant transformation (particularly if > 2 cm in size) and carcinomas elsewhere in stomach (because of dysplastic epithelium). Associated with pernicious anaemia.
3. **Hamartomatous** — characteristically multiple, small and relatively spare the antrum. Occur in 30% of Peutz–Jeghers syndrome, 40% of familiar polyposis coli and Gardner's syndrome.

SUBMUCOSAL NEOPLASMS

Smooth, well-defined filling defect, with a re-entry angle.

1. **Leiomyoma** — commonest by far. Can be very large with a substantial exogastric component. Central ulceration and massive haematemesis may occur.
2. **Lipoma** — can change shape with position of patient and may be relatively mobile on palpation.
3. **Neurofibroma** — NB. Leiomyomas and lipomas are more common, even in patients with generalized neurofibromatosis.
4. **Metastases** — Frequently ulcerate: 'bull's-eye' lesion (q.v.). Usually melanoma, but bronchus, breast, lymphoma, Kaposi's sarcoma and any adenocarcinoma may metastasize to stomach. Breast primary often produces a scirrhous reaction in the distal part of the stomach which is indistinguishable from linitis plastica (q.v.).

EXTRINSIC INDENTATION

1. **Pancreatic tumour/pseudocyst.**
2. **Splenomegaly/hepatomegaly.**
3. **Retroperitoneal tumours.**

OTHERS

1. **Nissen fundoplication** — may mimic a distorted mass in the fundus.

2. **Bezoar** — 'mass' may be mobile. Tricho- (hair) or phyto- (vegetable matter).
3. **Lymphoid hyperplasia** — innumerable, 1–3-mm diameter, round nodules in the antrum or antrum and body. Association with *H. pylori* gastritis.
4. **Pancreatic 'rest'** — ectopic pancreatic tissue causes a small filling defect, usually on the inferior wall of the antrum, and resembles a submucosal tumour. Central 'blob' of barium ('bull's-eye' or target lesion) in 50%.

Further Reading

An S.K., Han J.K., Kim Y.H. *et al.* (2001) Gastric mucosa-associated lymphoid tissue lymphoma: spectrum of findings at double contrast gastrointestinal examination with pathologic correlation. *RadioGraphics,* 21: 1491–504.

Cherukuri R., Levine M.S., Furth E.E. *et al.* (2000) Giant hyperplastic polyps in the stomach: radiographic findings in seven patients. *Am. J. Roentgenol.,* 175: 1445–8.

Gayer G., Jonas T., Apter S. *et al.* (1999) Bezoars in the stomach and small bowel — CT appearance. *Clin. Radiol.,* 54: 228–32.

Gore R.M. (1997) Gastric cancer. Clinical and pathologic features. *Radiol. Clin. North Am.,* 35(2): 295–310.

Gore R.M., Levine M.S., Ghahremani G.G. *et al.* (1997) Gastric cancer. Radiologic diagnosis. *Radiol. Clin. North Am.,* 35(2): 311–29.

Gossios K., Katsimbri P. & Tsianos E. (2000) CT features of gastric lymphoma. *Eur. Radiol.,* 10: 425–30.

Miller F.H., Kochman M.L., Talamonti M.S. *et al.* (1997) Gastric cancer. Radiologic staging. *Radiol. Clin. North Am.,* 35(2): 331–49.

Ripolles T., Garcia-Aguayo J., Martinez M.-J. *et al.* (2001) Gastrointestinal bezoars: sonographic and CT characteristics. *Am. J. Roentgenol.,* 177: 65–69.

Torigian D.A., Levine M.S., Gill N.S. *et al.* (2001) Lymphoid hyperplasia of the stomach: radiographic findings in five adult patients. *Am. J. Roentgenol.,* 177: 71–5.

6.19 THICK STOMACH FOLDS

Thickness greater than 1 cm.

INFLAMMATORY

1. **Gastritis** — localized or generalized fold thickening ± associated with inflammatory nodules (< 1 cm, mostly in the antrum), erosions and coarse areae gastricae.
2. **Zollinger–Ellison syndrome** — suspect if post-bulbar ulcers. Ulceration in both first and second parts of duodenum is suggestive, but ulceration distal to this is virtually diagnostic. Thick folds and small bowel dilatation may occur in response to excess acidity. Due to gastrinoma of non-beta cells of pancreas (no calcification, moderately vascular). 50% malignant — metastases to liver. (10% of gastrinomas may be ectopic — usually in medial wall of the duodenum.)
3. **Pancreatitis (acute).**
4. **Crohn's disease*** — mild thickening of folds with aphthoid ulceration may occur in up to 40% of Crohn's. However, these signs are subtle, and more obvious disease (i.e. deformity and narrowing of the antrum) only occurs in 2% of these.

INFILTRATIVE/NEOPLASTIC

1. **Lymphoma*** — usually non-Hodgkin's lymphoma and may be primary or secondary. Accounts for half of all gastrointestinal lymphomas. The predominant features of early disease are shallow ulceration or uneven mucosa with enlarged, radiating folds. Features which may suggest the diagnosis of advanced disease are: multiple masses or ulcerations, diffuse thickening of folds, extensive submucosal infiltration, extension across the pylorus or the gastro-oesophageal junction, large tumours over 10 cm in diameter and preservation of wall pliability.
2. **Carcinoma** — irregular folds with rigid wall.
3. **Pseudolymphoma** — benign reactive lymphoid hyperplasia. 70% have an ulcer near the centre of the area affected.
4. **Eosinophilic gastroenteritis.**

OTHERS

1. **Ménétrier's disease** — smooth folds predominantly on greater curve. Rarely extend into antrum. No rigidity or ulcers. 'Weep' protein sufficient to cause hypoproteinaemia (effusion, oedema, thick folds in small bowel). Commonly achlorhydric: cf. Zollinger–Ellison syndrome. In adults it pursues a chronic and unremitting course but in children resolution should be expected after weeks or months. In children the aetiology is likely to be CMV infection.
2. **Varices** — occur in fundus and usually associated with oesophageal varices.

Further Reading

An S.K., Han J.K., Kim Y.H. *et al.* (2001) Gastric mucosa-associated lymphoid tissue lymphoma: spectrum of findings at double contrast gastrointestinal examination with pathologic correlation. *RadioGraphics,* 21: 1491–504.

Coad N.A. & Shah K.J. (1986) Ménétrier's disease in childhood associated with cytomegalovirus infection: a case report and review of the literature. *Br. J. Radiol.,* 59: 615–20.

Gelfand D.W., Ott D.J. & Chen M.Y. (1999) Radiologic evaluation of gastritis and duodenitis. *Am. J. Roentgenol.,* 173: 357–61.

Hricak H., Thoeni R.F., Margulis A.R. *et al.* (1980) Extension of gastric lymphoma into the esophagus and duodenum. *Radiology,* 135: 309–12.

Sato T., Sakai Y., Ishiguro S. *et al.* (1986) Radiologic manifestations of early gastric lymphoma. *Am. J. Roentgenol.,* 146: 513–17.

6.20 LINITIS PLASTICA

NEOPLASTIC

1. **Gastric carcinoma.**
2. **Lymphoma*.**
3. **Metastases** — particularly breast.
4. **Local invasion** — pancreatic carcinoma.

INFLAMMATORY

1. **Corrosives** — can cause rigid stricture of antrum extending up to the pylorus.
2. **Radiotherapy** — can cause rigid stricture of antrum with some deformity. Mucosal folds may be thickened or effaced. Large antral ulcers can also occur.
3. **Granulomata** — Crohn's disease, TB.
4. **Eosinophilic enteritis** — commonly involves gastric antrum (causing narrowing and nodules) in addition to small bowel. Blood eosinophilia. Occasionally spares the mucosa, so needs full thickness biopsy for confirmation.

6.21 GASTROCOLIC FISTULA

INFLAMMATORY

1. **Peptic ulcer.**
2. **Crohn's disease*.**
3. **Pancreatitis (chronic).**
4. **Infections** — tuberculosis, actinomycosis.

NEOPLASTIC

1. **Carcinoma** — of stomach, colon or pancreas.
2. **Metastases.**

6.22 GASTRIC DILATATION

Gas- or food-filled stomach. Mottled translucencies (due to gas trapped in food residue) may be seen in gastric dilatation secondary to chronic obstruction. Resembles heavy faecal loading of the colon.

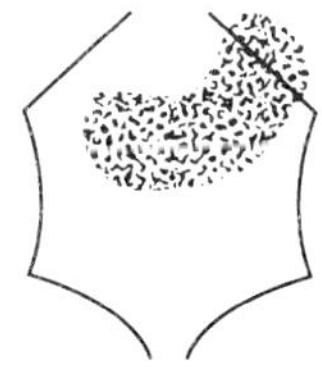

MECHANICAL OBSTRUCTION

1. **Fibrosis secondary to ulceration** — long history of dyspepsia.
2. **Malignancy** — shorter history, therefore dilatation is usually less marked. Often no abdominal pain.
3. **Volvulus** — 'organo-axial', associated with hiatus hernia. 'Vertical axis', not associated with hiatus hernia.
4. **Infantile hypertrophic pyloric stenosis** — the radiological signs on a barium meal are:
   (a) 'String sign' — barium in the narrowed pyloric canal.
   (b) 'Shoulder sign' — the pyloric 'tumour' indenting the barium-filled antrum.
   (c) 'Beak sign' — incomplete extension of the barium into the narrowed pyloric channel.
   (d) 'Double track sign' — parallel mucosal folds in the pyloric channel.

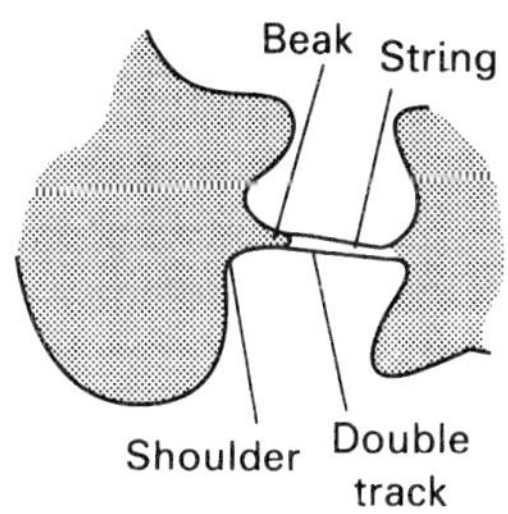

US has now largely replaced the barium meal for diagnosis.

5. **Proximal small bowel obstruction** — gastric and small bowel dilatation.
6. **Bezoar.**

PARALYTIC ILEUS

1. **Postoperative.**
2. **Post-vagotomy.**
3. **Drugs** — e.g. anticholinergics.
4. **Metabolic** — uraemia, hypokalaemia, etc.
5. **Acute gastric dilatation** — see 7.4.

6.23 'BULL'S-EYE' (TARGET) LESION IN THE STOMACH

Ulcer on apex of a nodule.

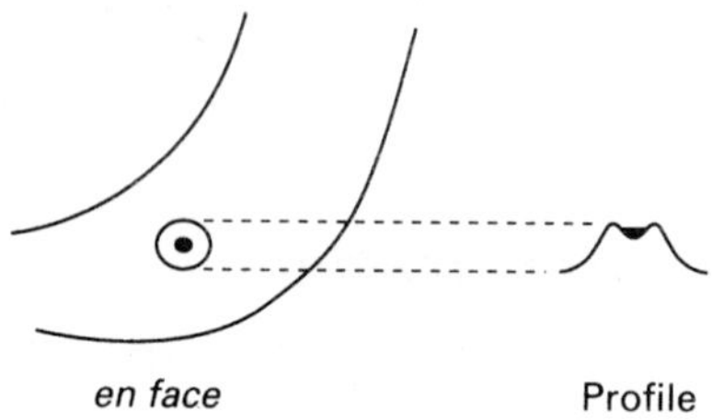

1. **Submucosal metastases** — may be multiple
   (a) Melanoma — commonest.
   (b) Lymphoma*.
   (c) Carcinoma — breast, bronchus, pancreas.
   (d) Carcinoid.
2. **Leiomyoma.**
3. **Pancreatic 'rest'** — ectopic pancreatic tissue. Usually on inferior wall of antrum. A central 'blob' of barium is seen in 50% — collects in primitive duct remnant. Can also occur in duodenum, jejunum, Meckel's diverticulum, liver, gallbladder and spleen.
4. **Neurofibroma** — may be multiple. Other stigmata of neurofibromatosis.

6.24 GAS IN THE STOMACH WALL

INTERSTITIAL GASTRIC EMPHYSEMA

Linear or curvilinear gas shadows in the wall of the stomach ± extension into the duodenum.

1. **Raised intragastric pressure** — obstruction and gastric distension.
2. **Post-gastroscopy.**
3. **Peptic ulceration** — with submucosal gas.
4. **Necrotizing enterocolitis.**

EMPHYSEMATOUS GASTRITIS

Due to gas-forming organisms in the stomach wall. Severe epigastric pain, haematemesis, prostration and toxaemic shock. Contracted stomach with mottled lucencies resembling interstitial emphysema.

1. **Diabetes.**
2. **Alcohol abuse.**
3. **Corrosive ingestion.**

CYSTIC PNEUMATOSIS

Mild symptoms; usually in elderly patients and often associated with chronic obstructive airways disease.

Further Reading

Colquhoun J. (1965) Intramural gas in hollow viscera. *Clin. Radiol.*, 16: 71–86.
Tuck J.S. & Boobis L.H. (1987) Case report: interstitial emphysema of the stomach due to perforated appendicitis. *Clin. Radiol.*, 38: 315–17.

6.25 COBBLESTONE DUODENAL CAP

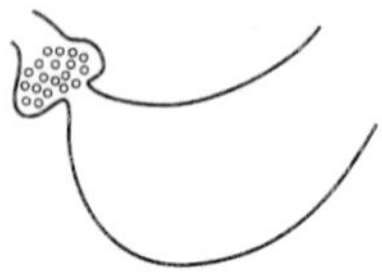

BIG 'POLYPOID'

1. **Oedema** — associated with an ulcer.
2. **Hypertrophied Brunner's glands** — can extend from pylorus to ampulla of Vater. Uniform in size. May occur in 25% of patients with end stage renal failure.
3. **Crohn's disease*** — involved in 2% and may rarely present here. Usually signs present in gastric antrum also.
4. **Varices** — base of cap. Decrease in size in erect position. Invariably associated with oesophageal varices.
5. **Lymphoma*.**
6. **Carcinoma.**

SMALL

1. **Duodenitis** — ± central flecks of barium.
2. **Nodular lymphoid hyperplasia** — pin-point (1–3 mm) nodules involving the entire duodenal loop. (Duodenum > jejunum.)
3. **Food residue/effervescent granules** — move around.
4. **Heterotopic gastric mucosa** — base of cap adjacent to pylorus.

Further Reading

Cassar-Pullicino V.N., Davies A.M., Hubscher S. *et al.* (1990) The nodular duodenum in chronic renal failure. *Clin. Radiol.*, 41: 326–30.

Gelfand D.W. (1994) Radiologic diagnosis of duodenitis. *Radiol. Clin. North Am.*, 32(6): 1253–8.

Schulman A. (1970) The cobblestone appearance of the duodenal cap, duodenitis and hyperplasia of Brunner's glands. *Br. J. Radiol.*, 43: 787–95.

6.26 DECREASED/ABSENT DUODENAL FOLDS

1. **Scleroderma*.**
2. **Crohn's disease*.**
3. **Strongyloides.**
4. **Cystic fibrosis*.**
5. **Amyloidosis.**

6.27 THICKENED DUODENAL FOLDS

INFLAMMATORY

1. **Duodenitis** — usually proximal to the ampulla of Vater.
2. **Pancreatitis.**
3. **Crohn's disease*** — occurs before aphthoid ulcers. Mild signs occur in duodenum in up to 40%, but severe involvement only occurs in 2%. Cap and proximal half of second part of duodenum predominantly affected.
4. **Zollinger–Ellison syndrome** — response to excess acidity.

NEOPLASTIC

1. **Lymphoma*.**
2. **Metastases** — particularly melanoma, breast, ovary, gastrointestinal tract (lung, kidney are rare).

INFILTRATIVE

1. **Amyloidosis** — bowel commonly involved (primary, generalized thickening; secondary, segmental thickening).
2. **Eosinophilic enteritis** — gastric antrum commonly involved. Blood eosinophilia.
3. **Mastocytosis** — dense bones. ± Gastric polyps.
4. **Whipple's disease.**

VASCULAR

1. **Intramural haematoma** — due to trauma. Common in the duodenum because it is fixed to the posterior abdominal wall. 'Stacked coins' appearance. An extensive haematoma may occur in bleeding diatheses.
2. **Ischaemia** — widespread changes can occur in vasculitis secondary to radiotherapy, collagen diseases and Henoch–Schönlein purpura.

OEDEMA

1. **Hypoproteinaemia** — nephrotic syndrome, cirrhosis or protein-losing enteropathy.
2. **Venous obstruction** — cirrhosis, Budd–Chiari syndrome or constrictive pericarditis.
3. **Lymphatic obstruction.**
4. **Angioneurotic oedema.**

INFESTATIONS

1. **Worms**
   (a) Hookworm (*Ankylostoma duodenale*) — the head of the worm produces an inflammatory reaction.
   (b) Tapeworm (*Taenia saginata* or *T. solium*) — has a similar effect on the duodenum. The worm may be visible as a filling defect during a barium study.
   (c) *Strongyloides* — similar appearance to giardiasis (see below). Strictures in chronic cases.
2. **Giardiasis** — predominantly affects the duodenum and proximal jejunum. Thickened, blunted and distorted mucosal folds. Hypermotility leads to rapid transit. Spasm produces narrowing. May be associated with nodular lymphoid hyperplasia or hypogammaglobulinaemia.

See also 6.31 and 6.32.

Further Reading

Clements R., Evans K.T. & Rhodes J. (1990) Coarse mucosal folds in the duodenum: a twenty-year follow-up. *Clin. Radiol.*, 41: 421–4.

Gelfand D.W., Ott D.J. & Chen M.Y. (1999) Radiologic evaluation of gastritis and duodenitis. *Am. J. Roentgenol.*, 173: 357–61.

Hwang J.-I., Chiang J.-H., Yu C. *et al.* (1998) Pictorial review: radiological diagnosis of duodenal abnormalities. *Clin. Radiol.*, 53: 323–32.

Reeder M.M. (1997) Radiological diagnosis of giardiasis. *Semin. Roentgenol.* , 32(4): 291–300.

Strouse P.J., Close B.J., Marshall K.W. *et al.* (1999) CT of bowel and mesenteric trauma in children. *RadioGraphics*, 19: 1237–50.

6.28 DILATED DUODENUM

MECHANICAL OBSTRUCTION

1. **Bands** — most frequent cause of neonatal duodenal obstruction. Associated with malrotation and midgut volvulus.
2. **Atresia, webs, stenosis** — often associated with Down's syndrome. 'Double bubble' sign in neonate due to dilated stomach and duodenum. Webs have a high incidence of incomplete rotation.
3. **Annular pancreas.**
4. **Superior mesenteric artery syndrome** — hold up of barium in third part of duodenum with some proximal dilatation and vigorous peristalsis (prior to muscle relaxant). Postprandial pain relieved by lying on left side. Associated with a plaster of Paris body cast. 20% have associated duodenal ulcer. Never occurs in obese people.

PARALYTIC ILEUS

Particularly due to pancreatitis.

SCLERODERMA*

Further Reading

Anderson J.R., Earnshaw P.M. & Fraser G.M. (1982) Extrinsic compression of the third part of the duodenum. *Clin. Radiol.*, 33: 75–81.

Traubici J. (2001) The double bubble sign. *Radiology,* 220: 463–4.

6.29 DILATED SMALL BOWEL

Calibre: proximal jejunum > 3.5 cm (4.5 cm if small bowel enema)
mid-small bowel > 3.0 cm (4.0 cm if small bowel enema)
ileum > 2.5 cm (3.0 cm if small bowel enema).

NORMAL FOLDS

1. **Mechanical obstruction** — ± dilated large bowel, depending on level of obstruction.
2. **Paralytic ileus** — dilated small and large bowel.
3. **Coeliac disease, tropical sprue, dermatitis herpetiformis** — can produce identical signs. Dilatation is the hallmark, and correlates well with severity, but it is relatively uncommon. ± Dilution and flocculation of barium. See 6.34.
4. **Scleroderma.**
5. **Iatrogenic** — postvagotomy and gastrectomy may produce dilatation due to rapid emptying of stomach contents. Dilatation may also occur proximal to a small bowel loop.

THICK FOLDS

1. **Ischaemia.**
2. **Crohn's disease*** — combination of obstructive and inflammatory changes.
3. **Radiotherapy.**
4. **Lymphoma*.**
5. **Zollinger–Ellison syndrome** — ileus due to excess acidity.
6. **Extensive small bowel resection** — compensatory dilatation and thickening of folds.
7. **Amyloidosis.**

Further Reading

Burkill G., Bell. & Healy J. (2001) Small bowel obstruction: the role of computed tomography in its diagnosis and management with reference to other imaging modalities. *Eur. Radiol.*, 11: 1405–22.

Boudiaf M., Soyer P., Terem C. *et al.* (2001) CT evaluation of small bowel obstruction. *RadioGraphics*, 21: 613–24.

6.30 STRICTURES IN THE SMALL BOWEL

1. **Adhesions** — angulation of bowel which is constant in site. Normal mucosal folds.
2. **Crohn's disease*** — ± ulcers and altered mucosal pattern.
3. **Ischaemia** — ulcers are rare. Evolution is more rapid than Crohn's ± long strictures.
4. **Radiation enteritis** — see 6.31.
5. **Tumours**
   (a) Lymphoma* — usually secondary to contiguous spread from lymph nodes. Primary disease may occur and is nearly always due to non-Hodgkin's lymphoma.
   (b) Carcinoid — although the appendix is the commonest site, these never metastasize. Of those occurring in small bowel, 90% are in ileum (mostly distal 2 feet), and 30% are multifocal. A fibroblastic response to infiltration produces a stricture ± mass. It is the commonest primary malignancy of small bowel, but only 30% metastasize (more likely if > 2 cm diameter) or invade. Carcinoid syndrome only develops with liver metastases — see 6.36.
   (c) Carcinoma — if duodenal lesions are included this is the most common primary malignancy of the small bowel and the duodenum is the most frequent site. Ileal lesions are rare (unless associated with Crohn's disease). Short segment annular stricture with mucosal destruction, ulcerating or polypoidal lesion. High incidence of second primary tumours.
   (d) Sarcoma — lymphosarcoma or leiomyosarcoma. Thick folds with an eccentric lumen. Leiomyosarcomas may present as a large mass displacing bowel loops with a large barium-filled cavity.
   (e) Metastases — usual sites of origin are malignant melanoma, ovary, pancreas, stomach, colon, breast, lung and uterus. Rounded deformities of the bowel wall with flattened mucosal folds. In patients with gynaecological malignancies, duodenal or jejunal obstructions are most likely due to metastases; most radiation-induced strictures are in the ileum.
6. **Enteric coated potassium tablets.**

Further Reading

Boudiaf M., Soyer P., Pelage J.-P. *et al.* (2000) CT of radiation-induced injury of the gastrointestinal tract: spectrum of findings with barium studies correlation. *Eur. Radiol.*, 10: 920–5.

Buckley J.A. & Fishman E.K. (1998) CT evaluation of small bowel neoplasia: spectrum of disease. *RadioGraphics*, 18: 379–92.

Buckley J.A., Jones B. & Fishman E.K. (1997) Small bowel cancer. Imaging features and staging. *Radiol. Clin. North Am.*, 35(2): 381–402.

Gore R.M. (1997) Small bowel cancer. Clinical and pathologic features. *Radiol. Clin. North Am.*, 35(2): 351–80.

Maglinte D.D. & Reyes B.L. (1997) Small bowel cancer — radiologic diagnosis. *Radiol. Clin. North Am.*, 35: 361–80.

6.31 THICKENED FOLDS IN NON-DILATED SMALL BOWEL — SMOOTH AND REGULAR

Fold thickness: jejunum > 2.5 mm
ileum > 2.0 mm

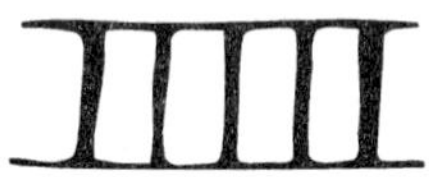

VASCULAR

1. **Intramural haematoma**

Homogeneous high attenuation wall on CT.

   (a) Trauma — commonest in duodenum, since fixed to posterior abdominal wall ('stacked coin' appearance).
   (b) Bleeding diathesis — commonly localized to a few loops.

2. **Ischaemia**
   (a) Acute — embolus, Henoch–Schönlein purpura. Can produce ileus. May perforate. Ulcers rare.
   (b) Chronic — vasculitis (collagen, radiotherapy), atheroma, fibromuscular dysplasia. Presents with postprandial pain, and malabsorption.

RADIOTHERAPY

Infrequently seen with tumour doses < 45 Gy. Underlying pathological process is endarteritis obliterans and concomitant arterial disease will exacerbate the damage. Majority of cases are secondary to treatment of female genital tract malignancy. Acute symptoms during radiotherapy do not correlate with the development of chronic radiation enteritis which may have a latent period of up to 25 years. Distal jejunum and ileum are the commonest sites.

1. **Acute** — thickening of valvulae conniventes and poor peristalsis. Ulceration is rare.
2. **Chronic** — most common signs are submucosal thickening of valvulae conniventes and/or mural thickening. Stenoses, adhesions, sinuses and fistulae may also occur. (The absence of ulceration, cobblestoning and asymmetry differentiate it from Crohn's disease.) May show homogeneous enhancement on contrast-enhanced CT.

OEDEMA

1. **Adjacent inflammation** — focal.
2. **Hypoproteinaemia** — e.g. nephrotic, cirrhosis, protein-losing enteropathy. Generalized.
3. **Venous obstruction** — e.g. cirrhosis, Budd–Chiari syndrome, constrictive pericarditis.
4. **Lymphatic obstruction** — e.g. lymphoma, retroperitoneal fibrosis, primary lymphangiectasia (child with leg oedema).
5. **Angioneurotic.**

EARLY INFILTRATION

1. **Amyloidosis** — gastrointestinal tract commonly involved. Primary amyloid tends to produce generalized thickening, whereas secondary amyloid produces focal lesions. Malabsorption is unusual.
2. **Eosinophilic enteritis** — focal or generalized. Gastric antrum frequently involved. No ulcers. Blood eosinophilia. Occasionally spare mucosa — therefore need full thickness biopsy for diagnosis.

COELIAC DISEASE

Thickening of folds is not common, and is probably a functional abnormality rather than true fold thickening. ± Jejunal dilatation.

ABETALIPOPROTEINAEMIA

Rare, inherited. Malabsorption, acanthocytosis, and CNS abnormality. ± Dilated bowel.

Further Reading

Ledermann H.P., Borner N., Strunk H. *et al.* (2000) Bowel wall thickening on transabdominal sonography. *Am. J. Roentgenol.*, 174: 107–17.

Mendelson R.M. & Nolan D.J. (1985) The radiological features of chronic radiation enteritis. *Clin. Radiol.*, 36: 141–8.

Rettenbacher T., Hollerweger A., Macheiner P. *et al.* (1999) Adult celiac disease: US signs. *Radiology*, 211: 389–94.

Strouse P.J., Close B.J., Marshall K.W. *et al.* (1999) CT of bowel and mesenteric trauma in children. *RadioGraphics*, 19: 1237–50.

Taylor P.M., Johnson R.J., Eddleston B. *et al.* (1990) Radiological changes in the gastrointestinal and genitourinary tract following radiotherapy for carcinoma of the cervix. *Clin. Radiol.*, 41: 165–9.

Tomei E., Marini M., Messineo D. *et al.* (2000) Computed tomography of the small bowel in adult celiac disease: the jejunoileal fold pattern reversal. *Eur. Radiol.*, 10: 119–22.

6.32 THICKENED FOLDS IN NON-DILATED SMALL BOWEL – IRREGULAR AND DISTORTED

Fold thickness: jejunum < 2.5 mm
ileum < 2.0 mm.

LOCALIZED

Inflammatory

1. **Crohn's disease*** — occurs before aphthoid ulcers.
2. **Zollinger–Ellison syndrome** — predominantly proximal small bowel. Dilatation may occur.

Neoplastic

1. **Lymphoma*.**
2. **Metastases** — particularly melanoma, breast, ovary and gastrointestinal tract.
3. **Carcinoid** — commonest primary malignant small bowel tumour. 90% in the ileum and mostly in the distal 60 cm. It is more common in the appendix, where it is a benign tumour.

Infective

1. **Tuberculosis** — can look identical to Crohn's disease, but predominant caecal involvement may help to distinguish it. Less than 50% have pulmonary tuberculosis.

WIDESPREAD

Infiltrative

1. **Amyloidosis.**
2. **Eosinophilic enteritis.**
3. **Mastocytosis** — may have superimposed small nodules, urticaria pigmentosa and sclerotic bone lesions.
4. **Whipple's disease** — flitting arthralgia, lymphadenopathy and sacroiliitis.

Inflammatory

1. **Crohn's disease*.**

Infestations

1. **Giardiasis** — associates with hypogammaglobulinaemia and nodular lymphoid hyperplasia.
2. ***Strongyloides*** — ± absent folds in chronic cases.

STOMACH ABNORMALITY WITH THICKENED SMALL BOWEL MUCOSAL FOLDS

1. **Lymphoma/metastases.**
2. **Zollinger–Ellison syndrome.**
3. **Ménétrier's disease.**
4. **Amyloidosis.**
5. **Eosinophilic enteritis.**

Further Reading

Goldberg H.I. & Sheft D.J. (1976) Abnormalities in small intestine contour and calibre. *Radiol. Clin. North Am.*, 14: 461–75.

6.33 MULTIPLE NODULES IN THE SMALL BOWEL

INFLAMMATORY

1. **Nodular lymphoid hyperplasia** — nodules 2–4 mm with normal fold thickness. Associated with hypogammaglobulinaemia (IgA and IgM). Produces malabsorption, and there is a high incidence of intestinal infections (particularly giardiasis, but *Strongyloides* and *Candida* may also occur). Can also affect the colon, where in children it may be a normal variant, but in adults it may be an early sign of Crohn's disease.
2. **Crohn's disease*** — 'cobblestone' mucosa but other characteristic signs present.

INFILTRATIVE

1. **Whipple's disease** — ± myriad of tiny (< 1 mm) nodules superimposed on thick folds.
2. **Waldenström's macroglobulinaemia** — ± myriad of tiny (< 1 mm) nodules. Folds usually normal, but may occasionally be thick.
3. **Mastocytosis** — nodules a little larger and folds usually thick.

NEOPLASTIC

1. **Lymphoma*** — can produce diffuse nodules (2–4 mm) of varying sizes. Ulceration in the nodules is not uncommon.
2. **Polyposis**
   (a) Peutz–Jeghers' syndrome — AD. Buccal pigmentation. Multiple hamartomas (± intussusception) 'carpeting' the small bowel. Can also involve the colon (30%) and stomach (25%). Not in themselves premalignant, but associated with carcinoma of stomach, duodenum and ovary.
   (b) Gardner's syndrome — predominantly in the colon. Occasionally has adenomas in small bowel.
   (c) Canada–Cronkhite syndrome — predominantly stomach and colon, but may affect the small bowel.
3. **Metastases** — on antimesenteric border. Particularly melanoma, breast, gastrointestinal tract and ovary. (Rarely bronchus and kidney.) ± Ascites.

INFECTIVE

1. **Typhoid** — hypertrophy of 'Peyer's patches'.
2. **Yersinia** — ± nodules in terminal ileum.

Further Reading

Marshak R.H., Lindner A.E. & Maklansky D. (1976) Immunoglobulin disorders of the small bowel. *Radiol. Clin. North Am.*, 14: 477–91.

6.34 MALABSORPTION

MUCOSAL

1. **Coeliac disease** — commonest cause of malabsorption. Not all have steatorrhoea; can present with iron or folate deficiency. Jejunal biopsy shows subtotal villous atrophy (this can also occur in Whipple's disease, primary lymphoma and chronic ulcerative enteritis). Jejunal dilatation is the hallmark, but is relatively uncommon. It correlates well with severity. Fold thickness is normal in uncomplicated coeliac disease. An increase in ileal fold pattern ± a decrease of jejunal folds, i.e. a reversal of the normal fold pattern, indicates longstanding disease and should heighten awareness to potential malignant complications. Other signs, which are occasionally demonstrable on a barium follow-through examination, are:
   (a) Dilution of barium, because of hypersecretion of fluid by the bowel.
   (b) Segmentation of the column of barium. This is most marked in the ileum.
   (c) Moulage sign. The appearance of barium in a featureless tube due to the complete effacement of mucosal folds.

   If bowel calibre increases while on a gluten-free diet suspect a complication, i.e. lymphoma, carcinoma or intussusception (rare and non-obstructive). Tropical sprue and dermatitis herpetiformis can present with identical appearances.

2. **Inflammation**
   (a) Crohn's disease*.
   (b) Radiotherapy — if there is widespread involvement.
   (c) Scleroderma* — due to hypomotility.
3. **Ischaemia** — can cause mild malabsorption if chronic and widespread.
4. **Infiltration**
   (a) Whipple's disease.
   (b) Mastocytosis.
   (c) Amyloidosis — particularly in primary amyloidosis, since generalized bowel involvement is more common.
   (d) Eosinophilic enteritis — blood eosinophilia is common.
5. **Lymphangiectasia** — child. Blocked lymphatics interfere with the transport of fat. Hypoproteinaemia due to protein loss into the gut is common.
6. **Parasites** — particularly *Giardia* and *Strongyloides* spp.

DIGESTIVE

1. **Gastrectomy.**
2. **Biliary obstruction.**
3. **Pancreatic dysfunction** — pancreatitis, cystic fibrosis, carcinoma and pancreatectomy.
4. **Disaccharidase deficiency** — lactase deficiency is the commonest.

ANATOMICAL

1. **Fistula** — even a small one to the colon allows bacterial colonization.
2. **Resection.**
3. **Stagnant loop/stricture.**
4. **Jejunal diverticulosis** — in the erect view may resemble obstruction with multiple fluid levels. However, the diverticula have smooth walls, i.e. no mucosal folds. Produces folate deficiency.

Further Reading

Bova J.G., Friedman A.C., Weser E. *et al.* (1985) Adaptation of the ileum in nontropical sprue: reversal of the jejunoileal fold pattern. *Am. J. Roentgenol.*, 144: 299–302.

Laws J.W. & Pitman R.G. (1960) The radiological investigation of the malabsorption syndromes. *Br. J. Radiol.*, 33: 211–22.

6.35 PROTEIN-LOSING ENTEROPATHY

Oedema in small bowel will occur if plasma albumin $< 20 \text{ g l}^{-1}$.

'MUCOSAL'

1. **Coeliac disease.**
2. **Ménétrier's disease.**
3. **Sprue.**

INFLAMMATORY

1. **Crohn's disease*.**
2. **Ulcerative colitis*.**
3. **Radiotherapy.**

ULCERATION

1. **Carcinoma stomach/colon.**
2. **Villous adenoma.**

VENOUS OBSTRUCTION

1. **Cirrhosis.**
2. **Inferior vena cava thrombosis.**
3. **Constrictive pericarditis.**

CHRONIC ARTERIAL OBSTRUCTION

LYMPHATIC OBSTRUCTION

1. **Lymphangiectasia.**
2. **Lymphoma*.**
3. **Retroperitoneal fibrosis** — see 8.32.

INFILTRATIVE

1. **Whipple's disease.**
2. **Eosinophilic enteritis.**

Further Reading

Marshak R.H., Wolf B.S., Cohen N. *et al.* (1961) Protein-losing disorders of the gastrointestinal tract: Roentgen features. *Radiology*, 77: 893–905.

6.36 LESIONS IN THE TERMINAL ILEUM

INFLAMMATORY

1. **Crohn's disease*.**
2. **Ulcerative colitis*** — 10% of those with total colitis have 'backwash' ileitis for up to 25 cm causing granular mucosa, ± dilatation. No ulcers.
3. **Radiation enteritis** — submucosal thickening of mucosal folds, mural thickening, symmetrical stenoses, adhesions, sinuses and fistulae. Ulceration and cobblestoning are not seen.

INFECTIVE

1. **Tuberculosis** — can look identical to Crohn's disease. Continuity of involvement with caecum and ascending colon can occur. Longitudinal ulcers are uncommon. Less than 50% have pulmonary TB. Caecum is predominantly involved — progressive contraction of caecal wall opposite the ileocaecal valve, and cephalad retraction of the caecum with straightening of the ileocaecal angle.
2. **Yersinia** — 'cobblestone' appearance and aphthoid ulcers. No deep ulcers and spontaneous resolution, usually within 10 weeks, distinguishes it from Crohn's disease.
3. **Actinomycosis** — very rare. Predominantly caecum. ± Associated bone destruction with periosteal reaction.
4. **Histoplasmosis** — very rare.

NEOPLASTIC

1. **Lymphoma*** — may look like Crohn's disease.
2. **Carcinoid** — appendiceal carcinoid tumours are the most common and are usually benign. Most ileal carcinoids originate in the distal ileum and are invariably malignant if > 2 cm. Radiological signs reflect the primary lesion (annular fibrotic stricture (± obstruction); intraluminal filling defect(s)), the mesenteric secondary mass (stretching of loops; rigidity and fixation), interference with the blood supply to the ileum by the secondary mass (thickening of mucosal folds) or the effects of fibrosis (sharp angulation of a loop; stellate arrangement of loops). The caecum may be involved and strictures may be multifocal.
3. **Metastases** — no ulcers.

ISCHAEMIA

A rare site. Thickened folds, 'cobblestone' appearance and 'thumb printing', but rapid progression of changes helps to discriminate it from Crohn's disease.

Further Reading

Boudiaf M., Soyer P., Pelage J.-P. *et al.* (2000) CT of radiation-induced injury of the gastrointestinal tract: spectrum of findings with barium studies correlation. *Eur. Radiol.*, 10: 920–5.
Calenoff I. (1970) Rare ileocaecal lesions. *Am. J. Roentgenol.*, 110: 343–51.
Jeffree M.A., Barter S.J., Hemingway A.P. *et al.* (1984) Primary carcinoid tumours of the ileum: the radiological appearances. *Clin. Radiol.*, 35: 451–5.
Lee I.-J., Ha H.K., Park C.M. *et al.* (2001) Abdominopelvic actinomycosis involving the gastrointestinal tract: CT features. *Radiology*, 220: 76–80.
Mendelson R.M. & Nolan D.J. (1985) The radiological features of chronic radiation enteritis. *Clin. Radiol.*, 36: 141–8.

6.37 COLONIC POLYPS

ADENOMATOUS

1. **Simple tubular adenoma, tubulovillous adenoma, villous adenoma** — these three form a spectrum both in size and degree of dysplasia. Villous adenoma is the largest, shows the most severe dysplasia and has the highest incidence of malignancy. Signs suggestive of malignancy are:
   (a) Size: < 5 mm — 0% malignant
   5 mm–1 cm — 1% malignant
   1–2 cm — 10% malignant
   > 2 cm — 50% malignant.
   (b) Sessile — base greater than height.
   (c) 'Puckering' of colonic wall at base of polyp.
   (d) Irregular surface.
   Villous adenomas are typically fronded, sessile and are poorly coated by barium because of their mucous secretion. May cause a protein-losing enteropathy or hypokalaemia.

2. **Familial polyposis coli and Gardner's syndrome** — AD. Both conditions may represent a spectrum of the same disease. Multiple adenomas of the colon which are more numerous in the distal colon and rectum. Colonic carcinoma develops in early adulthood (in 30% by 10 years after diagnosis and in 100% by 20 years). 60% of those who present with colonic symptoms already have a carcinoma. The carcinoma is multifocal in 50%. Extracolonic abnormalities may occur:
   (a) Hamartomas of the stomach (40%).
   (b) Gastric adenomas (more common in the Japanese).
   (c) Adenomas of the duodenum (25%).
   (d) Periampullary carcinoma (12%).
   (e) Jejunal and ileal polyps (in 60% of patients in the Japanese literature).
   (f) Mesenteric fibromatosis — a non-calcified soft-tissue mass which may displace bowel loops and produce mucosal irregularity from local invasion. US reveals a hypoechoic or hyperechoic mass and CT a homogeneous mass of muscle density.
   (g) Multiple osteomas, most frequently in the outer table of the skull, the angle of the mandible and frontal sinuses.
   (h) Dental abnormalities — hypercementomas, odontomas, dentigerous cysts, supernumerary teeth and multiple caries.
   (i) Multiple epidermoid cysts — usually on the legs, face, scalp and arms.
   (j) Pigmented lesions of the ocular fundus — in 90% of patients with Gardner's syndrome and other extracolonic manifestations.
   (k) Thyroid carcinoma in 0.6%.

HYPERPLASTIC

1. **Solitary/multiple** — most frequently found in rectum.
2. **Nodular lymphoid hyperplasia** — usually children. Filling defects are smaller than familial polyposis coli.

HAMARTOMATOUS

1. **Juvenile polyposis** — ± familial. Children under 10 years. Commonly solitary in the rectum.
2. **Peutz–Jeghers syndrome** — AD. 'Carpets' small bowel, but also affects colon and stomach in 30%. Increased incidence of carcinoma of stomach, duodenum and ovary.

INFLAMMATORY

1. **Ulcerative colitis*** — polyps can be seen at all stages of activity of the colitis (no malignant potential): acute – pseudopolyps (i.e. mucosal hyperplasia); chronic – sessile polyp (resembles villous adenoma); quiescent – tubular/filiform ('wormlike') and can show a branching pattern.
   Dysplasia in colitic colons is usually not radiologically visible. When visible it appears as a solitary nodule, several separate nodules (both non-specific) or as a close grouping of multiple adjacent nodules with apposed, flattened edges (the latter appearance being associated with dysplasia in 50% of cases).
2. **Crohn's disease*** — polyps less common than in ulcerative colitis.

INFECTIVE

1. **Schistosomiasis** — predominantly involves rectum. ± Strictures.
2. **Amoebiasis.**

OTHERS

1. **Canada–Cronkhite syndrome** — not hereditary. Predominantly affects stomach and colon, but can occur anywhere in bowel. Increased incidence of carcinoma of colon. Other features are alopecia, nail atrophy and skin pigmentation.
2. **Turcot's syndrome** — AR. Increased incidence of CNS malignancy.

Further Reading

Dodds W.J. (1976) Clinical and roentgen features of the intestinal polyposis syndromes. *Gastrointest. Radiol.*, 1: 127–42.

Harned R.K., Buck J.L., Olmsted W.W. *et al.* (1991) Extracolonic manifestations of the familial adenomatous polyposis syndromes. *Am. J. Roentgenol.*, 156: 481–5.

Hooyman J.R., MacCarty R.L., Carpenter H.A. *et al.* (1987) Radiographic appearance of mucosal dysplasia associated with ulcerative colitis. *Am. J. Roentgenol.*, 149: 47–51.

Morson B.C. (1984) The evolution of colorectal carcinoma. *Clin. Radiol.*, 35: 425–31.

Ott D.J. (1996) Barium enema: colorectal polyps and carcinoma. *Semin. Roentgenol.*, 31(2): 125–41.

6.38 COLONIC STRICTURES

NEOPLASTIC

1. **Carcinoma** — mucosal destruction and 'shouldering'. Often shorter than 6 cm.
2. **Lymphoma*.**

INFLAMMATORY

Tend to be symmetrical, smooth and tapered.

1. **Ulcerative colitis*** — usually requires extensive involvement for longer than 5 years. Commonest in sigmoid colon. May be multiple. Beware malignant complications — these are commonly irregular, annular strictures (30% are multiple). Risk factors are: total colitis, length of history (risk starts at 10 years and increases by 10% per decade), epithelial dysplasia on biopsy.
2. **Crohn's disease*** — strictures occur in 25% of colonic Crohn's disease, and 50% of these are multiple.
3. **Pericolic abscess** — can look malignant, but relative lack of mucosal destruction.
4. **Radiotherapy** — occurs several years after treatment. Commonest site is rectosigmoid colon, which appears smooth and narrow, and rises vertically out of pelvis due to thickening of surrounding tissue.

ISCHAEMIA

Infarction heals by stricture formation relatively rapidly. Commonest site is splenic flexure, but 20% occur in other sites. It can be extensive and has tapering ends.

INFECTIVE

1. **Tuberculosis** — commonest in ileocaecal region. Short, 'hourglass' stricture.
2. **Amoeboma** — more common in descending colon. Occurs in 2–8% of amoebiasis and is multiple in 50%. Rapid improvement after treatment with metronidazole.
3. **Schistosomiasis** — commonly rectosigmoid region. Granulation tissue forming after the acute stage (oedema, fold-thickening and polyps) may cause a stricture.
4. **Lymphogranuloma venereum** — sexually transmitted *Chlamydia*. Late complications are strictures which are characteristically long and tubular, and affect the rectosigmoid region. Fistulae may occur.

EXTRINSIC MASSES

Inflammatory, tumours (primary and secondary), and endometriosis.

CATHARTIC COLON

Pseudostrictures which alter their configuration during the barium enema. The colon may be atonic and dilated. Changes are initially in the ascending colon, but can progress to involve the entire colon.

Further Reading

Blakeborough A., Chapman A.H., Swift S. *et al.* (2001) Strictures of the sigmoid colon: barium enema evaluation. *Radiology,* 220: 343–8.

Gore R.M. (1997) Colorectal cancer. Clinical and pathologic features. *Radiol. Clin. North Am.,* 35(2): 403–38.

Levine M.S. (ed.) (2000) Colorectal cancer: diagnosis, screening, and staging. *Semin. Roentgenol.,* 35(4).

Simpkins K.C. and Young A.C. (1971) The differential diagnoses of large bowel strictures. *Clin. Radiol.,* 22: 449–57.

Smith C. (1997) Colorectal cancer. Radiologic diagnosis. *Radiol. Clin. North Am.,* 35(2): 439–56.

Thoeni R.F (1997) Colorectal cancer. Radiologic staging. *Radiol. Clin. North Am.,* 35(2): 457–85.

6.39 PNEUMATOSIS INTESTINALIS (GAS IN THE BOWEL WALL)

PRIMARY (15%)

1. **Pneumatosis coli** — cystic blebs of air. Can produce 'polypoid' filling defects on a barium enema. Some are associated with chronic obstructive airways disease.

SECONDARY (85%)

1. **Necrotizing enterocolitis** — in the neonate.
2. **Steroid and other immunosuppressive therapy.**
3. **Collagen disorders** — mainly scleroderma but also dermatomyositis and juvenile chronic arthritis.
4. **Leukaemia.**
5. **Colitis and enteritis** — ulcerative colitis (including toxic megacolon; see 6.40), Crohn's disease, ischaemia, severe gastroenteritis (particularly rotavirus) and CMV colitis and cryptosporidiosis in HIV infection.

Further Reading

Buonomo C. (1999) The radiology of necrotizing enterocolitis. *Radiol. Clin. North Am.*, 37(6): 1187–98.

Fenton L.Z. & Buonomo C. (2000) Benign pneumatosis in children. *Pediatr. Radiol.*, 30: 786–93.

Pear B.L. (1998) Pneumatosis intestinalis: a review. *Radiology*, 207: 13–29.

6.40 MEGACOLON IN AN ADULT

Colonic calibre greater than 5.5 cm.

NON-TOXIC (WITHOUT MUCOSAL ABNORMALITIES)

1. **Distal obstruction** — e.g. carcinoma.
2. **Ileus** — paralytic or secondary to electrolyte imbalance.
3. **Pseudo-obstruction** — symptoms and signs of large bowel obstruction but with no organic lesion identifiable by barium enema. A continuous, gas-filled colon with sharp, thin bowel wall, few fluid levels and gas or faeces in the rectum may differentiate from organic obstruction. Mortality is 25–30% and the risk of caecal necrosis and perforation is up to 15%.
4. **Purgative abuse.**

TOXIC (with severe mucosal abnormalities)

Deep ulceration and inflammation produce a neuromuscular degeneration. Thick oedematous folds and extensive sloughing of the mucosa leaves mucosal islands. The underlying causes produce similar plain film changes. The presence of intramural gas indicates that perforation is imminent.

1. **Inflammatory**
   (a) Ulcerative colitis*.
   (b) Crohn's disease*.
   (c) Pseudomembranous colitis.
2. **Ischaemic colitis.**
3. **Dysentery**
   (a) Amoebiasis.
   (b) *Salmonella.*

Further Reading

Gilchrist A.M., Mills J.O. & Russell C.F. (1985) Acute large-bowel pseudo-obstruction. *Clin. Radiol.*, 36: 401–4.

Kimura K., Stoopen M., Reeder M.M. *et al.* (1997) Amebiasis: modern diagnostic imaging with pathological and clinical correlation. *Semin. Roentgenol.*, 32(4): 250–75.

6.41 'THUMBPRINTING' IN THE COLON

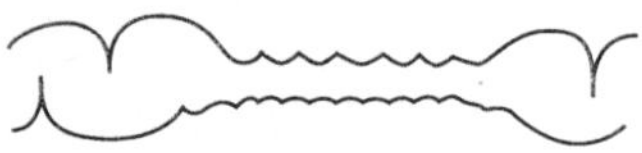

COLITIDES

1. **Ulcerative colitis*.**
2. **Crohn's disease*.**
3. **Ischaemic colitis** — commonest at the splenic flexure, but anywhere possible. Air insufflation may obliterate the 'thumbprinting'.
4. **Pseudomembranous colitis.**
5. **Amoebic colitis.**
6. **Schistosomiasis.**

NEOPLASTIC

1. **Lymphoma*.**
2. **Metastases.**

DIFFERENTIAL DIAGNOSIS

1. **Pneumatosis coli** — cysts may indent the mucosa, giving a similar appearance, but gas is seen in the wall.

Further Reading

Kimura K., Stoopen M., Reeder M.M. *et al.* (1997) Amebiasis: modern diagnostic imaging with pathological and clinical correlation. *Semin. Roentgenol.*, 32(4): 250–75.

6.42 APHTHOID ULCERS

Barium in a central ulcer surrounded by a halo of oedematous mucosa.

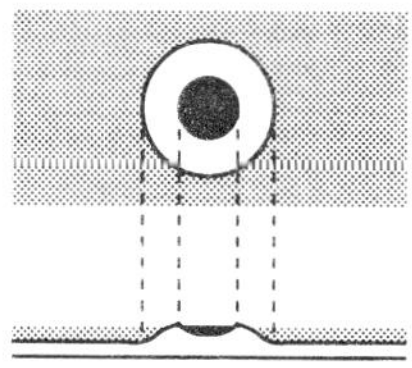

IN COLON

1. **Crohn's disease*** — the earliest sign in the terminal ileum and colon. Observed in 50% of patients.
2. ***Yersinia* enterocolitis.**
3. **Amoebic colitis.**
4. **Ischaemic colitis.**
5. **Behçet's disease** — mostly resembles Crohn's disease, but can occasionally simulate an idiopathic ulcerative proctocolitis.

IN SMALL BOWEL

1. **Crohn's disease*.**
2. ***Yersinia* enterocolitis.**
3. **Polyarteritis nodosa.**

Further Reading

Simpkins K.C. (1977) Aphthoid ulcers in Crohn's colitis. *Clin. Radiol.*, 28: 601–8.

6.43 ANTERIOR INDENTATION OF THE RECTOSIGMOID JUNCTION

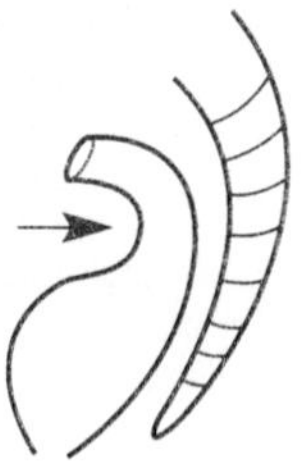

1. **Tumours**
   (a) Peritoneal metastases — common site. Particularly from stomach, colon, pancreas and ovary.
   (b) Primary pelvic tumour.
2. **Abscess.**
3. **Haematoma.**
4. **Ascites** — if in erect position.
5. **Endometriosis** — common site.
6. **Hydatid** — metastatic cyst from rupture of a peripheral hepatic cyst.
7. **Surgical** — sling repair for rectal prolapse.

Further Reading

Schulman A. & Fataar S. (1979) Extrinsic stretching, narrowing, and anterior indentation of the rectosigmoid junction. *Clin. Radiol.*, 30: 463–9.

6.44 WIDENING OF THE RETRORECTAL SPACE

The post-rectal soft-tissue space at S3–S5 is greater than 1.5 cm.

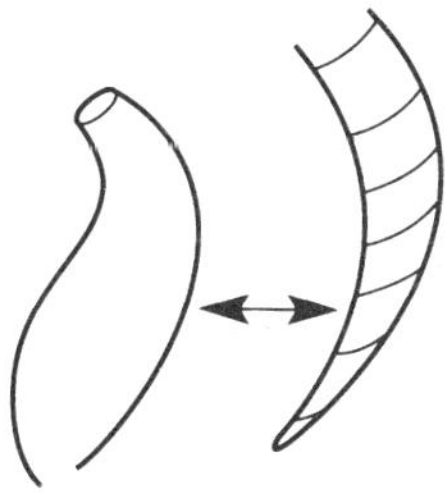

NORMAL VARIATION

40% of cases and these are mostly large or obese individuals.

INFLAMMATORY

1. **Ulcerative colitis*** — seen in 50% of these patients and the width increases as the disease progresses.
2. **Crohn's disease*** — the widening may diminish during the course of the disease.
3. **Radiotherapy.**
4. **Diverticulitis.**
5. **Abscess.**

NEOPLASTIC

1. **Carcinoma of the rectum.**
2. **Metastases to the rectum** — especially from prostate, ovary and bladder.
3. **Sacral tumours** — metastases, plasmacytoma, chordoma and, in children, sacrococcygeal teratoma.

OTHERS

1. **Anterior sacral meningocoele** — a sac containing CSF protrudes through a round or oval defect in the anterior wall of the sacrum. The diagnosis is confirmed by CT myelography or MRI.
2. **Pelvic lipomatosis.**
3. **Enteric duplication cysts.**

Further Reading

Teplick S.K., Stark P., Clark R.E. *et al.* (1978) The retrorectal space. *Clin. Radiol.*, 29: 177–84.

6.45 CT OF A RETROPERITONEAL CYSTIC MASS

PANCREAS

1. **Pseudocyst.**
2. **Cystadenoma/carcinoma.**
3. **von Hippel–Lindau.**

KIDNEY – see 8.21.

PARA-AORTIC CYSTIC NODES

1. **Testicular teratoma.**
2. **Carcinoma cervix.**

RETROPERITONEAL CYSTIC TUMOUR

1. **Lymphangioma.**
2. **Leiomyosarcoma.**
3. **Haemangiopericytoma.**

NB. Any tumour with a fatty content can appear cystic due to density averaging, e.g. neurofibroma.

OTHERS

1. **Haematoma** — late stage.
2. **Abscess.**
3. **Lymphocoele.**
4. **Meningocoele.**

Further Reading

Alpern M.B., Thorsen M.K., Kellman G.M. *et al.* (1986) C.T. appearances of haemangiopericytoma. *J. Comput. Assist. Tomogr.*, 10: 264–7.

Hes F.J. & Feldberg M.A. (1999) Von Hippel–Lindau disease: strategies in early detection (renal-, adrenal-, pancreatic masses). *Eur. Radiol.*, 9: 598–610.

Munechika H., Honda M., Kushihashi T. *et al.* (1986) Computed tomography of retroperitoneal cystic lymphangiomas. *J. Comput. Assist. Tomogr.*, 11: 116–9.

6.46 CT OF A MESENTERIC CYSTIC LESION

CYSTS

1. **Pancreatic pseudocyst.**
2. **Enteric duplication cyst.**
3. **Mesothelial cyst.**

TUMOUR

1. **Teratoma.**
2. **Cystic leiomyoma/sarcoma.**
3. **Cystic mesothelioma.**
4. **Lymphangioma.**

Further Reading

Aviv R.I., McHugh K., Hunt J. (2001) Angiomatosis of bone and soft tissue: a spectrum of disease from diffuse lymphangiomatosis to vanishing bone disease in young patients. *Clin. Radiol.*, 56; 184–90.

Ros P., Olmsted W., Moser R. *et al.* (1987) Mesenteric and omental cysts: histology classification with imaging correlation. *Radiology,* 164: 327–32.

Ruess L., Frazier A.A. & Sivit C.J. (1995) CT of the mesentery, omentum, and peritoneum in children. *RadioGraphics,* 15: 89–104.

6.47 MRI OF POST-RADIATION CHANGES IN THE PELVIS

	T_1W	T_2W	*Comments*
Bone marrow in sacrum	↑	↑	Due to fat deposition
Fibrous tissue	↓	↑	No gadolinium enhancement
Granulation tissue	↓	↑	Enhances with gadolinium; mimics tumour recurrence; can persist for several years
Bladder, rectum, muscle	Isointense	±↑	Thickened, oedematous neovascularity
Ovary/uterus	Isointense	↓	Atrophy
Fascial planes	↓	Variable	Thickened

Further Reading

Iyer R.B., Jhingran A., Sawaf H. *et al.* (2001) Imaging findings after radiotherapy to the pelvis. *Am. J. Roentgenol.*, 177: 1083–9.

Outwater E. & Kressel H.Y. (1992) Evaluation of gynaecologic malignancy by magnetic resonance imaging. *Radiol. Clin. North Am.*, 30: 789–806.

6.48 MRI OF FEMALE PELVIC PATHOLOGY

	T_1W	T_2W	*Comments*
Carcinoma of cervix	Isointense	↑	
Endometrial carcinoma	↓ (↑ if haemorrhage or retained fluid)	Variable, but usually ↑ compared to myometrium and junctional zone. (If ↓, looks like fibroid)	15–20% not visible (presumably superficial). Haemorrhage, metastases, leiomyosarcoma and endometrial hyperplasia can mimic
Gestational trophoblastic disease	Isointense (↑ if haemorrhage)	Usually ↑	May have signal voids +, due to marked vascularity. 30–50% have associated theca lutein cysts due to hormonal stimulation
Uterine fibroid			
non-degenerative	iso (↓ if Ca^{2+})	↓	
degenerative	iso, ↑	↑	
Uterine adenomyosis			
diffuse	±↑	±↑	Thickened junctional zone
focal	iso	↓	like fibroid
Ovarian carcinoma			Cannot distinguish benign from malignant
solid	Isointense	↑	
cystic	↓	↑	
Ovarian dermoid	↑ (fat)	↑ (fat)	± fluid/fluid levels
Ovarian fibroma	↓	↓	
Endometrioma	↑ (blood)	↓ (inhomogeneous)	Haemorrhage into ovarian carcinoma can mimic
Vaginal carcinoma	Isointense	Isointense, ↑	Only seen if vaginal outline is distorted. The rich perivaginal venous plexus can mask the tumour
Post-radiation change			
fibrous	↓	↓	No gadolinium enhancement
granulation	↓	↑	Gadolinium enhancement can persist for several years and mimic tumour

Further Reading

Outwater E. & Kressel H.Y. (1992) Evaluation of gynaecologic malignancy by magnetic resonance imaging. *Radiol. Clin. North Am.*, 30: 789–806.

6.49 SOMATOSTATIN RECEPTOR SCINTIGRAPHY

1. **Neuroendocrine tumours**
   (a) Pituitary tumours — growth hormone or thyroid-stimulating hormone, secreting or non-functioning.
   (b) Gastrinoma, insulinoma, glucagonoma. Some insulinomas are negative, as are exocrine pancreatic tumours.
   (c) Paragangliomas — it is important to image the whole body.
   (d) Neuroblastoma and phaeochromocytoma — MIBG preferred for phaeochromocytoma because of kidney accumulation of octreotide.
   (e) Medullary thyroid carcinoma. Poor results for metastases in the liver, or for intrathyroidal tumours.
   (f) Carcinoid tumour — liver metastases may be difficult to visualize.
   (g) Small cell lung cancer.
2. **Brain tumours, especially meningiomas and astrocytomas.**
3. **Breast cancer.**
4. **Lymphomas.**
5. **Sarcoidosis.**
6. **Autoimmune diseases** — thyroid in Graves' disease and joints in rheumatoid arthritis.
7. **False positive**
   (a) Lung uptake after irradiation or bleomycin.
   (b) Recent operation sites.
8. **Visualization of normal organs**
   (a) Pituitary, thyroid.
   (b) Spleen, liver (occasionally gallbladder).
   (c) Kidneys, urinary bladder.
   (d) Nasal region and lung hila with the common cold.

Further Reading

Krenning E.R., Kwekkeboom D.G., Bakker W.H. *et al.* (1993) Somatostatin receptor scintigraphy with [^{111}In-DTPA-D-Phe] and [^{123}-Tyr^{3}]-octreotide: the Rotterdam experience with more than 1000 patients. *Eur. J. Nucl. Med.* 20: 716–31.

6.50 LOCALIZATION OF GASTROINTESTINAL BLEEDING

1. **Ulcers** — benign or malignant.
2. **Vascular lesions** — telangiectasia, haematoma, fistula, angiodysplasia.
3. **Tumours** — leiomyoma, adenoma.
4. **Inflammatory lesions** — gastritis, duodenitis.
5. **Varices** — oesophageal or stomach.
6. **Surgical anastomosis.**
7. **Meckel's diverticulum** (q.v.).
8. **Intussusception.**
9. **Metastatic disease.**
10. **Diverticula.**
11. **False positive**
    (a) Renal tract, liver, spleen, small bowel vascularity.
    (b) Uterus.
    (c) Accessory spleen.
    (d) Marrow uptake of colloid, especially if irregular.

TECHNIQUES:

1. ^{99}mTc-labelled red blood cells. Labelling efficiency is important, as false positive scans can result from accumulations of free pertechnetate.
2. ^{99}mTc-colloid. Used to be a commonly used alternative to labelled red cells, but a number of studies have shown it to be a less sensitive tracer for detecting bleeding sites, hence it is not recommended. Colloids are rapidly extracted from the circulation, so bleeding occurring only within 10 minutes or so of injection can be detected. Also localizes intensely in liver and spleen, masking upper GI bleeding sites.

Further Reading

Holder L.E. (2000) Radionuclide imaging in the evaluation of acute gastrointestinal bleeding. *RadioGraphics*, 20: 1153–9.

Silberstein E.B. & McAfee J.G. (eds) (1984) *Differential Diagnosis in Nuclear Medicine.* New York: McGraw-Hill, pp. 191–3.

6.51 MECKEL'S DIVERTICULUM

Technique: ^{99m}Tc pertechnetate.

MECKEL'S DIVERTICULUM

Appears at the same time as the stomach, and the activity increases in intensity with the stomach. May change in position during the study and may empty its contents into the bowel.

GASTROINTESTINAL BLEEDING

Any blood leaking into the bowel would be apparent, although it would not show the rounded appearance of a Meckel's diverticulum.

FALSE POSITIVE RESULTS

1. **Physiological**
   (a) Gastric emptying.
   (b) Renal tract — pelvis, ureter, bladder diverticulum.
   (c) Iliac vessels.
   (d) Uterus.
2. **Pathological**
   (a) Ectopic gastric mucosa in the small bowel.
   (b) Infection — for example, acute appendicitis.
   (c) Intussusception.
   (d) Haemangioma of the bowel — gradual reduction in activity.

FALSE NEGATIVE

1. **No ectopic gastric mucosa in the diverticulum.**
2. **Hidden by bladder or stomach.**

Further Reading

Merrick M.V. (1986) In: P.J. Robinson (ed.), *Nuclear Gastroenterology.* Edinburgh: Churchill Livingstone, pp. 163–8.

6.52 LOCALIZATION OF INFECTION

Technique: ^{111}In leucocytes or ^{99m}Tc HMPAO leucocytes.

1. **Collection of pus.**
2. **False positive**
   (a) Surgical scars.
   (b) Drip sites and drainage tubes.
   (c) i.v. injection sites.
   (d) Lung accumulation in early images.
   (e) Gastrointestinal bleeding.
   (f) Sites of bone marrow aspiration.
   (g) Swallowed white blood cells from lung, sinuses, mouth.
   (h) Fractures within the first 2 weeks.
   (i) Inflammatory arthritis.
   (j) Biliary and renal tract (hexamethylpropyleneamineoxime (HMPAO only).
3. **False negative**
   (a) Walled-off avascular pus.
   (b) Chronic inflammatory (lymphocytic) reaction.
   (c) Acute osteomyelitis — especially spinal.
   (d) Chronic infection of joint prosthesis.
   (e) Agranulocytosis.
4. **Inflammatory bowel disease** — uptake at 2 h and reduces by 24 h. Image at 1 h using ^{99m}Tc hexamethylpropyleneamineoxime (HMPAO)
   (a) Crohn's disease.
   (b) Ulcerative colitis.
   (c) Infective colitis.
5. **Infected prosthesis.**
6. **Sinusitis.**
7. **Acute infarcts** — including bowel, myocardial, cerebral.
8. **Myocarditis.**
9. **Rejected transplant** — kidney.
10. **Pancreatitis.**
11. **Infected tumour** — especially bronchial.

Further Reading

Mello A.M., Blake K. & McDougall I.R. (1992) Cold lesions on indium^{111} white blood cell scintigraphy. *Semin. Nucl. Med.* 22: 292–4.

Palestro C.J., Love C., Tronco G.G. *et al.* (2000) Role of radionuclide imaging in the diagnosis of postoperative infection. *RadioGraphics,* 20: 1649–60.

6.53 GALLIUM UPTAKE

Technique: imaging 24 h after ^{67}Ga injection for inflammatory lesions; up to 72 h for tumour.

INFLAMMATORY

1. **Inflammation or abscess.**
2. **Sarcoidosis** — lacrimal and salivary gland uptake are typical.
3. **Diffuse lung disease** — interstitial fibrosis, scleroderma, asbestosis.
4. **Heart** — myocarditis, pericarditis, systemic lupus erythematosus.

TUMOURS

1. **Lymphoma*** — positive in 90% of patients and 80% of affected sites.
2. **Bronchial carcinoma** — (90%). Used for staging.
3. **Gastrointestinal tumours** — (20%).
4. **Hepatoma.**
5. **Other malignant tumours.**

NORMAL VARIANTS

1. **Nasopharynx.**
2. **Bowel** — diffuse or outlining the colon.
3. **Breast** — often due to antiemetics or oral contraceptives. Intense uptake if recent breastfeeding.

Further Reading

Rehm P.K. (2001) Radionuclide evaluation of patients with lymphoma. *Radiol. Clin. North Am.*, 39(5): 957–78.

7 Gallbladder, liver, spleen and pancreas

7.1 NON-VISUALIZATION OF THE GALLBLADDER

DURING ORAL CHOLECYSTOGRAPHY

1. **Technical failures**
   (a) No fatty meal prior to taking of contrast medium.
   (b) Tablets not taken or taken at the wrong time.
   (c) Vomiting or diarrhoea.
   (d) Failure to fast after taking contrast medium.
   (e) Films taken too early or too late.
   (f) Bilirubin greater than 34 mmol l^{-1}.
2. **Previous cholecystectomy.**
3. **Ectopic gallbladder** — confirmed by taking a film of the entire abdomen.
4. **Cholecystitis.**
5. **Cystic duct obstruction.**

DURING INTRAVENOUS CHOLANGIOGRAPHY

1. **Technical failures**
   (a) Contrast medium given too rapidly — renal excretion is seen.
   (b) Bilirubin greater than 50 mmol l^{-1}.
2. **Previous cholecystectomy.**
3. **Ectopic gallbladder.**
4. **Cystic duct obstruction.**
5. **Cholecystitis.**

7.2 FILLING DEFECT IN THE GALLBLADDER

MULTIPLE

1. **Calculi** — 30% are radio-opaque. Freely mobile.
2. **Cholesterosis ('strawberry' gallbladder)** — characteristically multiple fixed mural filling defects.

SINGLE AND SMALL

1. **Calculus.**
2. **Adenomyomatosis** — three characteristic signs.
   (a) Fundal nodular filling defect.
   (b) Stricture — anywhere in the gallbladder. Sharply localized or a diffuse narrowing. More prominent following contraction after a fatty meal.
   (c) Rokitansky–Aschoff sinuses — may only be visible after gallbladder contraction.

SINGLE AND LARGE

1. **Calculus.**
2. **Carcinoma** — difficult to diagnose as the radiological presentation is usually with a non-functioning gallbladder. Nearly always associated with gallstones and, therefore, if filling does occur it is indistinguishable from them. Cross-sectional imaging demonstrates a mass replacing the gallbladder (40–65%), focal or diffuse gallbladder wall thickening (20–30%) or an intraluminal polypoid mass (15–25%).

Further Reading

Levy A.D., Murkata L.A. & Rohrmann C.A. Jr (2001) Gallbladder carcinoma: radiologic–pathologic correlation. *RadioGraphics*, 21: 295–314.

7.3 GAS IN THE BILIARY TRACT

Irregularly branching gas shadows which do not reach to the liver edge, probably because of the direction of bile flow. The gallbladder may also be outlined.

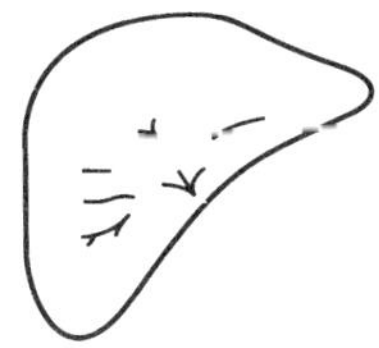

WITHIN THE BILE DUCTS

Incompetence of the sphincter of ODDI

1. **Following sphincterotomy.**
2. **Following passage of a gallstone.**
3. **Patulous sphincter in the elderly.**

Postoperative

1. **Cholecystoenterostomy.**
2. **Choledochoenterostomy.**

Spontaneous biliary fistula

1. **Passage of a gallstone directly from an inflamed gallbladder into the bowel** — 90% of spontaneous fistulae. 57% erode into the duodenum and 18% into the colon. May result in a gallstone ileus.
2. **Duodenal ulcer perforating into the common bile duct** — 6% of spontaneous fistulae.
3. **Malignancy or trauma** — 4% of spontaneous fistulae.

WITHIN THE GALLBLADDER

1. **All of the above.**
2. **Emphysematous cholecystitis** — due to gas-forming organisms and associated with diabetes in 20% of cases. There is intramural and intraluminal gas but, because there is usually cystic duct obstruction, gas is present in the bile ducts in only 20%. The erect film may show an air–bile interface.

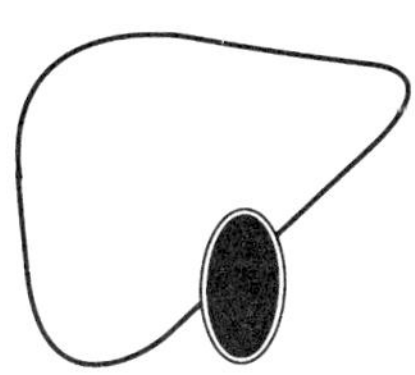

7.4 GAS IN THE PORTAL VEINS

Gas shadows which extend to within 2 cm of the liver capsule because of the direction of blood flow in the portal veins. Gas may also be present in the portal and mesenteric veins and the bowel wall.

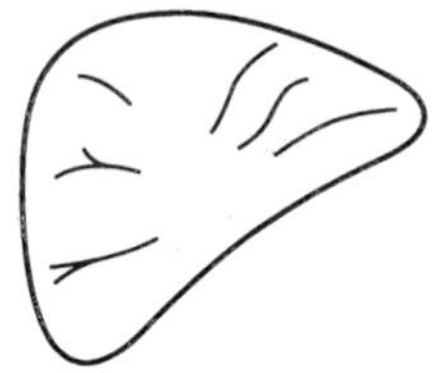

CHILDREN

1. **Necrotizing enterocolitis** — 10% develop gas in the portal vein. Necrotic bowel wall allows gas or gas-forming organisms into the portal circulation. The finding of portal vein gas is of serious significance.
2. **Umbilical vein catheterization** — with the inadvertent injection of air.
3. **Erythroblastosis fetalis.**

ADULTS

1. **Mesenteric infarction** — the majority of patients die soon after gas is seen in the portal veins.
2. **Air embolus during double contrast barium enema** — this has been observed during the examination of severely ulcerated colons and is not associated with a fatal outcome.
3. **Acute gastric dilatation** — in bed-ridden young people. May recover following decompression with a nasogastric tube.

Further Reading

Benson M.B. (1985) Adult survival with intrahepatic portal venous gas secondary to acute gastric dilatation with a review of portal venous gas. *Clin. Radiol.*, 36: 441–3.

Mindelzun R. & McCort J.J. (1980) Hepatic and perihepatic radiolucencies. *Radiol. Clin. North Am.*, 18: 221–38.

Radin D.R., Roson R.S. & Halls J.M. (1987) Acute gastric dilatation: a rare cause of portal venous gas. *Am. J. Roentgenol.*, 148: 279–80.

Sisk P.B. (1961) Gas in the portal venous system. *Radiology*, 77: 103–6.

Wiot J.F. & Felson B. (1961) Gas in the portal venous system. *Am. J. Roentgenol.*, 86: 920–9.

7.5 SEGMENTAL ANATOMY OF THE LIVER

25% of colorectal carcinomas have liver secondaries at presentation. Of these, 10% have surgically resectable disease. Surgeons need to know the number, size, location and proximity to vessels.

The liver is divided into segments in the horizontal plane by the right and left main portal veins, and in the vertical plane by the right, middle and left hepatic veins.

Upper Segments: above the level of the right and left portal veins.

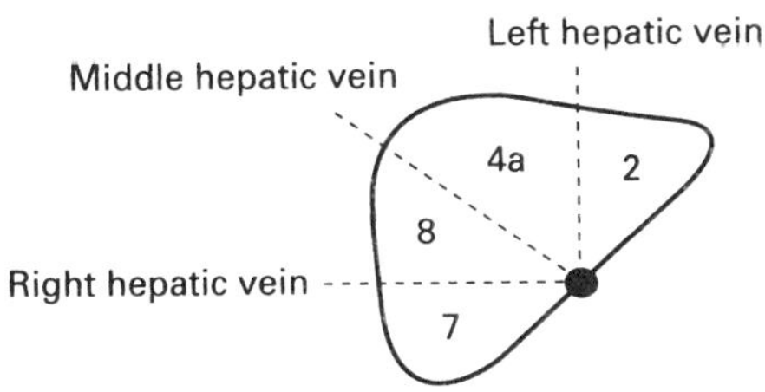

Caudate lobe is segment 1

Lower Segments: below the evel of the right and left portal veins.

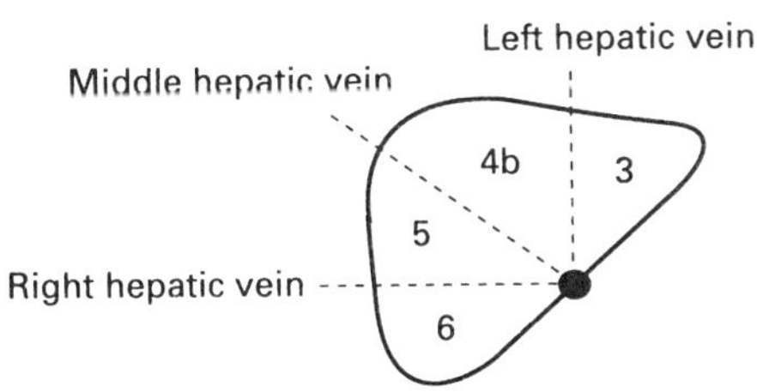

Further Reading

Nelson R.C., Chezmer J.L., Sugarbaker P.H. *et al.* (1990) Preoperative localisation of focal liver lesions to specific liver segments. *Radiology*, 176: 86–94.

Vauthey J.N. (1998) Liver Imaging – a surgeon's perspective. *Radiol. Clin. North Am.*, 36: 445–57.

7.6 HEPATOMEGALY

NEOPLASTIC

1. **Metastases.**
2. **Hepatoma.**
3. **Lymphoma*** — secondary involvement occurs in up to 50% of patients with systemic lymphoma, but is frequently occult. Primary hepatic lymphoma is very rare.

RAISED VENOUS PRESSURE

1. **Congestive cardiac failure.**
2. **Constrictive pericarditis.**
3. **Tricuspid stenosis.**
4. **Budd–Chiari syndrome.**

DEGENERATIVE

1. **Cirrhosis** — especially alcoholic.
2. **Fatty infiltration.**

MYELOPROLIFERATIVE DISORDERS

1. **Polycythaemia rubra vera.**
2. **Myelofibrosis.**

INFECTIVE

1. **Viral** — infectious and serum hepatitis; infectious mononucleosis.
2. **Bacterial** — abscess; brucellosis.
3. **Protozoal** — amoebic abscess, malaria, trypanosomiasis and kala-azar.
4. **Parasitic** — hydatid.

STORAGE DISORDERS

1. **Amyloid.**
2. **Haemochromatosis.**
3. **Gaucher's disease.**
4. **Niemann–Pick disease.**

CONGENITAL

1. **Riedel's lobe.**
2. **Polycystic disease*.**

Further Reading

Lewall D.B. (1998) Hydatid disease: biology, pathology, imaging and classification. *Clin. Radiol.*, 53: 863–74.

7.7 HEPATIC TUMOURS IN CHILDREN

Feature	*Hepatoblastoma*	*Hepatocellular carcinoma*
Age	Usually < 5 years old	Usually > 5 years old
Sex	M >> F	M > F
Associated conditions	Beckwith–Wiedemann syndrome, hemihypertrophy	
Associated liver disease	No	↑ incidence (cirrhosis, glycogen storage disease 1, tyrosinaemia, biliary atresia and chronic hepatitis)
Presentation	Mass ± pain. Hormone production may lead to male sexual precocity, polycythaemia, hypoglycaemia, hyperlipidaemia or hypercalcaemia. ± Signs of chronic liver disease	
↑ Serum alpha-fetoprotein	Almost all	Most
Multifocal	Less likely	More likely
Location	Right lobe >> left lobe	Right lobe > left lobe, but in most both lobes are involved
Resectability at diagnosis	More likely	Less likely
Relative prognosis	Better	Worse
Ultrasound	Very variable; usually non-homogenous increased echoes	
CT	Non-homogeneous low attenuation with some enhancement	
MRI	↓ Signal on T_1W and ↑ signal on T_2W. Tumour invasion of vessels is seen best by this modality	
Metastases	Lungs (in 10% at diagnosis), abdominal lymph nodes and skeleton	

Modified from Cohen (1992).

1. **Hepatoblastoma**
2. **Hepatocellular carcinoma**

} there are no major imaging differences between these two tumours but clinical differences, particularly age, may enable prebiopsy differentiation. (See above table).

3. **Haemangioendothelioma** — often present in the newborn period with hepatomegaly and congestive cardiac failure. ± Skin haemangiomas (50%) ± consumptive coagulopathy (thrombocytopenia). Unifocal or multifocal, well-defined or diffuse. Typical pattern of enhancement on CT with early rim enhancement and variable delayed 'filling-in' of the centre of the tumour over next 30 minutes. On MRI the lesions have a non-specific hypointense T_1W and hyperintense T_2W appearance with variable areas of T_1W hypointensity corresponding to fibrosis and haemosiderin deposition. ^{99m}Tc-labelled red cells will accumulate in this tumour. In the neonate, this and cavernous haemangioma may be considered together.
4. **Stage IV-S neuroblastoma** — diffuse and infiltrating. Lesions in bone and bone marrow, ↑ urinary VMAs and positive MIBG scan.
5. **Adenoma** — solitary or multiple, occurring spontaneously or complicating glycogen storage disease, Fanconi's anaemia treated with anabolic steroids, and teenagers on the oral contraceptive pill. Hypodense on CT. Variable appearance on MRI.

DIFFERENTIAL DIAGNOSIS

1. **Focal nodular hyperplasia** — a wide spectrum of appearances.
2. **Simple cyst.**
3. **Choledochal cyst.**
4. **Abscess.**

Further Reading

Burrows P.E., Dubois J. & Kassarjian A. (2001) Pediatric hepatic vascular anomalies. *Pediatr. Radiol.*, 3: 533–45.

Cheon J.-E., Kim W.S., Kim I.-O. *et al.* (1998) Radiological features of focal nodular hyperplasia of the liver in children. *Pediatr. Radiol.*, 28: 878–83.

Cohen M.D. (1992) *Imaging of Children with Cancer,* Ch. 3. St Louis: Mosby Year Book, pp. 20–42.

Donnelly L.F. & Bissett G.S. III (1998) Pediatric hepatic imaging. *Radiol. Clin. North Am.*, 36(2): 413–27.

Helmberger T.K., Ros P.R., Mergo P.J. *et al.* (1999) Pediatric liver neoplasms: a radiologic–pathologic correlation. *Eur. Radiol.*, 9: 1339–47.

Pobiel R.S. & Bisset G.S. III (1995) Pictorial essay: imaging of liver tumours in the infant and child. *Pediatr. Radiol.*, 25: 495–506.

7.8 HEPATIC CALCIFICATION

MULTIPLE AND SMALL

1. **Healed granulomas** — tuberculosis, histoplasmosis and, less commonly, brucellosis and coccidioidomycosis. Usually < 2 cm. May be solitary. May be calcified granulomas in other organs.

CURVILINEAR

1. **Hydatid** — liver is the commonest site of hydatid disease. Most cysts are in the right lobe and are clinically silent but may cause pain, a palpable mass or a thrill. Calcification in 20–30% and, although calcification does not necessarily indicate death of the parasite, extensive calcification favours an inactive cyst. Calcification of daughter cysts produces several rings of calcification.
2. **Abscess** — especially amoebic abscess when the right lobe is most frequently affected.
3. **Calcified (porcelain) gallbladder** — strong association with gallbladder carcinoma.

LOCALIZED IN MASS

1. **Metastases** — calcification is uncommon but colloid carcinoma of the rectum, colon or stomach calcify most frequently. It may be amorphous, flaky, stippled or granular and solitary or multiple. Calcification may follow radiotherapy or chemotherapy.
2. **Adenoma** — rare. Calcifications are punctate, stippled or granular. Often placed eccentrically within a complex heterogeneous mass.

SUNRAY SPICULATION

1. **Haemangioma** — calcification in 10% (on AXR) to 20% (on CT). Phleboliths may also occur but are uncommon.
2. **Metastases** — infrequently in metastases from colloid carcinomas.
3. **Adenoma.**

DIFFUSE INCREASED DENSITY

1. **Haemochromatosis***.

Further Reading

Hale H.L., Husband J.E., Gossios K. *et al.* (1998) CT of calcified liver metastases in colorectal carcinoma. *Clin. Radiol.*, 53: 735–41.

Paley M.R. & Ros P.R. (1998) Hepatic calcification. *Radiol. Clin. North Am.*, 36(2): 391–8.

Stoupis C., Taylor H.M., Paley M.R. *et al.* (1998) The rocky liver: radiologic–pathologic correlation of calcified hepatic masses. *RadioGraphics*, 18: 675–85.

7.9 FETAL OR NEONATAL LIVER CALCIFICATION

PERITONEAL

1. **Meconium peritonitis** — the commonest cause of neonatal abdominal calcification. US reveals intra-abdominal solid or cystic masses with calcified walls.
2. **Plastic peritonitis due to ruptured hydrometrocolpos** — similar appearance to meconium peritonitis but US may demonstrate a dilated, fluid-filled uterus and vagina.

PARENCHYMAL

1. **Congenital infections** — TORCH complex (toxoplasmosis, rubella, cytomegalovirus, herpes simplex) and varicella. Randomly scattered nodular calcification. Often calcification elsewhere and other congenital abnormalities.
2. **Tumours** — haemangioma, hamartoma, hepatoblastoma, teratoma and metastatic neuroblastoma. Complex mass on US.

VASCULAR

1. **Portal vein thromboemboli** — subcapsular branching calcification.
2. **Ischaemic infarcts** — branching calcifications but distributed throughout the liver.

Further Reading

Brugman S.M., Bjelland J.J., Thomason J.E. *et al.* (1979) Sonographic findings with radiologic correlation in meconium peritonitis. *J. Clin. Ultrasound,* 7: 305–6.

Friedman A.P., Haller J.O., Boyer B. *et al.* (1981) Calcified portal vein thromboemboli in infants: radiography and ultrasonography. *Radiology,* 140: 381–2.

Nguyen D.L. & Leonard J.C. (1986) Ischaemic hepatic necrosis: a cause of fetal liver calcification. *Am. J. Roentgenol.,* 147: 596–7.

Schackelford G.D. & Kirks D.R. (1977) Neonatal hepatic calcification secondary to transplacental infection. *Radiology,* 122: 753–7.

7.10 JAUNDICE IN INFANCY

ANATOMICAL ABNORMALITIES

1. **Biliary atresia** — 1 in 15 000 live births. Three types: I (focal), extremely rare; II (intrahepatic), uncommon; III (extrahepatic), which is subdivided into subtype 1 (66%) with a bile duct remnant at the porta hepatis and subtype 2 (34%) with no bile duct. Subtype 2 is associated with multiple congenital abnormalities (polysplenia, intestinal malrotation, azygos continuation of the IVC, situs inversus and preduodenal portal vein).
   US:
   (a) A normal-sized gallbladder that contracts following a fatty meal excludes the diagnosis.
   (b) Absence of, or a small, gallbladder favours the diagnosis but a normal gallbladder may be seen in 10% of cases.
   (c) Liver echogenicity is normal or increased.
   (d) A triangular or tubular echogenic structure (due to fibrous tissue) at the porta hepatis is specific for extrahepatic biliary atresia.
   TBIDA scan:
   (a) Normal uptake by hepatocytes but no excretion into the bowel suggests the diagnosis but is not diagnostic since alpha-1-antitrypsin may show similar appearances. Operative cholangiography is indicated.
2. **Choledochal cyst** — may present in the neonatal period or at a later age. Classification is:
   I (80–90%) Fusiform or focal dilatation of the common bile duct ± common hepatic duct.
   II (2%) Diverticulum of the common bile duct.
   III (2–5%) Outpouching of the common bile duct in the wall of thc second part of the duodenum — a choledochocoele.
   IVa Dilatation of the common bile duct and focal dilatations of the intrahepatic ducts.
   IVb Focal dilatations of the common bile duct.
   V Focal dilatations of the intrahepatic bile ducts (Caroli's disease).
   US:
   (a) Anechoic structure which communicates with the biliary tree and is separate from the gallbladder.
   TBIDA scan:
   (a) Photopenic area which accumulates tracer on delayed images.

Complications:
(a) Calculi.
(b) Pancreatitis.
(c) Intrahepatic abscesses.
(d) Biliary cirrhosis.
(e) Portal hypertension.
(f) Malignancy — 4–28%; in the cyst in 3%.

3. **Alagille syndrome** — AD with variable expressivity. Dysmorphic facies, eye abnormalities, cardiovascular abnormalities, especially peripheral pulmonary stenosis or hypoplasia, hypoplasia of intrahepatic bile ducts, butterfly vertebrae, radioulnar synostosis.

METABOLIC DEFECTS

e.g. Alpha-1-antitrypsin deficiency, galactosaemia, tyrosinaemia.

INFECTIONS

1. **Neonatal hepatitis** — possibly secondary to reovirus.
   US:
   (a) Liver echogenicity and size normal or increased.
   (b) Normal bile ducts and gall bladder, although gallbladder may be small when hepatocellular function is poor and bile flow is reduced.
   TBIDA scan:
   (a) May have delayed uptake by hepatocytes.
   (b) Normal excretion into bowel but may be little, if any, if hepatocyte function is severely impaired.

Further Reading

Gubernick J.A., Rosenburg H.K., Ilaslan H. *et al.* (2000) US approach to jaundice in infants and children. *RadioGraphics,* 20: 173–95.
Kim O.H., Chung H.J. & Choi B.G. (1995) Imaging of the choledochal cyst. *RadioGraphics,* 15: 69–88.

7.11 ULTRASOUND LIVER – GENERALIZED HYPOECHOIC

1. **Acute hepatitis** — mild hepatitis has normal echo pattern.
2. **Diffuse malignant infiltration.**

7.12 ULTRASOUND LIVER – GENERALIZED HYPERECHOIC (Bright liver)

1. **Fatty infiltration.**
2. **Cirrhosis.**
3. **Hepatitis** — particularly chronic.
4. **Infiltration/deposition** — malignant, granulomata (e.g. TB, brucellosis, sarcoidosis), glycogen storage disease.

Further Reading

Vilgrain V. (2001) Ultrasound of diffuse liver disease and portal hypertension. *Eur. Radiol.*, 11: 1563–77.

7.13 ULTRASOUND LIVER – FOCAL HYPERECHOIC

1. **Metastases** — gastrointestinal tract, ovary, pancreas, urogenital tract.
2. **Capillary haemangioma.**
3. **Adenoma** — particularly if associated haemorrhage.
4. **Focal nodular hyperplasia** — may be hyperechoic.
5. **Focal fatty infiltration.**
6. **Debris within lesion** — e.g. abscess, haematoma.
7. **Hepatoma** — can be hyperechoic or hypoechoic.

Further Reading

Harvey C.J. & Albrecht T. (2001) Ultrasound of focal liver lesions. *Eur. Radiol.*, 11: 1578–93.
Hosten N., Puls R., Bechstein W.O. *et al.* (1999) Focal liver lesions: Doppler ultrasound. *Eur. Radiol.*, 9: 428–35.
Nisenbaum H.L. & Rowling S.E. (1995) Ultrasound of focal hepatic lesions. *Semin. Roentgenol.*, 30(4): 324–46.

7.14 ULTRASOUND LIVER — FOCAL HYPOECHOIC

1. **Metastasis** — including cystic metastases (e.g. ovary, pancreas, stomach, colon).
2. **Lymphoma*.**
3. **Hepatoma** — can be hypoechoic or hyperechoic.
4. **Cysts** — benign, hydatid. Hydatid cysts can be classified according to their sonographic pattern. Type I, (commonest) uncomplicated unilocular cyst; Type II, a cyst with a split wall, i.e. a detached endocyst membrane; Type III, a cyst containing daughter cysts; Type IV, a cyst with a predominantly heterogeneous solid echo pattern with thick membranes and a few daughter cysts; Type V, a calcified cyst.
5. **Abscess** — ± hyperechoic wall due to fibrosis, ± surrounding hypoechoic rim due to oedema. Gas produces areas of very bright echoes.
6. **Haematoma** — acute stage.
7. **Cavernous haemangioma.**

Further Reading

Haddad M.C., Birjawa G.A., Khouzami R.A. *et al.* (2001) Unilocular hepatic echinococcal cysts: sonography and computed tomography findings. *Clin. Radiol.*, 56: 746–50.

Harvey C.J. & Albrecht T. (2001) Ultrasound of focal liver lesions. *Eur. Radiol.*, 11: 1578–93.

Hosten N., Puls R., Bechstein W.O. *et al.* (1999) Focal liver lesions: Doppler ultrasound. *Eur. Radiol.*, 9: 428–35.

Lewall D.B. (1998) Hydatid disease: biology, pathology, imaging and classification. *Clin. Radiol.*, 53: 863–74.

Nisenbaum H.L. & Rowling S.E. (1995) Ultrasound of focal hepatic lesions. *Semin. Roentgenol.*, 30(4): 324–46.

Pedrosa I., Saiz A., Arrazola J. *et al.* (2000) Hydatid disease: radiologic and pathologic features and complications. *RadioGraphics*, 20: 795–817.

7.15 ULTRASOUND LIVER – PERIPORTAL HYPERECHOIC

1. **Air in biliary tree.**
2. **Schistosomiasis.**
3. **Cholecystitis.**
4. **Recurrent pyogenic cholangitis (oriental).**

Further Reading

Chau E.M., Leong L.L. & Chan F.L. (1987) Recurrent pyogenic cholangitis: ultrasound evaluation compared with endoscopic retrograde cholangiopancreatography. *Clin. Radiol.*, 38: 79–85.

7.16 PERIPORTAL HYPOECHOGENICITY (COLLAR SIGN) ON ULTRASOUND/ PERIPORTAL LOW ATTENUATION ON CT

1. **Orthotopic liver transplant rejection** — particularly when the peripheral and central parts of the liver are affected. May also be observed in non-rejecting liver transplants; severed lymphatic channels and tracking of extrahepatic fluid contribute to the sign.
2. **Congestive hepatomegaly.**
3. **Malignant lymphatic obstruction.**
4. **Blunt abdominal trauma** — localized or widespread but many with this sign may have no other evidence of hepatic injury or even any intra-abdominal injury. Probably due to distended periportal lymphatics and lymphoedema associated with elevated central venous pressure following vigorous i.v. fluid replacement. Related to the severity of injury and associated with a higher mortality.
5. **Cholangitis.**
6. **Viral hepatitis.**

Further Reading

Kaplan S.B., Sumkin J.H., Campbell W.L. *et al.* (1989) Periportal low-attenuation areas on CT: value as evidence of liver transplant rejection. *Am. J. Roentgenol.*, 152: 285–7.

Patrick L.E., Ball T.I., Atkinson G.O. *et al.* (1992) Pediatric blunt abdominal trauma: periportal tracking at CT. *Radiology,* 183: 689–91.

Shanmuganathan K., Mirvis S.E. & Amoroso M. (1993) Periportal low density on CT in patients with blunt trauma: association with elevated venous pressure. *Am. J. Roentgenol.,* 160: 279–83.

Siegel M.J. & Herman T.E. (1992) Periportal low attenuation at CT in childhood. *Radiology,* 183: 685–8.

Sivit C.J., Taylor G.A., Eichelberger M.R. *et al.* (1993) Significance of periportal low-attenuation zones following blunt trauma in children. *Pediatr. Radiol.*, 23: 388–90.

7.17 THICKENED GALLBLADDER WALL

>3 mm — excluding the physiological, contracted (empty) gallbladder.

1. **Cholecystitis.**
2. **Hepatitis.**
3. **Hypoalbuminaemia.**
4. **Cirrhosis.**
5. **Congestive heart failure.**
6. **Renal failure.**

In infants also consider bright echoes around the gallbladder due to NEC.

Further Reading

Avni E.F., Rypens F., Cohen E. *et al.* (1991) Pericholecystic hyperechogenicities in necrotizing enterocolitis: a specific sonographic sign? *Pediatr. Radiol.*, 21: 179–81.

Kim P.N., Ha H.K., Kim Y.H. *et al.* (1998) US findings in xanthogranulomatous cholecystitis. *Clin. Radiol.*, 53: 290–2.

Patriquin H.B., DiPietro M., Barber F.E. *et al.* (1983) Sonography of thickened gallbladder wall: causes in children. *Am. J. Roentgenol.*, 141: 57–60.

7.18 CT LIVER – FOCAL HYPODENSE LESION PRE-INTRAVENOUS CONTRAST MEDIUM

	Appearances post intravenous contrast
1. **Malignant tumours** – e.g. hepatoma, metastases, lymphoma, haemangiosarcoma, intrahepatic cholangiocarcinoma	± Irregular patchy enhancement
2. **Benign tumours** (a) Haemangioma — usually well defined, in right lobe of liver, ± multiple. Technetium99m-labelled red blood cells may help make diagnosis (b) Adenoma — often young woman, related to use of oral contraceptive. Usually only slightly hypodense, and can be hyperdense due to predisposition to acute haemorrhage. Very rarely transforms to hepatoma	 75% Peripheral enhancement, 10% central enhancement, 74% progressively isodense on delayed scan, 24% partially isodense on delayed scan, 2% remain hypodense on delayed scan. 85% Hyperdense during arterial phase but rapidly (45 s–1 min) become iso or hypodense
3. **Cyst** — benign hepatic, polycystic, hydatid, von Hippel–Lindau. Water density if large enough. Small cysts can have higher density and apparently ill defined walls due to partial volume effect	Margins more clearly demarcated
4. **Abscess** (a) Pyogenic (b) Fungal — immunosuppressed, multiple small lesions, can effect spleen (c) Amoebic – ± crescent of low attenuation just peripheral to wall of abscess	 ± Peripheral enhancement may not show any peripheral enhancement. ± Peripheral enhancement
5. **Focal nodular hyperplasia** — usually only slightly hypodense. Often young female, asymptomatic unless large when pressure effects produce pain. Can contain sufficient functioning Kupffer cells to be normal or even increased in uptake on technetium 99m sulphur colloid scan which can help to discriminate it from other lesions, such as adenomas	Most are hyperdense during arterial phase but rapidly (45 s–1 min) becomes iso or hypodense, ± stellate central low density due to scar, but this is not specific and occurs in adenomas, haemangiomas and fibrolamellar hepatomas
6. **Focal fatty infiltration** — occasionally rounded in appearance, but usually diffuse or 'geographical' in distribution	No change
7. **Vascular** — infarction, laceration, old haematoma	No change
8. **Biliary tree dilatation** — Caroli's, choledochal cyst	No change

Further Reading

Brancatelli G., Federle M.P., Grazioloi L. *et al.* (2001) Focal nodular hyperplasia: CT findings with emphasis on multiphasic helical CT in 78 patients. *Radiology,* 219: 61–8.

Carlson S.K., Johnson C.D., Bender C.E. *et al.* (2000) CT of focal nodular hyperplasia of the liver. *Am. J. Roentgenol.,* 174: 705–12.

Farman J., Javors B., Chao P. *et al.* (1987) C.T. demonstration of giant choledochal cysts in adults. *J. Comput. Assist. Tomogr.,* 11: 771–4.

Grazioli L., Federle M.P., Brancatelli G. *et al.* (2001) Hepatic adenomas: imaging and pathologic findings. *RadioGraphics,* 21: 877–94.

Jacobs J.E. & Birnbaum B.A. (1995) Computed tomography imaging of focal hepatic lesions. *Semin. Roentgenol.,* 30(4): 308–23.

Kawamoto S., Soyer P.A., Fishman E.K. *et al.* (1998) Non-neoplastic liver disease: evaluation with CT and MR imaging. *RadioGraphics,* 18: 827–48.

Kehagias D., Moulopoulos L., Antoniou A. *et al.* (2001) Focal nodular hyperplasia: imaging findings. *Eur. Radiol.,* 11: 201–12.

Kimura K., Stoopen M., Reeder M.M. *et al.* (1997) Amebiasis: modern diagnostic imaging with pathological and clinical correlation. *Semin. Roentgenol.,* 32(4): 250–75.

Lewall D.B. (1998) Hydatid disease: biology, pathology, imaging and classification. *Clin. Radiol.,* 53: 863–74.

Maher M.M., McDermott S.R., Fenlon H.M. *et al.* (2001) Imaging of primary non-Hodgkin's lymphoma of the liver. *Clin. Radiol.,* 56: 295–301.

Mortele K.J. & Ros P.R. (2001) Cystic focal liver lesions in the adult: differential CT and MR imaging features. *RadioGraphics,* 21: 895–910.

Rademaker J., Widjaja A. & Galanski M. (2000) Hepatic hemangiosarcoma: imaging findings and differential diagnosis. *Eur. Radiol.,* 10: 129–33.

Yates C.K. & Streight R.A. (1986) Focal fatty infiltration of the liver simulating metastatic disease. *Radiology,* 159: 83–4.

7.19 CT LIVER – FOCAL HYPERENHANCING LESION

DURING THE ARTERIAL PHASE

1. **Hepatocellular carcinoma.**
2. **Haemangioma.**
3. **Focal nodular hyperplasia.**
4. **Adenoma.**
5. **Metastases** — particularly carcinoid and pancreatic islet cell. Most metastases are hypovascular.

DURING THE PORTAL VEIN PHASE

1. **Haemangioma.**
2. **Hepatocellular carcinoma** — unusually. Most are iso- or low-attenuation during this phase.
3. **Venous collaterals** — from an obstructed SVC to the IVC via hepatic veins.

DURING THE EQUILIBRIUM PHASE

1. **Haemangioma** — because of progressive fill-in.
2. **Cholangiocarcinoma.**
3. **Solitary fibrous tumour.**
4. **Treated metastases.**

Further Reading

Carlson S.K., Johnson C.D., Bender C.E. *et al.* (2000) CT of focal nodular hyperplasia of the liver. *Am. J. Roentgenol.,* 174: 705–12.

Shanmuganathan K. & Mirvis S.E. (1998) CT scan evaluation of blunt hepatic trauma. *Radiol. Clin. North Am.,* 36: 399–411.

Valls C., Andia E., Sanchez A. *et al.* (1999) Hyperenhancing focal liver lesions: differential diagnosis with helical CT. *Am. J. Roentgenol.,* 173: 605–11.

Vilgrain V., Boulos L., Vullierme M.-P. *et al.* (2000) Imaging of atypical haemangiomas of the liver with pathologic correlation. *RadioGraphics,* 20: 379–97.

7.20 CT LIVER — FOCAL HYPERDENSE LESION

PRE-INTRAVENOUS CONTRAST

1. **Calcification in:**
   (a) Metastasis — usually colorectal, but ovary, stomach, islet cell pancreas also possible.
   (b) Primary tumour — hepatoma, hepatoblastoma, haemangioendothelioma.
   (c) Infective lesion — hydatid, tuberculous granuloma.
2. **Acute haemorrhage** — post-traumatic or bleed into a vascular tumour, e.g. adenoma.

POST-INTRAVENOUS CONTRAST

1. **Hypervascular masses**
   (a) Metastases — carcinoid, renal cell carcinoma, islet cell pancreas and phaeochromocytoma.
   (b) Adenoma
   (c) Focal nodular hyperplasia
   } enhancement only seen during arterial phase, i.e. within 1 minute of injection. After this they may appear hypodense.
2. **Vascular abnormalities** — e.g. arterioportal shunts which may occur in hepatoma.

Further Reading

Paley M.R. & Ros P.R. (1998) Hepatic metastases. *Radiol. Clin. North Am.*, 36(2): 349–63.

7.21 CT LIVER — GENERALIZED LOW DENSITY PRE-INTRAVENOUS CONTRAST MEDIUM

Assess by comparing liver with spleen. Also intrahepatic vessels stand out as 'high' density against low density background of liver, but aorta shows normal soft-tissue density indicating the apparent high density of the intrahepatic vessels is not due to intravenous contrast.

1. **Fatty infiltration** — early cirrhosis, obesity, parenteral feeding, bypass surgery, malnourishment, cystic fibrosis, steroids, Cushing's, late pregnancy, carbon tetrachloride exposure, chemotherapy, high-dose tetracycline, and glycogen storage disease.
2. **Malignant infiltration.**
3. **Budd–Chiari**
   (a) Acute — big low-density liver with ascites. After intravenous contrast there is patchy enhancement of the hilum of the liver due to multiple collaterals, and non-visualization of the hepatic veins and/or IVC.
   (b) Chronic — atrophied patchy low-density liver with sparing and hypertrophy of caudate lobe. Post-intravenous contrast scans show similar signs as the acute stage.
4. **Amyloid** — no change after intravenous contrast.

Further Reading

Halversen R.A., Korobkin M., Ram P.C. *et al.* (1982) C.T. appearance of focal fatty infiltration of the liver. *Am. J. Roentgenol.*, 139: 277–81.

Mathieu D., Vasile N., Menu Y. *et al.* (1987) Budd Chiari syndrome: Dynamic C.T. *Radiology,* 165: 409–13.

Suzuki S., Takizawa K., Nakajima Y. *et al.* (1986) C.T. findings in hepatic and splenic amyloidosis. *J. Comput. Assist. Tomogr.,* 10: 332–4.

Vogelzang R.L., Anscheutz S.L. & Gore R.M. (1987) Budd–Chiari syndrome: C.T. observations. *Radiology,* 163: 329–33.

Yates C.K. & Streight R.A. (1986) Focal fatty infiltration of the liver simulating metastatic disease. *Radiology,* 159: 83–4.

7.22 CT LIVER – GENERALIZED INCREASE IN DENSITY PRE-INTRAVENOUS CONTRAST MEDIUM

Assess by comparing liver with spleen. Also intrahepatic vessels stand out as low-density against high-density background of liver.

1. **Haemochromatosis** — may be an associated hepatoma present.
2. **Haemosiderosis.**
3. **Iron overload** — e.g. from large number of blood transfusions.
4. **Glycogen storage disease** — liver may be increased or decreased in density.
5. **Amiodarone treatment** — contains iodine. Can also cause pulmonary interstitial and alveolar infiltrates.

Further Reading

Butler S. & Smathers R.L. (1985) Computed tomography of amiodarone pulmonary toxicity. *J. Comput. Assist. Tomogr.*, 9: 375–6.

7.23 CT LIVER – PATCHY AREAS OF LOW-DENSITY POST-INTRAVENOUS CONTRAST MEDIUM

1. **Cirrhosis.**
2. **Hepatitis.**
3. **Portal vein thrombosis.**
4. **Budd–Chiari** — chronic.
5. **Lymphoma infiltration*.**
6. **Sarcoidosis*.**

Further Reading

Dodd G.D. III, Baron R.L., Oliver J.H. III *et al.* (1999) Spectrum of imaging findings of the liver in end-stage cirrhosis: part I, gross morphology and diffuse abnormalities. *Am. J. Roentgenol.*, 173: 1031–6.

Dodd G.D. III, Baron R.L., Oliver J.H. III *et al.* (1999) Spectrum of imaging findings of the liver in end-stage cirrhosis: part II, focal abnormalities. *Am. J. Roentgenol.*, 173: 1185–92.

7.24 MRI LIVER

	T_1W	T_2W	*Gadolinium*
Hepatocellular carcinoma	↓, iso or ↑ (due to fat degeneration)	↑	↑
Metastases	↓	↑	±↑
Haemangioma	↓	↑ ++ = to CSF at long TE	↑ (like CT)
Adenoma	↑	↓	
Focal nodular hyperplasia			
central scar	↓	↑+	↑
margins	isointense	↑	±↑
Regenerating nodule	↓, isointense	↓	
Haemochromatosis/iron deposition	↓	↓++	

Further Reading

Bartolozzi C., Cioni D., Donati F. *et al.* (2001) Focal liver lesions: MR imaging–pathologic correlation. *Eur. Radiol.*, 11: 1374–88.

Bartolozzi C., Lencioni R., Donati F. *et al.* (1999) Abdominal MR: liver and pancreas. *Eur. Radiol.*, 9: 1496–1512.

del Pilar Fernandez M. & Redvanly R.D. (1998) Primary hepatic malignant neoplasms. *Radiol. Clin. North Am.*, 36: 333–48.

Kawamoto S., Soyer P.A., Fishman E.K. *et al.* (1998) Non-neoplastic liver disease: evaluation with CT and MR imaging. *RadioGraphics*, 18: 827–48.

Mergo P.J. & Ros P.R. (1998) Benign lesions of the liver. *Radiol. Clin. North Am.*, 36: 319–30.

Mergo P.J. & Ros P.R. (1998) Imaging of diffuse liver disease. *Radiol. Clin. North Am.*, 36(2): 365–75.

Paley M.R. & Ros P.R. (1998) Hepatic metastases. *Radiol. Clin. North Am.*, 36: 349–62.

Ralls P.W. (1998) Focal inflammatory disease of the liver. *Radiol. Clin. North Am.*, 36: 377–88.

Robinson P.J. (2000) Imaging liver metastases: current limitations and future prospects. *Br. J. Radiol.*, 73: 234–41.

Schnall M. (1995) Magnetic resonance imaging of focal liver lesions. *Semin. Roentgenol.*, 30(4): 347–61.

Sica G.T., Ji H. & Ros P.R. (2000) CT and MR imaging of hepatic metastases. *Am. J. Roentgenol.*, 174: 691–8.

Siegelman E.S. & Outwater E.K. (1998) Magnetic resonance imaging of focal and diffuse hepatic disease. *Semin. Ultrasound CT MRI*, 19(1): 2–34.

7.25 MRI LIVER – FOCAL HYPERINTENSE LESION ON T_1W

NB. Most lesions are hypointense on T_1W.

1. **Fat** — lipomas, angiomyolipomas, focal fatty deposits, surgical defect packed with omental fat, occasionally hepatomas undergo fatty degeneration.
2. **Blood** — in the acute stage due to methaemoglobin (which is paramagnetic).
3. **Proteinaceous material** — occurs in dependent layer of fluid/fluid levels in abscesses and haematomas due to increased concentration of hydrated protein molecules.
4. **Melanoma metastases** — ?Due to paramagnetic effect of melanin or associated haemorrhage.
5. **Chemical** — gadolinium, lipiodol (contains fat).
6. **'Relative'** — i.e. normal signal intensity liver surrounded by low signal intensity liver which may occur with iron deposition (haemochromatosis, i.v. ferrite particles), cirrhosis (unclear aetiology, but a regenerating nodule within a cirrhotic area may appear artifactually hyperintense), oedema.
7. **Artefact** — pulsation artefact from abdominal aorta can produce a periodic 'ghost' artefact along the phase-encoded direction which can be hypointense or hyperintense depending on the phase.

Further Reading

Lee M.J., Hahn P.F., Saini S. *et al.* (1992) Differential diagnosis of hyperintense liver lesions on T_1W MR images. *Am. J. Roentgenol.*, 159: 1017–20.

7.26 MRI LIVER – RINGED HEPATIC LESIONS

One or several layers which may be a component of the lesion itself or a response of the liver to the presence of the adjacent lesion.

1. **Capsules of 1° liver tumours** — a low signal ring (because of collagen and best seen on T_1W) may be seen in 25–40% but does not differentiate between benign and malignant. A peritumoral halo of high signal on T_2W is seen in 30% of 1° tumours and more closely correlates with malignancy.
2. **Metastases** — halo of high signal on T_2W or with central liquefaction to give an even higher centre and a 'target' lesion. A peritumoral halo or a target on T_2W distinguishes metastasis from cavernous haemangioma.
3. **Subacute haematoma** — low-signal rim on T_1W and T_2W (because of iron) with an inner bright ring on T_1W (because of methaemoglobin).
4. **Hydatid cyst** — T_2W high-signal cyst contents with a low-signal capsule. The capsule is not well seen on T_1W.
5. **Amoebic abscess** — prior to treatment incomplete concentric rings of variable intensity, better seen on T_2W than T_1W. During antibiotic treatment, T_1W and T_2W images show the development of four concentric zones because of central liquefaction and resolution of hepatic oedema.

Further Reading

Elizondo G., Weissleder R., Stark D.D. *et al.* (1987) Amebic liver abscess – diagnosis and treatment evaluation with MR imaging. *Radiology,* 165: 795–800.

Hahn P.F., Stark D.D., Saini S. *et al.* (1990) The differential diagnosis of ringed hepatic lesions in MR imaging. *Am. J. Roentgenol.,* 154: 287–90.

Hoff F.L., Aisen A.M., Walden M.E. *et al.* (1987) MR imaging in hydatid disease of the liver. *Gastrointest. Radiol.,* 12: 39–42.

Wittenberg J., Stark D.D., Forman B.H. *et al.* (1988) Differentiation of hepatic metastases from hepatic hemangiomas and cysts by using MR imaging. *Am. J. Roentgenol.,* 151: 79–84.

7.27 SPLENOMEGALY

Splenomegaly should be suspected in children if the spleen is more than 1.25 times longer than the adjacent kidney.

HUGE SPLEEN

1. **Chronic myeloid leukaemia.**
2. **Myelofibrosis.**
3. **Malaria.**
4. **Kala-azar.**
5. **Gaucher's disease.**
6. **Lymphoma*.**

MODERATELY LARGE SPLEEN

1. **All of the above.**
2. **Storage diseases.**
3. **Haemolytic anaemias.**
4. **Portal hypertension.**
5. **Leukaemias.**

SLIGHTLY LARGE SPLEEN

1. **All of the above.**
2. **Infections**
   (a) Viral — infectious hepatitis, infectious mononucleosis.
   (b) Bacterial — septicaemia, brucellosis, typhoid and tuberculosis.
   (c) Rickettsial — typhus.
   (d) Fungal — histoplasmosis.
3. **Sarcoidosis*.**
4. **Amyloidosis.**
5. **Rheumatoid arthritis (Felty's syndrome)*.**
6. **Systemic lupus erythematosus*.**

Further Reading

Gorg C., Weide R. & Schwerk W.B. (1997) Malignant splenic lymphoma: sonographic patterns, diagnosis and follow-up. *Clin. Radiol.*, 52: 535–40.

Loftus W.K. & Metrewelli C. (1998) Ultrasound assessment of mild splenomegaly: spleen/kidney ratio. *Pediatr. Radiol.*, 28: 98–100.

Paterson A., Frush D.P., Donnelly L.F. *et al.* (1999) A pattern-oriented approach to splenic imaging in infants and children. *RadioGraphics*, 19: 1465–85.

Robertson F., Leander P. & Ekberg O. (2001) Radiology of the spleen. *Eur. Radiol.*, 11: 80–95.

7.28 SPLENIC CALCIFICATION

CURVILINEAR

1. **Splenic artery atherosclerosis** — including splenic artery aneurysm.
2. **Cyst** — hydatid or post-traumatic.

MULTIPLE SMALL NODULAR

1. **Phleboliths** — may have small central lucencies.
2. **Haemangioma** — phleboliths.
3. **Tuberculosis.**
4. **Histoplasmosis.**
5. **Brucellosis.**
6. **Sickle-cell anaemia*.**

DIFFUSE HOMOGENEOUS OR FINELY GRANULAR

1. **Sickle-cell anaemia*.**
2. ***Pneumocystis carinii.***

SOLITARY GREATER THAN 1 CM

1. **Healed infarct or haematoma.**
2. **Healed abscess.**
3. **Tuberculosis.**

Further Reading

McCall I.W., Vaidya S. & Serjeant G.R. (1981) Splenic opacification in homozygous sickle cell disease. *Clin. Radiol.*, 32: 611–15.

7.29 CT SPLEEN – FOCAL LOW DENSITY LESION

1. **Lymphoma*.**
2. **Metastases.**
3. **Haemangioma.**
4. **Abscess** — fungal abscesses are small and multifocal.

7.30 PANCREATIC CALCIFICATION

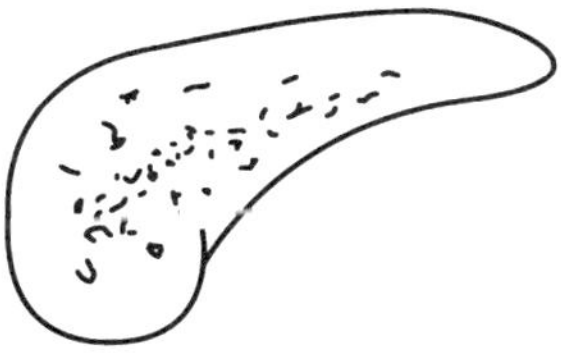

Alcoholic chronic pancreatitis
Hyperparathyroidism
Kwashiorkor

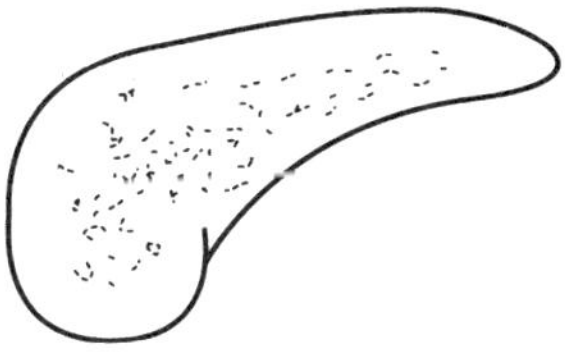

Cystic fibrosis

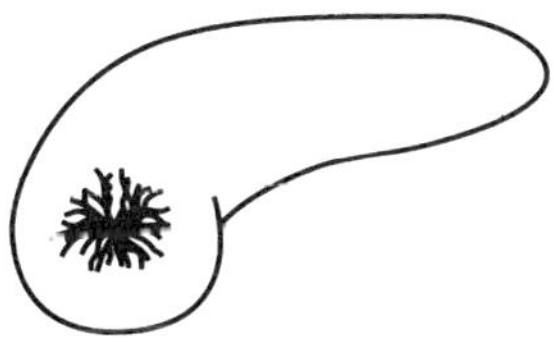

Cystadenocarcinoma

1. **Alcoholic pancreatitis** — calcification, which is almost exclusively due to intraductal calculi, is seen in 20–40% (compared with 2% of gallstone pancreatitis). Usually after 5–10 years of pain. Limited to head or tail in 25%. Rarely solitary. Calculi are numerous, irregular and generally small.
2. **Pseudocyst** — 12–20% exhibit calcification which is usually similar to that seen in chronic pancreatitis but may be curvilinear rim calcification.
3. **Carcinoma of the pancreas** — although for all practical purposes adenocarcinoma does not calcify there is an increased incidence of pancreatic cancer in chronic pancreatitis and the two will be found concurrently in about 2% of cases.
4. **Hyperparathyroidism*** — pancreatitis occurs as a complication of hyperparathyroidism in 10% of cases and 30% of these show calcification which is similar to that observed in chronic pancreatitis. 70% have nephrocalcinosis or urolithiasis and this should suggest the diagnosis.
5. **Cystic fibrosis*** — calcification occurs late in the disease when there is advanced pancreatic fibrosis associated with diabetes mellitus. Calcification is typically finely granular.
6. **Kwashiorkor** — pancreatic lithiasis is a frequent finding and appears before adulthood. Its pattern is similar to chronic alcoholic pancreatitis.

7. **Hereditary pancreatitis** — AD. 60% show calcification which is typically rounded and often larger than in other pancreatic diseases. 20% die from pancreatic malignancy. The diagnosis should be considered in young, non-alcoholic patients.
8. **Tumours** — calcification is observed in 10% of cystadenomas and cystadenocarcinomas. It is non-specific but occasionally 'sunburst'. The rare cavernous lymphangioma contains phleboliths in and adjacent to it.
9. **Idiopathic.**

Further Reading

Lesniak R.J., Hohenwalter M.D. & Taylor A.J. (2002) Spectrum of causes of pancreatic calcifications. *Am. J. Roentgenol.,* 178: 79–86.

Ring E.J., Eaton S.B., Ferrucci J.T. *et al.* (1973) Differential diagnosis of pancreatic calcification. *Am. J. Roentgenol.,* 117: 446–52.

7.31 CT OF PANCREAS – FOCAL MASS

1. **Adenocarcinoma** — 60% head, 10% body, 5% tail, 20% diffuse. 40% are isodense on pre-contrast scan, but most of these show reduced density on a post-contrast scan. Virtually never contain calcification. The presence of metastases (nodes, liver) or invasion around vascular structures (SMA, coeliac axis, portal and splenic vein) helps to distinguish this from focal pancreatitis.
2. **Focal pancreatitis** — usually in head of pancreas. Can contain calcification, but if not may be difficult to distinguish from carcinoma.
3. **Metastasis** — e.g. breast, lung, stomach, kidney, thyroid.
4. **Islet cell tumour** — equal incidence in head, body and tail. 80% are functioning and so will present at a relatively small size. 20% are non-functioning and so are larger and more frequently contain calcification at presentation. In general, functioning islet cell tumours, other than insulinomas, are often malignant, whereas 75% of non-functioning tumours are benign.

(a) Beta cell:
Insulinoma — 90% benign, 10% multiple, 80% < 2 cm in diameter. Usually isodense with marked contrast enhancement. Can calcify.

(b) Non-beta cell:
Gastrinoma — 60% malignant, 30% benign adenoma, 10% hyperplasia. 90% located in pancreas, 5% duodenum, occasionally stomach and splenic hilum. Shows marked contrast enhancement. Multiple adenomas seen as part of multiple endocrine adenopathy I syndrome (pituitary, parathyroid and pancreatic adenomas).
Glucagonoma — usually > 4 cm, since endocrine disturbance is often less marked.

5. **Mucinous cystadenoma and cystadenocarcinoma** — majority of cases have a large central cyst surrounded by smaller cysts, usually in body or tail. Calcification may be more common in the malignant lesions. The thick walls may help to distinguish from pseudocysts. Usually in females aged over 60 years.
6. **Pancreatic abscess** — infected phlegmon/pseudocyst. Occurs in 3% of those with pancreatitis.

Further Reading

Breatnach E.S., Han S.Y., Rahatzad M.T. *et al.* (1985) C.T. evaluation of glucagonomas. *J. Comput. Assist. Tomogr.*, 9: 25–9.

Coley S.C., Strickland N.H., Walker J.D. *et al.* (1997) Spiral CT and the pre-operative assessment of pancreatic carcinoma. *Clin. Radiol.*, 52: 24–30.

Grogan J.R., Saeian K., Taylor A.J. *et al.* (2001) Making sense of mucin-producing pancreatic tumors. *Am. J. Roentgenol.*, 176: 921–9.

Mergo P.J., Helmberger T.K., Buetow P.C. *et al.* (1997) Pancreatic neoplasms: MR imaging and pathologic correlation. *RadioGraphics,* 17: 281–301.

Procacci C., Carbognin G., Accordini S. *et al.* (2001) CT features of malignant mucinous cystic tumors of the pancreas. *Eur. Radiol.*, 11: 1626–30.

Robinson P.J. & Sheridan M.B. (2000) Pancreatitis: computed tomography and magnetic resonance imaging. *Eur. Radiol.*, 10: 401–8.

Scott J., Martin I., Redhead D. *et al.* (2000) Mucinous cystic neoplasms of the pancreas: imaging features and diagnostic difficulties. *Clin. Radiol.*, 55: 187–92.

Vaughn D.D., Jabra A.A. & Fishman E.K. (1998) Pancreatic disease in children and young adults: evaluation with CT. *RadioGraphics,* 18: 1171–87.

7.32 NON-VISUALIZATION OF THE GALLBLADDER WITH TBIDA

NO BOWEL ACTIVITY

1. **Common bile duct obstruction** — of any cause.
2. **Severe hepatitis.**
3. **Opiates** — because of their effect on the sphincter of Oddi.

WITH BOWEL ACTIVITY

1. **Acute cholecystitis.**
2. **Chronic cholecystitis** — usually fills after 1 hour.
3. **Cholecystectomy.**
4. **Inadequate fasting** — including i.v. feeding.
5. **Biliary pancreatitis.**
6. **Severe diffuse hepatocellular disease.**

Further Reading

Lecklitner M.L. & Growcock G. (1984) Hepatobiliary scintigraphy: non-visualization of activity in the area of the gallbladder associated with intestinal activity. *Semin. Nucl. Med.*, 14: 345–6.

8 Adrenals, urinary tract and testes

8.1 ADRENAL CALCIFICATION

CHILD

1. **Cystic disease** — usually the result of haemorrhage which may be secondary to birth trauma, infection, haemorrhagic disorders or arterial or venous thromboses. Partial or complete ring-like calcification is observed initially but this later becomes compact as the cyst collapses. Frequently asymptomatic.
2. **Neuroblastoma** — in 50% of cases on plain films; 90% on CT. Ill-defined, stippled and non-homogeneous. Lymph node and liver metastases can also calcify.
3. **Ganglioneuroma** — similar appearance to neuroblastoma, but only 20% are within the adrenal.
4. **Wolman's disease** — a rare AR lipoidosis. Hepatomegaly, splenomegaly and adrenomegaly with punctate cortical adrenal calcification is pathognomonic.

ADULT

1. **Cystic disease** — similar to that seen in the child. Bilateral in 15% of cases.
2. **Carcinoma** — irregular punctate calcifications. Average size of tumour is 14 cm and there is frequently displacement of the ipsilateral kidney.
3. **Addison's disease** — now most commonly due to autoimmune disease or metastasis. In the past, when tuberculosis was a frequent cause, calcification was a common finding.
4. **Ganglioneuroma** — 40% occur over the age of 20 years. Slightly flocculent calcifications in a mass which is usually asymptomatic. If the tumour is large enough there will be displacement of the adjacent kidney and/or ureter.
5. **Inflammatory** — primary tuberculosis and histoplasmosis.

6. **Phaeochromocytoma** — calcification is rare but when present is usually an 'egg-shell' pattern.

Further Reading

Queloz J.M., Capitanio M.A. & Kirkpatrick J.A. (1972) Wolman's disease. Roentgen observations in three siblings. *Radiology,* 104: 357–9.

8.2 CT OF ADRENAL MASSES

Length of limbs is variable: can be up to 4 cm. Width of limb is normally less than 1 cm. The right adrenal lies behind inferior vena cava and above right kidney, i.e. not on same slice as the kidney. The left adrenal lies in front of upper pole of left kidney, i.e. on same slice as the kidney — do not mistake upper pole of left kidney for an adrenal mass.

STRUCTURES MIMICKING LEFT ADRENAL MASS

1. **Upper pole of left kidney.**
2. **Gastric diverticulum** — give oral contrast.
3. **Splenic lobulation/accessory spleen** — give intravenous contrast, should enhance to the same level as the body of the spleen.
4. **Large mass in tail of pancreas** — give intravenous contrast, pancreatic mass usually displaces splenic vein posteriorly, whereas adrenal mass displaces it anteriorly.

FUNCTIONING TUMOURS

1. **Conn's adenoma** — accounts for 70% of Conn's syndrome. Usually small, 0.5–1.5 cm. Homogeneous, relatively low density due to build up of cholesterol. 30% of Conn's syndrome due to hyperplasia which can occasionally be nodular and mimic an adenoma.

2. **Phaeochromocytoma** — usually large, > 5 cm, with marked contrast enhancement (beware hypertensive crisis with i.v. contrast medium). 10% malignant, 10% bilateral, 10% ectopic (of these 50% are located around the kidney, particularly renal hilum. If CT does not detect, MIBG isotope scan may be helpful), 10% multiple (usually part of multiple endocrine adenopathy II (MEA II) syndrome). Associated with neurofibromatosis, von Hippel–Lindau and MEA II.
3. **Cushing's adenoma** — accounts for 10% of Cushing's syndrome. Usually over 2 cm. 40% show slight reduction in density. 80% of Cushing's syndrome due to excess ACTH from pituitary tumour or ectopic source (oat cell carcinoma, pancreatic islet cell, carcinoid, medullary carcinoma of thyroid, thymoma) which causes adrenal hyperplasia not visible on CT scan. Other 10% of Cushing's syndrome due to adrenal carcinoma. The possibilities for adrenal mass in Cushing's syndrome are:
   (a) Functioning adenoma/carcinoma.
   (b) Coincidental non-functioning adenoma.
   (c) Metastasis from oat cell primary.
   (d) Nodular hyperplasia, which occurs in 20% of Cushing's syndrome due to pituitary adenoma.
4. **Adrenal carcinoma** — 50% present as functioning tumours (Cushing's 35%, Cushing's with virilization 20%, virilization 20%, feminization 5%).

MALIGNANT TUMOURS

1. **Metastases** — may be bilateral, usually greater than 2–3 cm, irregular outline with patchy contrast enhancement. Recent haemorrhage into a vascular metastasis (e.g. melanoma) can give a patchy high density on pre-contrast scan. In patients without a known extra-adrenal primary tumour the vast majority of adrenal masses are benign; even in the presence of a known primary malignant tumour many adrenal masses will still be benign.
2. **Carcinoma** — Typical features are: (a) >5 cm; (b) central areas of low attenuation due to tumour necrosis; (c) calcification; and (d) hepatic, nodal or venous spread.
3. **Lymphoma** — 25% also involve kidneys at autopsy. Lymphadenopathy will be seen elsewhere.
4. **Neuroblastoma** — greater than 5 cm. Calcification in 90%. Extends across midline. Nodes commonly surround and displace the aorta and inferior vena cava.

BENIGN

1. **Non-functioning adenoma** — occurs in 5% at autopsy. Usually relatively small (50% less than 2 cm), homogeneous and well-defined.
2. **Angiomyolipoma** — occurs in 0.2% at autopsy. Usually 1–2 cm. May contain fat density.
3. **Cyst** — well-defined, water density.
4. **Post-traumatic haemorrhage** — homogeneous, hyperdense. Occurs in 25% of severe trauma, 20% bilateral, 85% on right. Adrenal haemorrhage can also occur in vascular metastases, anticoagulant treatment, and severe stress (e.g. surgery, sepsis, burns, hypotension).

Further Reading

Francis I.R. & Korobkin M. (1996) Pheochromocytoma. *Radiol. Clin. North Am.*, 34(6): 1101–12.

Korobkin M., Francis I.R., Kloos R.T. *et al.* (1996) The incidental adrenal mass. *Radiol. Clin. North Am.*, 34(5): 1037–54.

Mayo-Smith W., Boland G.W., Noto R.B. *et al.* (2001) State-of-the-art adrenal imaging. *RadioGraphics*, 21: 995–1012.

Pender S.M., Boland G.W. & Lee M.J. (1998) The incidental nonhyperfunctioning adrenal mass: an imaging algorithm for characterization. *Clin. Radiol.*, 53: 796–804.

8.3 META-IODO-BENZYL-GUANIDINE (MIBG) IMAGING

NORMAL

1. **Myocardium.**
2. **Liver and spleen.**
3. **Bladder.**
4. **Adrenal glands** — more marked with ^{123}I MIBG.
5. **Salivary glands.**
6. **Nasopharynx.**
7. **Thyroid.**
8. **Colon.**

ABNORMAL

1. **Phaeochromocytoma.**
2. **Neuroblastoma.**
3. **Carcinoid tumour.**
4. **Paraganglioma.**
5. **Medullary thyroid carcinoma.**
6. **Ganglioneuroma.**

Further Reading

McEwan A.H., Shapiro B., Sisson J.C. *et al.* (1985). Radioiodobenzylguanidine for the scintigraphic localisation and therapy of adrenergic tumours. *Semin. Nucl. Med.*, 15: 132–53.

Standalick R.C. (1992) The biodistribution of metaiodobenzylguanidine. *Semin. Nucl. Med.*, 22: 46–7.

8.4 LOSS OF A RENAL OUTLINE ON THE PLAIN FILM

Not necessarily associated with a non-visualized kidney after intravenous contrast medium.

1. **Technical factors** — e.g. poor radiography, overlying faeces, etc.
2. **Congenital absence** — 1:1000 live births. Increased incidence of extrarenal abnormalities (ventricular septal defect, meningomyelocoele, intestinal tract strictures, imperforate anus, skeletal abnormalities and unicornuate uterus). The normal solitary kidney may approach twice normal size.
3. **Displaced or ectopic kidney** — presacral, crossed ectopia or intrathoracic.
4. **Perinephric haematoma** — obliteration of the perirenal fat. ± Other signs of trauma, e.g. fractured transverse processes.
5. **Perinephric abscess** — scoliosis concave to the affected side. May be associated with gas in the perirenal tissues. ± Localized ileus.
6. **Tumour** — when perinephric fat is replaced by tumour.
7. **Postnephrectomy** — rare because residual perinephric fat preserves an apparent renal outline. Surgical resection of twelfth rib is usually evident.

8.5 RENAL CALCIFICATION

CALCULI (see 8.6)

DYSTROPHIC CALCIFICATION DUE TO LOCALIZED DISEASE

Usually one kidney or part of one kidney.

1. **Infections**
   (a) Tuberculosis — variable appearance of nodular, curvilinear or amorphous calcification. Typically multifocal with calcification elsewhere in the urinary tract.
   (b) Hydatid — the cyst is usually polar and calcification is curvilinear or heterogeneous.
   (c) Xanthogranulomatous pyelonephritis.
   (d) Abscess.
2. **Carcinoma** — in 6% of carcinomas. Usually amorphous or irregular, but occasionally curvilinear.
3. **Aneurysm** — of the renal artery. Curvilinear.

NEPHROCALCINOSIS

Parenchymal calcification associated with a diffuse renal lesion (i.e. dystrophic calcification) or metabolic abnormality, e.g. hypercalcaemia (metabolic or metastatic calcification). May be medullary or cortical.

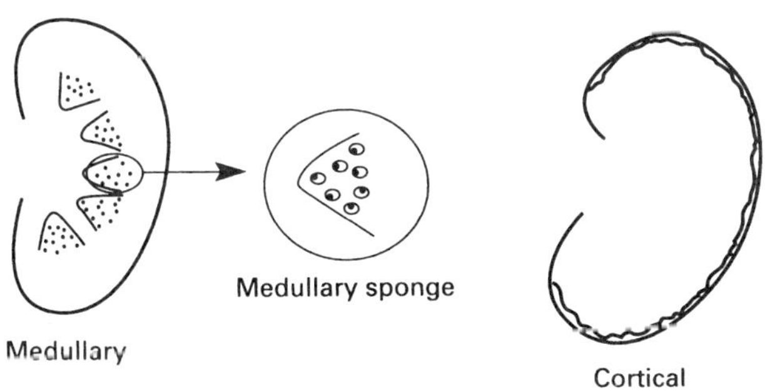

Medullary (pyramidal)

The first three causes account for 70% of cases.

1. **Hyperparathyroidism*.**
2. **Renal tubular acidosis** — may be associated with osteomalacia or rickets. Calcification tends to be more severe than that due to other causes. It is the commonest cause in children. Almost always a distal tubular defect.

3. **Medullary sponge kidney** — a variable portion of one or both kidneys contains numerous small medullary cysts which communicate with tubules and therefore opacify during excretion urography. The cysts contain small calculi, giving a 'bunch of grapes' appearance. Big kidneys. ± Multiple cysts or large medullary cystic cavities which may be > 2 cm in diameter. (Although not strictly a cause of nephrocalcinosis, because it comprises calculi in ectatic ducts, it is included here because of the plain film findings which simulate nephrocalcinosis.)
4. **Renal papillary necrosis** — calcification of necrotic papillae. See 8.25.
5. **Causes of hypercalcaemia or hypercalciuria**
   (a) Milk-alkali syndrome.
   (b) Idiopathic hypercalciuria.
   (c) Sarcoidosis*.
   (d) Hypervitaminosis D.
6. **Preterm infants** — in up to two-thirds. Risk factors include extreme prematurity, severe respiratory disease, gentamicin use and high urinary oxalate and urate excretion. 50% resolve spontaneously.
7. **Primary hyperoxaluria** — rare. AR. 65% present below 5 years of age (younger than the other causes). Radiologically — nephrocalcinosis (generally diffuse and homogeneous but may be patchy), recurrent nephrolithiasis, dense vascular calcification, osteopenia or renal osteodystrophy and abnormal metaphyses (dense and/or lucent bands).

Cortical

1. **Acute cortical necrosis** — classically 'tramline' calcification.
2. **Chronic glomerulonephritis** — rarely.
3. **Chronic transplant rejection.**

Further Reading

Daniel W.W., Hartman G.W., Witten D.M. *et al.* (1972) Calcified renal masses. *Radiology,* 103: 503–8.
Day D.L., Scheinman J.I. & Mahan I. (1986) Radiological aspects of primary hyperoxaluria. *Am. J. Roentgenol.,* 146: 395–401.
Gedroyc W.M. & Saxton H.M. (1988) More medullary sponge variants. *Clin. Radiol.,* 39: 423–5.
Lalli A.F. (1982) Renal parenchyma calcifications. *Semin. Roentgenol.,* 17 (2): 101–12.
Narendra A., White M.P., Rolton, H.A. *et al.* (2001) Nephrocalcinosis in preterm babies. *Arch. Dis. Child. Fetal Neonatal Ed.,* 85: F207–213.
Wrong O.M. & Feest T.G. (1976) Nephrocalcinosis. *Adv. Med.,* 12: 394–406.

8.6 RENAL CALCULI

OPAQUE

Calcium phosphate/calcium oxalate, calcium oxalate, calcium phosphate/magnesium ammonium phosphate and calcium phosphate. Calcium oxalate stones are more opaque than triple phosphate stones.

POORLY OPAQUE

Cystine (in cystinuria).

NON-OPAQUE

Uric acid, xanthine and matrix (mucoprotein).

CALCIUM-CONTAINING

1. **With normocalcaemia** — obstruction, urinary tract infection, prolonged bed rest, 'horseshoe' kidney, vesical diverticulum, renal tubular acidosis, medullary sponge kidney and idiopathic hypercalciuria.
2. **With hypercalcaemia** — hyperparathyroidism, milk-alkali syndrome, excess vitamin D, idiopathic hypercalcaemia of infancy and sarcoidosis.

PURE CALCIUM OXALATE DUE TO HYPEROXALURIA

1. **Primary hyperoxaluria** — rare. AR. 65% present below 5 years of age. Radiologically — nephrocalcinosis (generally diffuse and homogeneous but may be patchy), recurrent nephrolithiasis, dense vascular calcification, osteopenia or renal osteodystrophy and abnormal metaphyses (dense and/or lucent bands).
2. **Enteric hyperoxaluria** — due to a disturbance of bile acid metabolism. Mainly in patients with small bowel disease, either Crohn's disease or surgical resection.

URIC ACID

1. **With hyperuricaemia** — gout, myeloproliferative disorders and during the treatment of tumours with antimitotic agents.
2. **With normouricaemia** — idiopathic or associated with acid, concentrated urine (in hot climate and in ileostomy patients).

XANTHINE

Due to a failure of normal oxidation of purines.

MATRIX

Rare. In poorly functioning, infected urinary tracts.

Further Reading

Banner M.P. & Pollack H.M. (1982) Urolithiasis in the lower urinary tract. *Semin. Roentgenol.*, 17(2): 140–8.
Day D.L., Scheinman J.I. & Mahan J. (1986) Radiological aspects of primary hyperoxaluria. *Am. J. Roentgenol.*, 146: 395–401.
Elkin M. (1983) Calcification in the urinary tract. In: Baker S.R. & Elkin M (eds). *Plain Film Approach to Abdominal Calcifications.* Philadelphia: Saunders, pp. 39–46.
Singh E.O. & Malek R.S. (1982) Calculus disease in the upper urinary tract. *Semin. Roentgenol.*, 17(2): 113–32.
Thornbury J.R. & Parker T.W. (1982) Ureteral calculi. *Semin. Roentgenol.*, 17(2): 133–9.

8.7 GAS IN THE URINARY TRACT

Gas shadows which conform to the position and shape of the bladder, ureters or pelvicalyceal systems.

GAS INSIDE THE BLADDER

1. **Vesicointestinal fistula** — diverticular disease, carcinoma of the colon or rectum and Crohn's disease.
2. **Cystitis** — due to gas-forming organisms and fermentation, especially in diabetics. Usually *Escherichia coli*. Clostridial infections are rare and usually secondary to septicaemia.
3. **Following instrumentation.**
4. **Penetrating wounds.**

GAS IN THE BLADDER WALL

1. **Emphysematous cystitis** — usually in diabetics.

GAS IN THE URETERS AND PELVICALYCEAL SYSTEMS

1. **Any cause of gas in the bladder.**
2. **Ureteric diversion** — into the colon or bladder.
3. **Fistula** — Crohn's disease or perforated duodenal ulcer.
4. **Infection** — usually in diabetics. Gas may also be present in the renal parenchyma and retroperitoneal tissues.

Further Reading

Rodriguez-de-Velasquez A., Yoder I.C., Velasquez P.A. *et al.* (1995) Imaging the effects of diabetes on the genitourinary system. *RadioGraphics,* 15: 1051–68.

Roy C., Pfleger D.D., Tuchmann C.M. *et al.* (2001) Emphysematous pyelitis. Findings in five patients. *Radiology,* 218: 647–50.

8.8 NON-VISUALIZATION OF ONE KIDNEY DURING EXCRETION UROGRAPHY

1. **Absent kidney** — congenital absence or postnephrectomy.
2. **Ectopic kidney.**
3. **Chronic obstructive uropathy.**
4. **Infection** — pyonephrosis, xanthogranulomatous pyelonephritis or tuberculosis.
5. **Tumour** — an avascular tumour completely replacing the kidney or preventing normal function of residual renal tissue by occluding the renal vein or pelvis.
6. **Renal artery occlusion** — including trauma.
7. **Renal vein occlusion** — see 8.27.
8. **Multicystic kidney** — see 8.22.

8.9 UNILATERAL SCARRED KIDNEY

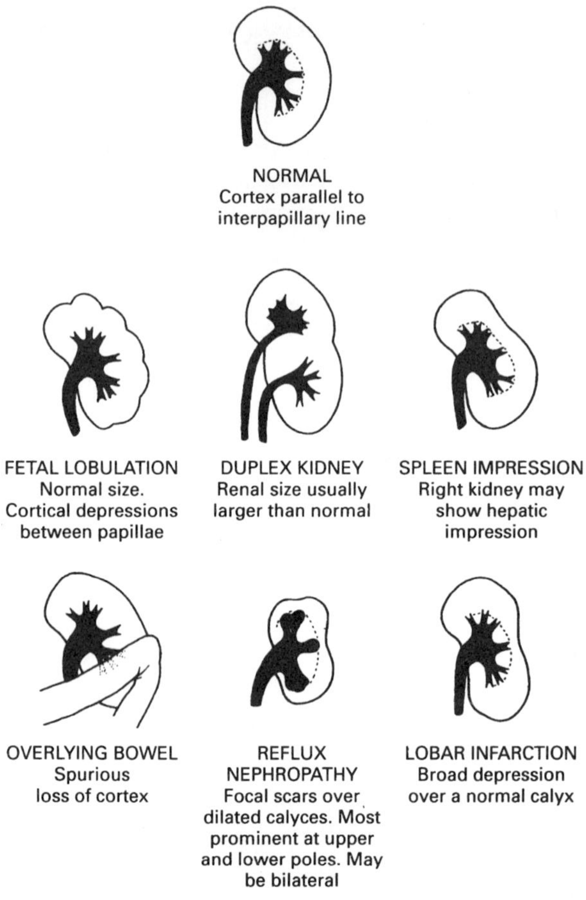

Redrawn from Taylor C.M. & Chapman S. (1989) *Handbook of Renal Investigations in Children.* London: Wright. By kind permission of the publisher.

1. **Reflux nephropathy** — a focal scar over a dilated calyx. Usually multifocal and may be bilateral. Scarring is most prominent in the upper and lower poles. Minimal scarring, especially at a pole, may produce decreased cortical thickness with a normal papilla and is then indistinguishable from lobar infarction.

2. **Tuberculosis** — calcification differentiates it from the other members of this section.
3. **Lobar infarction** — a broad contour depression over a normal calyx. Normal interpapillary line.
4. **Renal dysplasia** — a forme fruste multicystic kidney. Dilated calyces. Indistinguishable from chronic pyelonephritis. Arteriography outlines a small threadlike renal artery.

DIFFERENTIAL DIAGNOSIS

1. **Persistent fetal lobulation** — lobules overlie calyces with interlobular septa between the calyces. Normal size kidney.

Further Reading

Davidson A.J. (1977) *Radiological Diagnosis of Renal Parenchymal Disease,* Ch. 4. Philadelphia: Saunders, pp. 47–68.

8.10 UNILATERAL SMALL SMOOTH KIDNEY

In all these conditions chronic unilateral disease is associated with compensatory hypertrophy of the contralateral kidney.

WITH A DILATED COLLECTING SYSTEM

1. **Post-obstructive atrophy** — ± thinning of the renal cortex and if there is impaired renal function this will be revealed by poor contrast medium density in the collecting system.

WITH A SMALL-VOLUME COLLECTING SYSTEM

This is a sign of diminished urinary volume and, together with global cortical thinning, delayed opacification of the calyces, increased density of the opacified collecting system and delayed wash-out following oral fluids or diuretics, indicates ischaemia.

1. **Ischaemia due to renal artery stenosis** — ureteric notching is due to enlarged collateral vessels and differentiates this from the other causes in this group. See 8.26.
2. **Radiation nephritis** — at least 23 Gy over 5 weeks. The collecting system may be normal or small. Depending on the size of the radiation field both, one or just part of one kidney may be affected. There may be other sequelae of radiotherapy, e.g. scoliosis following radiotherapy in childhood.
3. **End result of renal infarction** — due to previous severe trauma involving the renal artery or renal vein thrombosis. The collecting system does not usually opacify during excretion urography.

WITH FIVE OR LESS CALYCES

1. **Congenital hypoplasia** — the pelvicalyceal system is otherwise normal.

Further Reading

Davidson A.J. (1977) *Radiological Diagnosis of Renal Parenchymal Disease,* Ch. 5. Philadelphia: Saunders, pp. 69–95.

8.11 BILATERAL SMALL SMOOTH KIDNEYS

1. **Generalized arteriosclerosis** — normal calyces.
2. **Chronic glomerulonephritis** — normal calyces. Reduced nephrogram density and poor calyceal opacification.
3. **Chronic papillary necrosis** (see 8.25) — with other signs of necrotic papillae.
4. **Arterial hypotension** — distinguished by the time relationship to the contrast medium injection and its transient nature.
5. **Cause of unilateral small smooth kidneys occurring bilaterally** — e.g. obstructive uropathy or renal artery stenosis.

Further Reading

Davidson A.J. (1977) *Radiological Diagnosis of Renal Parenchymal Disease,* Ch. 6. Philadelphia: Saunders, pp. 96–131.

8.12 UNILATERAL LARGE SMOOTH KIDNEY

1. **Compensatory hypertrophy.**
2. **Obstructed kidney** } dilated calyces.
3. **Pyonephrosis** } dilated calyces.
4. **Duplex kidney** — female:male, 2:1. Equal incidence on both sides and 20% are bilateral. Incomplete more common than complete. Only 50% are bigger than the contralateral kidney; 40% are the same size; 10% are smaller.
5. **Tumour** — see 8.16 and 8.17.
6. **Crossed fused ectopia** — may be associated with anorectal anomalies and renal dysplasia. No kidney on the contralateral side and ureter crosses the midline.
7. **Multicystic kidney** — see 8.22.
8. **Acute pyelonephritis** — impaired excretion of contrast medium. ± Increasingly dense nephrogram. Attenuated calyces but may have non-obstructive pelvicalyceal or ureteric dilatation. Completely reversible within a few weeks of clinical recovery.
9. **Trauma** — haematoma or urinoma.
10. **Renal vein thrombosis** — see 8.27.
11. **Acute arterial infarction.**
12. **Adult polycystic disease*** — asymmetrical bilateral enlargement, but 8% of cases are unilateral. Lobulated rather than completely smooth.

Further Reading

Pickhardt P.J., Lonergan G.J., Davis C.J. Jr. *et al.* (2000) Infiltrative renal lesions: radiologic–pathologic correlation. *RadioGraphics*, 20: 215–43.

8.13 BILATERAL LARGE SMOOTH KIDNEYS

It is often difficult to distinguish, radiologically, the members of this group from one another. The appearance of the nephrogram may be helpful — see 8.24. Associated clinical and radiological abnormalities elsewhere are often more useful, e.g. in sickle-cell anaemia, Goodpasture's disease and acromegaly.

PROLIFERATIVE AND NECROTIZING DISORDERS

1. **Acute glomerulonephritis.**
2. **Polyarteritis nodosa.**
3. **Wegener's granulomatosis.**
4. **Goodpasture's disease.**
5. **Systemic lupus erythematosus*.**

DEPOSITION OF ABNORMAL PROTEINS

1. **Amyloid** — renal involvement in 80% of secondary and 35% of primary amyloid. Chronic deposition results in small kidneys.
2. **Multiple myeloma*.**

ABNORMAL FLUID ACCUMULATION

1. **Acute tubular necrosis.**
2. **Acute cortical necrosis** — may show an opacified medulla and outer rim with non-opacified cortex. Cortical calcification is a late finding.

NEOPLASTIC INFILTRATION

1. **Leukaemia and lymphoma.**

INFLAMMATORY CELL INFILTRATION

1. **Acute interstitial nephritis.**

MISCELLANEOUS

1. **Renal vein thrombosis** (see 8.27).
2. **Acute renal papillary necrosis** (see 8.25).
3. **Polycystic disease*** — infantile form has smooth outlines.
4. **Acute urate nephropathy.**

5. **Sickle-cell anaemia*.**
6. **Bilateral hydronephrosis.**
7. **Medullary sponge kidneys** — with 'bunch of grapes' calcification.
8. **Acromegaly* and gigantism** — as part of the generalized visceromegaly.

Further Reading

Davidson A.J. (1977) *Radiological Diagnosis of Renal Parenchymal Disease,* Ch. 7, Philadelphia: Saunders, pp. 132–61.

8.14 LOCALIZED BULGE OF THE RENAL OUTLINE

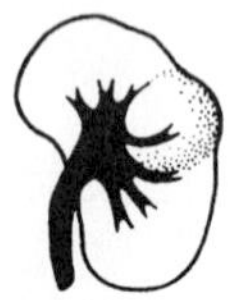

RENAL CYST
US confirms typical echo-free cyst

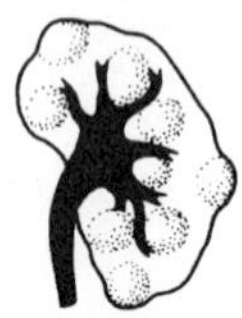

MULTIPLE RENAL CYSTS
e.g. adult type polycystic disease. Spider leg deformity of calyces

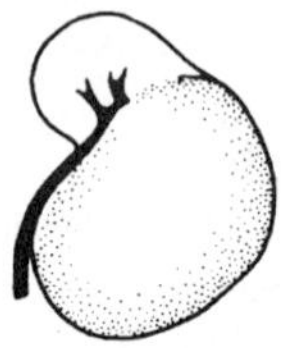

TUMOUR
Replacement of much or all of normal renal tissue

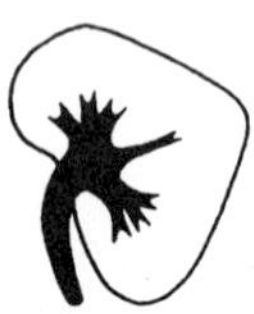

DROMEDARY HUMP
Left sided variant

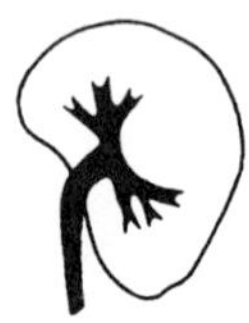

PROMINENT SEPTUM OF BERTIN
Increased activity on Tc-DMSA scanning

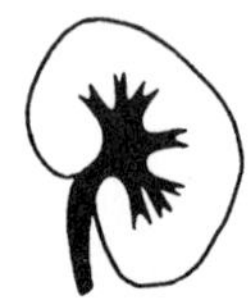

HILAR LIP
Hyperplasia of parenchyma adjacent to the renal hilum. Normal on Tc-DMSA scan

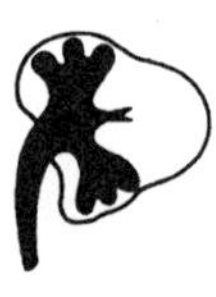

PSEUDOTUMOUR IN REFLUX NEPHROPATHY
Hypertrophy of unscarred renal parenchyma

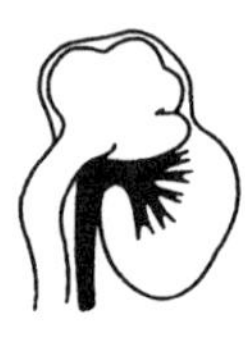

DUPLEX KIDNEY WITH HYDRONEPHROTIC UPPER MOIETY
Drooping flower appearance

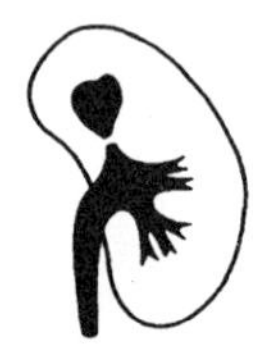

DILATATION OF A SINGLE CALYX
Most commonly due to extrinsic compression by an intrarenal artery (Fraley syndrome)

Redrawn from Taylor C.M. & Chapman S. (1989) *Handbook of Renal Investigations in Children.* London: Wright. By kind permission of the publisher.

1. **Cyst** — well-defined nephrographic defect with a thin wall on the outer margin. Beak sign. Displacement and distortion of smooth-walled calyces without obliteration.
2. **Tumour** — mostly renal cell carcinoma in adults and Wilms' tumour in children. See 8.16 and 8.17.
3. **Fetal lobulation** — the lobule directly overlies a normal calyx. Normal interpapillary line. See 8.9.
4. **Dromedary hump** — on the midportion of the lateral border of the kidney. The arc of the interpapillary line parallels the renal contour.
5. **Splenic impression** — on the left side only. This produces an apparent bulge inferiorly.
6. **Enlarged septum of Bertin** — overgrowth of renal cortex from two adjacent renal lobules. Excretion urography shows a pseudomass with calyceal splaying and associated short calyx ± attempted duplication. Tc-DMSA accumulates normally or in excess. On US echogenicity is usually similar to normal renal cortex but may be of increased echogenicity.
7. **Localized hypertrophy** — e.g. adjacent to an area of pyelonephritic scarring.
8. **Acute focal nephritis (lobar nephronia)** — usually an ill-defined hypoechoic mass on US, but may be hyperechoic. CT shows an ill-defined, low attenuation, wedge-shaped mass with reduced contrast enhancement.
9. **Abscess** — loss of renal outline and psoas margin on the control film. Scoliosis concave to the involved side. Initially there is no nephrographic defect, but following central necrosis there will be a central defect surrounded by a thick irregular wall. Adjacent calyces are displaced or effaced.
10. **Non-functioning moiety of a duplex** — usually a hydronephrotic upper moiety. Delayed films may show contrast medium in the upper moiety calyces. Lower moiety calyces have 'drooping flowers' appearance.

Further Reading

Felson B. & Moskowitz M. (1969) Renal pseudotumours. The regenerated nodule and other lumps, bumps and dromedary humps. *Am. J. Roentgenol.*, 107: 720–9.

Hardwick D. & Hendry G.M.A. (1984) The ultrasonic appearances of the septa of Bertin in children. *Clin. Radiol.*, 34: 107–12.

Kawashima A., Goldman S.M. & Sandler C.M. (1996) The indeterminate renal mass. *Radiol. Clin. North Am.*, 34(5): 997–1015.

Levitin A & Becker J.A. (1995) Tumorlike conditions of the kidney. *Semin. Roentgenol.*, 30(2): 185–99.

8.15 CORTICAL DEFECTS IN RADIONUCLIDE RENAL IMAGES

1. **Scars** — note that apparent scars present during infection may resolve later. Oblique views are required.
2. **Hydronephrosis.**
3. **Trauma** — subcapsular or intrarenal.
4. **Renal cysts.**
5. **Carcinoma.**
6. **Infarct or ischaemia.**
7. **Abscesses.**
8. **Metastases.**
9. **Wilms' tumour.**

Further Reading

Fogelman I. & Maisey M. (1988) *An Atlas of Clinical Nuclear Medicine.* London: Martin Dunitz, pp. 217–373.

8.16 RENAL NEOPLASMS IN AN ADULT

MALIGNANT

1. **Renal cell carcinoma** — 90% of adult malignant tumours. Bilateral in 10% and an increased incidence of bilaterality in polycystic kidneys and von Hippel–Lindau disease. A mass lesion (showing irregular or amorphous calcification in 10% of cases). Calyces are obliterated, distorted and/or displaced. Half-shadow filling defect in a calyx or pelvis. Arteriography shows a typical pathological circulation in the majority.

2. **Transitional cell carcinoma** — usually papilliferous. May obstruct or obliterate a calyx or obstruct a whole kidney. Seeding may produce a second lesion further down the urinary tract. Bilateral tumours are rare. Calcification in 2%.
3. **Squamous cell carcinoma** — ulcerated plaque or stricture. 50% are associated with calculi. There is usually a large parenchymal mass before there is any sizeable intrapelvic mass. No calcification. Avascular at arteriography.
4. **Leukaemia/lymphoma** — bilateral large smooth kidneys. Thickened parenchyma with compression of the pelvicalyceal systems.
5. **Metastases** — not uncommon. Usually multiple. Bronchus, breast and stomach.

BENIGN

1. **Hamartoma** — usually solitary but often multiple and bilateral in tuberous sclerosis. Diagnostic appearance on the plain film of radiolucent fat (but only observed in 9%). Other signs are of any mass lesion, and angiography does not differentiate from renal cell carcinoma.
2. **Adenoma** — usually small and frequently multiple. Majority are found at autopsy. Hypovascular at arteriography.
3. **Others** — myoma, lipoma, haemangioma and fibroma are all rare.

Further Reading

Helenon O., Correas J.M., Balleyguier C. *et al.* (2001) Ultrasound of renal tumours. *Eur. Radiol.*, 11: 1890–1901.

Hes E.J. & Feldberg M.A. (1999) Von Hippel–Lindau disease: strategies in early detection (renal-, adrenal-, pancreatic masses). *Eur. Radiol.*, 9: 598–610.

Meilstrup J.W., Mosher T.J., Dhadha R.S. *et al.* (1995) Other renal tumours. *Semin. Roentgenol.*, 30(2): 168–84.

Patel U. (1999) Small and indeterminate renal masses: characterisation and management. *CME Journal Radiology*, 1: 47–55.

Ramchandani P. & Pollack H.M. (1995) Tumors of the urothelium. *Semin. Roentgenol.*, 30(2): 149–67.

8.17 PRIMARY RENAL NEOPLASMS IN CHILDHOOD

1. **Wilms' tumour** — $8/10^6$ children. 80% present in the first 3 years. Bilateral in 5%. Associated abnormalities: cryptorchidism (3%), hypospadias (2%), hemihypertrophy (2%), sporadic aniridia (1%) [30% of those with aniridia and 10% of those with Beckwith–Wiedemann syndrome (macroglossia, organomegaly, exomphalos ± hemihypertrophy) develop Wilms' tumour]. 90% have favourable histology. 2° → lungs and liver. 5% have tumour thrombus in the IVC or right atrium. Hypertension in 25%.
   Plain film: bulging flank (75%), loss of renal outline (66%), enlargement of renal outline (33%), displacement of bowel gas (50%), loss of psoas outline (33%), calcification (10%).
   Ultrasound: large well-defined mass, greater echogenicity than liver. Solid with haemorrhage/necrosis. Lack of IVC narrowing on inspiration suggests occlusion.
   CT: large, well-defined, low attenuation, heterogeneous with foci of even lower attenuation due to necrosis. Minimal enhancement compared with the residual rind of functioning renal tissue.
   MRI: inhomogeneous, low signal (T_1W), high signal (T_2W). Inhomogeneous enhancement compared with residual renal tissue.
2. **Nephroblastomatosis** — nephrogenic rests which maintain the potential for malignant induction to Wilms' tumour. Nephrogenic tests in 40% of unilateral and 99% of bilateral Wilms' tumours. May be: *perilobar*: most common, at the lobar surface; *intralobar*: anywhere in the cortex or medulla, or combined.
   Ultrasound: hypoechoic.
   CT: low attenuation and non-enhancing (therefore best shown on contrast-enhanced images).
   MRI: similar signal to renal cortex. Non-enhancing (therefore best shown on contrast-enhanced images).
3. **Congenital mesoblastic nephroma** — most common solid renal tumour in the newborn. Mean age at diagnosis is $3\frac{1}{2}$ months. No recurrence when diagnosed in first 3 months. Indistinguishable from Wilms' tumour but some demonstrate function.
4. **Clear cell sarcoma** — 4–6% of childhood renal tumours. Presentation at 3–5 years. Poor prognosis with early 2° (to bone; usually lytic but may be sclerotic). Never bilateral. No specific imaging features of the primary tumour.

5. **Rhabdoid tumour of kidney** — 2% of childhood renal tumours. Presentation at 3 months to $4\frac{1}{2}$ years (50% in first year). Most malignant renal tumour with extrarenal extension or haematogenous 2° (to brain or bone) often present at diagnosis. Association with midline posterior fossa tumours. Hypercalcaemia sometimes present. Imaging of the primary tumour is similar to Wilms' tumour.
6. **Multilocular cystic nephroma** — presents 3 months to 4 years. Multiple cysts of varying size. Thin septae. Thick septae, nodules or a large solid component suggest Wilms' tumour with cystic degeneration. Resection is curative and local recurrence is rare. Differential diagnosis is a multicystic dysplastic kidney but this affects the entire kidney.
   Ultrasound and CT: cystic with thin septae.
   MRI: round collections of variable signal intensity suggesting haemorrhage or proteinaceous material.
7. **Renal cell carcinoma** — rare. Differentiating features from Wilms' tumour are: older age at presentation (mean 11–12 years), calcification is more common (25%) and more homogeneous, smaller at the time of diagnosis and haematuria is more common. Poorer prognosis compared with Wilms' tumour. Similar imaging findings. Association with von Hippel–Lindau disease and tuberous sclerosis*.
8. **Angiomyolipoma** — in 50–80% of patients with tuberous sclerosis*. 50% of patients with angiomyolipomas have tuberous sclerosis. Multiple bilateral tumours which are usually small.
   Ultrasound, CT and MRI: fat densities within the tumours. NB. Fat may occasionally be identified within Wilms' tumour.

Further Reading

Cohen M.D. (1992) Genitourinary tumours. In: *Imaging of Children with Cancer*, Ch. 4. St Louis: Mosby Year Book, pp. 52–88.

Geller E., Smergel E.M. & Lowry P.A. (1997) Renal neoplasms of childhood. *Radiol. Clin. North Am.* 34(6): 1081–1100.

Lowe L.H., Isuani B.H., Heller R.M. *et al.* (2000) Pediatric renal masses: Wilms tumor and beyond. *RadioGraphics*, 20: 1585–1603.

Navoy J.F., Royal S.A., Vaid Y.N. *et al.* (1995) Wilms' tumor: unusual manifestations. *Pediatr. Radiol.*, 25: S76–86.

Rohrschneider W.K., Weirich A., Rieden K. *et al.* (1998) US, CT and MR imaging characteristics of nephroblastomatosis. *Pediatr. Radiol.*, 28: 435–43.

Scott D.J., Wallace W.H. & Hendry G.M. (1999) With advances in medical imaging can the radiologist reliably diagnose Wilms' tumours? *Clin. Radiol.*, 54: 321–7.

8.18 MRI OF RENAL MASSES

MRI is not tissue-specific and it is usually not possible to differentiate benign from malignant lesions.

	T_1W	*T_2W*	*Comment*
Simple cysts	↓	↑	Wall not visible. If haemorrhage, infection or debris present the cyst may appear to be 'solid'
Abscess	Variable ↓ ± areas of ↑	↑	
Renal cell carcinoma	Iso or ↓ ± ↑ in areas containing clear cells	↑, iso	Can miss lesions < 3 cm but vascular anatomy well shown
Lymphoma	↓ homogeneous	slightly ↑	
Angiomyolipoma	↑ (fat content)	↑ (fat content)	

Further Reading

Krestin P. (1999) Genitourinary MR: kidneys and adrenal glands. *Eur. Radiol.*, 9: 1705–14.

8.19 CT KIDNEY — FOCAL HYPODENSE LESION

TUMOURS

1. **Malignant**
   (a) Renal cell carcinoma — usually inhomogeneous and irregular if large.
   (b) Metastases.
   (c) Lymphoma — usually late-stage Non-Hodgkin's lymphoma; only 5% at initial staging. 70% multiple and bilateral. Usually rounded in appearance.
   (d) Transitional cell carcinoma — can infiltrate and mimic renal cell carcinoma.
   (e) Wilms' — see 8.17.
2. **Benign**
   (a) Oncocytoma — adenoma arising from proximal tubular cells. Round, well-defined, homogeneous (usually high density pre-contrast, low density post-contrast), ± central stellate low-density scar if tumour bigger than 3 cm.
   (b) Angiomyoplipoma — well-defined containing fat densities. Association with tuberous sclerosis.

INFLAMMATION

1. **Abscess** — thick irregular walls ± perirenal fascial thickening, but this can occur in malignancy.
2. **Xanthogranulomatous pyelonephritis** — obstructing calculus seen in 80% cases leading to chronic sepsis, perinephric fluid collections and fistula formation.
3. **Acute focal bacterial nephritis** — wedge-shaped low density ± radiating striations after intravenous contrast.

VASCULAR

1. **Infarcts** — well-defined, peripheral, wedge-shaped.

CYST — see 8.20 and 8.21.

Further Reading

Ishikawa I., Saito Y., Onouchi Z. *et al.* (1985) Delayed contrast enhancement in acute focal bacterial nephritis: C.T. features. *J. Comput. Assist. Tomogr.*, 9 (5): 894–7.
Neirius D., Braedel H.U., Schindler E. *et al.* (1988) Computed tomographic and angiographic findings in renal oncocytoma. *Br. J. Radiol.*, 61: 1019–25.
Quinn M.J., Hartman D.S., Friedman A.C. *et al.* (1984) Renal oncocytoma: new observations. *Radiology*, 153: 49–53.
Rabushka L.S., Fishman E.K., Goldman S.M. *et al.* (1994) Pictorial review: computed tomography of renal inflammatory disease. *Urology*, 44: 473–80.
Sheth S., Scatarige J.C., Horton K.M. *et al.* (2001) Current concepts in the diagnosis and management of renal cell carcinoma: role of multidetector CT and three-dimensional CT. *RadioGraphics*, 21: S237–54.
Urban B.A. & Fishman E.K. (2000) Renal lymphoma: CT patterns with emphasis on helical CT. *RadioGraphics*, 20: 197–212.
Yuh B.I. & Cohan R.H. (1999) Different phases of renal enhancement: role in detecting and characterizing renal masses during helical CT. *Am. J. Roentgenol.*, 173: 747–55.

8.20 CLASSIFICATION OF RENAL CYSTS

(After Elkin & Bernstein, 1969).

RENAL DYSPLASIA

1. **Multicystic kidney** — see 8.22.
2. **Focal and segmental cystic dysplasia.**
3. **Multiple cysts associated with lower urinary tract obstruction** — usually posterior urethral valves in males.

POLYCYSTIC DISEASE*

1. **Autosomal recessive polycystic kidney disease.**
2. **Autosomal dominant polycystic kidney disease.**

CORTICAL CYSTS

1. **Simple cyst** — unilocular. Increase in size and number with age.
2. **Multilocular cystic nephroma** — see 8.17.
3. **Syndromes associated with cysts** — Zellweger's syndrome, tuberous sclerosis, Turner's syndrome, von Hippel–Lindau disease, trisomy 13 and 18.
4. **End-stage renal disease and haemodialysis** — in 8–13% of patients in renal failure not on dialysis; 10–20% of patients after 1–3 years of dialysis; >90% of patients after 5–10 years of dialysis. Diagnosis based on finding at least 3–5 cysts in each kidney. Cysts are of variable size and occur in cortex and medulla. Increased incidence of renal cell carcinoma, particularly when on dialysis.

MEDULLARY CYSTS

1. **Calyceal cysts (diverticulum)** — small, usually solitary cyst communicating via an isthmus with the fornix of a calyx.
2. **Medullary sponge kidney** — bilateral in 60–80%. Multiple, small, mainly pyramidal cysts which opacify during excretion urography and contain calculi.
3. **Papillary necrosis** — see 8.25.
4. **Juvenile nephronophthisis (medullary cystic disease)** — usually presents with polyuria and progressive renal failure. Positive family history. Normal or small kidneys. US shows a few medullary or corticomedullary cysts, loss of corticomedullary differentiation and increased parenchymal echogenicity.

MISCELLANEOUS INTRARENAL CYSTS

1. **Inflammatory**
   (a) Tuberculosis.
   (b) Calculus disease.
   (c) Hydatid.
2. **Neoplastic** — cystic degeneration of a carcinoma.
3. **Traumatic** — intrarenal haematoma.

EXTRAPARENCHYMAL RENAL CYSTS

1. **Parapelvic cyst** — located in or near the hilum, but does not communicate with the renal pelvis and therefore does not opacify during urography. Simple or multilocular; single or multiple, unilateral or bilateral. It compresses the renal pelvis and may cause hydronephrosis.

2. **Perinephric cyst** — beneath the capsule or between the capsule and perinephric fat. Secondary to trauma, obstruction or replacement of haematoma. It may compress the kidney, pelvis or ureter, leading to hydronephrosis or causing displacement of the kidney.

Further Reading

Choyke P.L. (1996) Inherited cystic diseases of the kidney. *Radiol. Clin. North Am.*, 34(5): 925–46.

Choyke P.L. (2000) Acquired cystic kidney disease. *Eur. Radiol.*, 10: 1716–21.

Elkin M. & Bernstein J. (1969) Cystic diseases of the kidney — radiological and pathological considerations. *Clin. Radiol.*, 20: 65–82.

Levine E. (1996) Acquired cystic kidney disease. *Radiol. Clin. North Am.*, 34(5): 947–64.

Pedrosa I., Saiz A., Arrazola L. *et al.* (2000) Hydatid disease: radiologic and pathologic features and complications. *RadioGraphics*, 20: 795–817.

Saunders A.J., Denton E., Stephens S. *et al.* (1999) Cystic kidney disease presenting in infancy. *Clin. Radiol.*, 54: 370–6.

Tattersall D.J. & Moore N.R. (2002) Von Hippel–Lindau disease: MRI of abdominal manifestations. *Clin. Radiol.*, 57: 85–92.

8.21 CT RENAL CYSTS

See also 8.20.

1. **Simple** — thin-walled, no enhancement. Occasionally haemorrhage can occur within one, producing a round hyperdense lesion.
2. **Malignant** — 5% of renal cell carcinomas are cystic. Suspect if thick walls or separations but this may just indicate previous infection/haemorrhage in cyst.
3. **Polycystic** — associated with hepatic cysts in approximately 60% of cases. Haemorrhage into cysts relatively common, so may be of varying density. Associated with increased incidence of renal cell carcinoma.
4. **Haemodialysis-related cysts** — cysts develop in approximately 50% of long-term haemodialysis patients, but can involute after a successful renal transplant. 7% incidence of associated renal cell carcinoma.
5. **von Hippel–Lindau** — associated pancreatic, hepatic cysts and renal cell carcinoma and phaeochromocytoma.
6. **Hydatid** — affected in 10% of cases. ± Curvilinear calcification in wall.
7. **Multicystic** — usually detected in infancy.
8. **Cystic hamartoma** — usually large with thick capsule and septations.

Further Reading

Beggs I (1985) The radiology of hydatid disease. *Am. J. Roentgenol.*, 145: 639–48.

Cho C., Friedland G.W. & Swenson R.S. (1984) Acquired renal cystic disease and renal neoplasms in haemodialysis patients. *Urol. Radiol.*, 6: 153–7.

Jennings C.M. & Games P.A. (1988) The abdominal manifestation of von Hippel–Lindau disease and a radiological screening protocol for an affected family. *Clin. Radiol.*, 39: 363–7.

8.22 RENAL MASS IN THE NEWBORN AND YOUNG INFANT

1. **Hydronephrosis** (q.v.) — unilateral or bilateral.
2. **Multicystic kidney** — unilateral, but 30% have an abnormal contralateral kidney (mostly pelviureteric junction obstruction). Non-functioning, multilobulated kidney. Rarely, nephrographic crescents and late pooling of contrast medium in cysts is observed. Curvilinear calcification is characteristic but only seen occasionally. US reveals multiple cysts of unequal size. The commonest renal mass in the first year of life.
3. **Polycystic kidneys** (see Polycystic disease*) — bilateral. Poor renal excretion. Striated nephrogram with no visualization of calyces. Highly echogenic on US.
4. **Renal vein thrombosis** (q.v.) — unilateral or bilateral.
5. **Nephroblastomatosis or mesoblastic nephroma** — see 8.17.
6. **Renal ectopia.**

Further Reading

Merten D.F. & Kirks D.R. (1985) Diagnostic imaging of paediatric abdominal masses. *Pediatr. Clin. North Am.*, 32: 1397–425.

8.23 HYDRONEPHROSIS IN A CHILD

1. **Pelviureteric junction obstruction** — more common on the left side. 20% bilateral. Due to stricture, neuromuscular inco-ordination or aberrant vessels. Contralateral kidney is dysplastic in 25% of cases and absent in 12%.
2. **Bladder outflow obstruction** (q.v.) — bilateral upper tract dilatation.
3. **Ureterovesical obstruction** — more common in males and more common on the left side. May be bilateral.
4. **Reflux without obstruction.**
5. **Associated with urinary tract infection** — but no obstruction or reflux. ? Represents atony.
6. **Neurogenic.**

Further Reading

Lebowitz R.L. & Griscom N.T. (1977) Neonatal hydronephrosis: 146 cases. *Radiol. Clin. North Am.*, 15: 49–59.

8.24 NEPHROGRAPHIC PATTERNS

IMMEDIATE FAINT PERSISTENT NEPHROGRAM

1. **Proliferative/necrotizing disorders** — e.g. acute glomerulonephritis. See 8.13.
2. **Renal vein thrombosis.**
3. **Chronic severe ischaemia.**

IMMEDIATE DISTINCT PERSISTENT NEPHROGRAM

1. **Acute tubular necrosis** — in 60% of cases.
2. **Other causes of acute renal failure.**
3. **Acute-on-chronic renal failure.**
4. **Acute hypotension** — uncommonly.

INCREASINGLY DENSE NEPHROGRAM

1. **Acute obstruction** — including urate nephropathy.
2. **Acute hypotension.**
3. **Acute tubular necrosis** — in 30% of cases.
4. **Acute pyelonephritis.**
5. **Multiple myeloma.**
6. **Renal vein thrombosis.**
7. **Acute glomerulonephritis.**
8. **Amyloid.**
9. **Acute papillary necrosis** — and rarely chronic papillary necrosis.

RIM NEPHROGRAM

1. **Severe hydronephrosis** — scalloped nephrogram with a negative pyelogram.
2. **Acute complete arterial occlusion** — smooth nephrogram from cortical perfusion by capsular arteries.

STRIATED NEPHROGRAM

1. **Acute ureteric obstruction.**
2. **Infantile polycystic disease** — contrast medium in dilated tubules.

3. **Medullary sponge kidney** — in the medulla only. Parallel or fan-shaped streaks radiating from the papilla to the periphery of the kidney.
4. **Acute pyelonephritis.**

Further Reading

Newhouse J.H. & Pfister R.C. (1979) The nephrogram. *Radiol. Clin. North Am.*, 17: 213–26.

Saunders H.S., Dyer R.B., Shifrin R.Y. *et al.* (1995) The CT nephrogram: implications for evaluation of urinary tract disease. *RadioGraphics*, 15: 1069–85.

8.25 RENAL PAPILLARY NECROSIS

1. Normal — small kidneys with smooth outlines.
2. Bilateral in 85% with multiple papillae affected.
3. Papillae may show:
   (a) Enlargement (early).
   (b) Partial sloughing — a fissure forms and may communicate with a central irregular cavity.
   (c) Total sloughing — the sloughed papillary tissue may: (i) fragment and be passed in the urine; (ii) cause ureteric obstruction; (iii) remain free in a calyx; or (iv) remain in the pelvis and form a ball calculus.
   (d) Necrosis-in-situ — the papilla is shrunken and necrotic but has not separated.
4. Calyces will appear dilated following total sloughing of a papilla.
5. Calcification and occasionally ossification of a shrunken, necrotic papilla. If marginal, it appears as a calculus with a radiolucent centre.

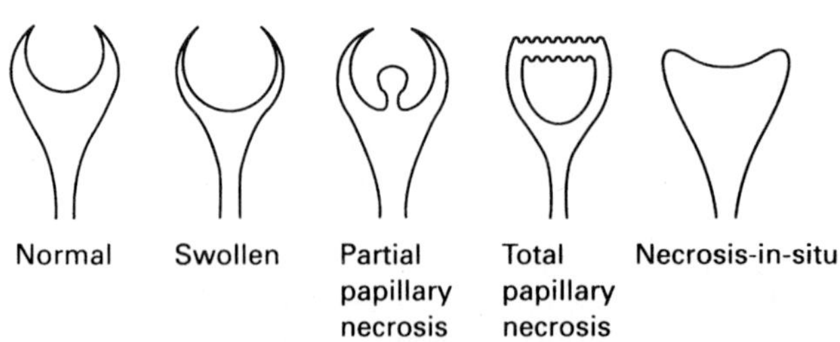

A useful mnemonic is *ADIPOSE*:

A Analgesics — phenacetin and aspirin.
D Diabetes.
I Infants in shock.
P Pyelonephritis.
O Obstruction.
S Sickle-cell disease.
E Ethanol.

However, diabetes, analgesics and sickle-cell anaemia are the most important, with diabetes the most frequent cause.

Further Reading

Hare W.S.C. and Poynter J.D. (1974) The radiology of renal papillary necrosis as seen in analgesic nephropathy. *Clin. Radiol.*, 25: 423–43.

8.26 RENAL-INDUCED HYPERTENSION

SIGNS OF UNILATERAL RENAL ARTERY STENOSIS ON IVU

1. Unilateral delay of 1 minute or more in the appearance of opacified calyces.
2. Small, smooth kidney
   - left more than 1.5 cm shorter than the right.
   - right more than 2 cm shorter than the left.
3. Increased density of opacified calyces.
4. Ureteric notching by collateral vessels.

SIGNS OF UNILATERAL RENAL ARTERY STENOSIS ON ACE INHIBITOR RENAL SCINTIGRAPHY

1. Low probability suggested by a normal study.
2. Intermediate probability when: (a) small kidney contributing $< 30\%$ of total renal function; (b) time to maximum activity (T_{max}) ≤ 2 minutes, and shows no change following administration of ACE inhibitor; and (c) bilateral symmetrical cortical retention of tracer.
3. High probability when unilateral parenchymal retention, indicated by: (a) a change in the 20-minute/peak uptake ratio ≥ 0.15, delayed excretion of tracer into the renal pelvis > 2 minutes, or increase in the T_{max} of ≥ 2 minutes or 40% after administration of ACE inhibitor.
4. Decreased sensitivity when bilateral renal artery stenosis, impaired renal function, urinary obstruction or long-term ACE therapy.

SIGNS OF UNILATERAL RENAL ARTERY STENOSIS ON DOPPLER SONOGRAPHY

1. Peak velocity in the renal artery > 100 cm/s.
2. Renal artery velocity $> 3.5 \times$ aortic velocity.
3. Tardus-parvus waveform — slope of the systolic upstroke < 3 m/s^2 and acceleration time (time from onset of systole to peak systole) > 0.07 s.
4. Turbulent flow in the post-stenotic renal artery.

RENAL ARTERY

1. **Arteriosclerosis** — 66% of renovascular causes. Stenosis of the proximal 2 cm of the renal artery; less frequently the distal artery or early branches at bifurcations. More common in males.
2. **Fibromuscular dysplasia** — 33% of renovascular causes. Stenoses ± dilatations which may give the characteristic 'string of beads' appearance. Mainly females less than 40 years. Bilateral in 60% of cases.
3. **Thrombosis/embolism.**
4. **Arteritis** — polyarteritis nodosa, thromboangiitis obliterans. Takayasu's disease, syphilis, congenital rubella or idiopathic.
5. **Neurofibromatosis*** — coarctation of the aorta. ± Stenoses of other arteries. ± Intrarenal arterial abnormalities.
6. **Trauma.**

7. **Aneurysm** — of the aorta or the renal artery.
8. **Arteriovenous fistula** — traumatic, congenital or a stump fistula following nephrectomy.
9. **Extrinsic compression** — neoplasm, aneurysm or lymph nodes.

CHRONIC BILATERAL PARENCHYMAL DISEASE

1. **Chronic glomerulonephritis.**
2. **Reflux nephropathy.**
3. **Adult polycystic disease*.**
4. **Diabetic glomerulosclerosis.**
5. **Connective tissue disorders** — systemic lupus erythematosus, scleroderma and polyarthritis nodosa.
6. **Radiotherapy.**
7. **Hydronephrosis.**
8. **Analgesic nephropathy.**
9. **Renal vein thrombosis.**

UNILATERAL PARENCHYMAL DISEASE

Much less common as a cause of hypertension.

1. **Reflux nephropathy.**
2. **Hydronephrosis.**
3. **Tumours** — hypertension is more common with Wilms' tumour than with renal cell carcinoma. The rare juxtaglomerular cell tumour secretes renin.
4. **Tuberculosis.**
5. **Xanthogranulomatous pyelonephritis.**
6. **Radiotherapy.**
7. **Renal vein thrombosis.**

Further Reading

Kawashima A., Sandler C.M., Ernst R.D. *et al.* (2000) CT evaluation of renovascular disease. *RadioGraphics*, 20: 1321–40.

Mitty H.A., Shapiro R.S., Parsons R.B. *et al.* (1996) Renovascular hypertension. *Radiol. Clin. North Am.*, 34(5): 1017–36.

Rankin S., Saunders A.J., Cook G.J. *et al.* (2000) Renovascular disease. *Clin. Radiol.*, 55: 1–12.

Soulez G., Oliva V.L., Turpin S. *et al.* (2000) Imaging of renovascular hypertension: respective values of renal scintigraphy, renal Doppler US, and MR angiography. *RadioGraphics*, 20: 1355–68.

8.27 RENAL VEIN THROMBOSIS

Unilateral or bilateral.

The ultrasound findings (after Cremin *et al.*, 1991) are:

1st week

1. Globular renal enlargement.
2. Increase in echogenicity which may be more prominent in the cortex.
3. Loss of corticomedullary differentiation.
4. Echogenic streaks in the direction of the interlobular vessels.
5. Loss of definition of normal renal sinus echoes.

2nd week

1. Diffuse renal enlargement is more obvious.
2. Diffuse 'snow storm' appearance of increased echogenicity.
3. Loss of corticomedullary differentiation.
4. Mixed hyperechoic areas (haemorrhage) and hypoechoic areas (oedema and/or resolving hemorrhage).
5. Thrombus in main renal vein or IVC.

Late

1. Kidney returns to normal size or becomes small and atrophic.
2. Calcification may occur in kidney or IVC.

Conventional radiography findings are:

Sudden occlusion

1. Large non-functioning kidney which, over a period of several months, becomes small and atrophic.
2. Retrograde pyelography reveals thickened parenchyma (due to oedema) with elongation and compression of the major calyces.
3. Arteriography shows stretching and separation of arterial branches with decreased flow and a poor persistent nephrogram. No opacification of the renal vein.

Gradual occlusion

1. Large kidney.
2. Nephrogram may be normal, poor persistent or increasingly dense.
3. Thickened parenchyma with elongation of major calyces.
4. Ureteric notching due to venous collaterals.

CHILDREN

1. **Dehydration and shock** — especially in infants delivered of diabetic mothers.
2. **Nephrotic syndrome.**
3. **Cyanotic heart disease.**

ADULTS

1. **Extension of renal cell carcinoma into the renal vein.**
2. **Local compression by tumour or retroperitoneal nodes.**
3. **Extension of thrombus from the IVC.**
4. **Trauma.**
5. **Secondary to renal disease** — especially amyloid and chronic glomerulonephritis with nephrotic syndrome.

Further Reading

Cremin B.J., Davey H. & Oleszczuk-Raszke K. (1991) Neonatal renal venous thrombosis: sequential ultrasonic appearances. *Clin. Radiol.*, 44: 52–5.

8.28 NON-VISUALIZATION OF A CALYX

1. **Technical factors** — incomplete filling during excretion urography.
2. **Tumour** — most commonly a renal cell carcinoma (adult) or Wilms' tumour (child).
3. **Obstructed infundibulum** — due to tumour, calculus or tuberculosis.
4. **Duplex kidney** — with a non-functioning upper or lower moiety. Signs suggesting a non-functioning upper moiety are:
   (a) Fewer calyces than the contralateral kidney. This sign is only reliable in unilateral duplication. (Calyceal distribution is symmetrical in 80% of normal individuals.)
   (b) A shortened upper calyx which does not reach into the upper pole.
   (c) The upper calyx of the lower moiety may be deformed by a dilated upper pole pelvis.
   (d) The kidney may be displaced downward by a dilated upper moiety pelvis. The appearances mimic a space-occupying lesion in the upper pole.
   (e) The upper pole may be rotated laterally and downward by a dilated upper moiety pelvis and the lower pole calyces adopt a 'drooping flower' appearance.
   (f) Lateral displacement of the entire kidney by a dilated upper moiety ureter.
   (g) The lower moiety ureter may be displaced or compressed by the upper pole ureter, resulting in a series of scalloped curves.
   (h) The lower moiety renal pelvis may be displaced laterally and its ureter then takes a direct oblique course to the lumbosacral junction.
5. **Infection** — abscess or tuberculosis.
6. **Partial nephrectomy** — with a surgical defect in the twelfth rib.

Further Reading

Fernbach S.K., Feinstein K.A., Spencer K. *et al.* (1997) Ureteral duplication and its complications. *RadioGraphics,* 17: 109–27.

8.29 RADIOLUCENT FILLING DEFECT IN THE RENAL PELVIS OR A CALYX

TECHNICAL FACTORS

1. **Incomplete filling during excretion urography.**
2. **Overlying gas shadows.**

EXTRINSIC WITH A SMOOTH MARGIN

1. **Cyst** — see 8.20.
2. **Vascular impression** — an intrarenal artery producing linear transverse or oblique compression lines and most commonly indenting an upper pole calyx, especially on the right side.
3. **Renal sinus lipomatosis** — most commonly in older patients with a wasting disease of the kidney. Fat in the renal hilum produces a relative lucency and narrows and elongates the major calyces.
4. **Collateral vessels** — most commonly ureteric artery collaterals in renal artery stenosis. Multiple small irregularities in the pelvic wall.

INSEPARABLE FROM THE WALL AND WITH SMOOTH MARGINS

1. **Blood clot** — due to trauma, tumour or bleeding diathesis. May be adherent to the wall or free in the lumen. Change in size or shape over several days.
2. **Papilloma** — solitary or multiple.
3. **Pyeloureteritis cystica** — due to chronic infection. Multiple well-defined submucosal cysts project into the lumen of the pelvis and/or ureter.

ARISING FROM THE WALL WITH AN IRREGULAR MARGIN

1. **Transitional cell carcinoma**
2. **Squamous cell carcinoma** } see 8.16.
3. **Renal cell carcinoma** }
4. **Squamous metaplasia (cholesteatoma)** — occurs rarely in association with chronic irritation from a calculus. Indistinguishable from tumour and may be premalignant.

IN THE LUMEN

1. **Blood clot.**
2. **Lucent calculus** — see 8.6.
3. **Sloughed papilla.**
4. **Air** — see 8.7.

Further Reading

Brown R.C., Jones M.C., Boldus R. *et al.* (1973) Lesions causing radiolucent defects in the renal pelvis. *Am. J. Roentgenol.,* 119: 770–8.

8.30 DILATED CALYX

WITH A NARROW INFUNDIBULUM

1. **Stricture** — tumour, calculus or tuberculosis.
2. **Extrinsic impression by an artery** — most commonly a right upper pole calyx (Fraley syndrome).
3. **Hydrocalycosis** — may be a congenital anomaly. Can only be safely diagnosed in childhood when calculus, tumour and tuberculosis are uncommon.

WITH A WIDE INFUNDIBULUM

1. **Post-obstructive atrophy** — generally all the calyces are affected and associated with parenchymal thinning.
2. **Megacalyces** — dilated calyces ± a slightly dilated pelvis. ± Stones. Increased number of calyces: 20–25 (normal 8–12). Because of the large volume collecting system full visualization during urography is delayed. Normal cortical thickness and good renal function differentiate it from post-obstructive atrophy.
3. **Polycalycosis** — rare. ± Ureteric abnormalities.

Further Reading

Talner L.B. & Gittes R.F. (1974) Megacalyces, further observations and differentiation from obstructive renal disease. *Am. J. Roentgenol.,* 121: 473–86.

8.31 DILATED URETER

OBSTRUCTION

Within the lumen

1. **Calculus** — see 8.6.
2. **Blood clot.**
3. **Sloughed papilla.**

In the wall

1. **Oedema or stricture due to calculus.**
2. **Tumour** — carcinoma or papilloma.
3. **Tuberculous stricture** — a particular hazard during the early weeks of treatment.
4. **Schistosomiasis** — especially the distal ureter. ± Calcification in the ureter or bladder.
5. **Post-surgical trauma** — e.g. a misplaced ligature.
6. **Ureterocoele.**
7. **Megaureter** — symmetrical tapered narrowing above the ureterovesical junction.

Outside the wall

1. **Retroperitoneal fibrosis** (q.v.).
2. **Carcinoma of cervix, bladder or prostate.**
3. **Retrocaval ureter** — right side only. Distal ureter lies medial to the dilated proximal portion.

VESICOURETERIC REFLUX

NO OBSTRUCTION OR REFLUX

1. **Postpartum** — more common on the right side.
2. **Following relief of obstruction** — most commonly calculus of prostatectomy.
3. **Urinary tract infection** — due to the effect of P fimbriated *E. coli* on the urothelium.
4. **Primary non-obstructive megaureter** — children > adults. The juxtavesical segment of ureter is of normal calibre but fails to transmit an effective peristaltic wave.

Further Reading

Mostbeck G.H., Zontsich T. & Turetschek K. (2001) Ultrasound of the kidney: obstruction and medical diseases. *Eur. Radiol.*, 11: 1878–89.

8.32 RETROPERITONEAL FIBROSIS

1. Ureteric obstruction of variable severity. 75% bilateral.
2. Tapering lumen or complete obstruction — usually at L4–5 level and never the extreme lower end.
3. Medial deviation of the ureters — more significant if there is a right-angled step in the course of the ureter rather than a gentle drift. The position of the ureters is frequently normal.
4. Easy retrograde catheterization of ureter(s).
5. Retroperitoneal, periaortic mass that envelops the aorta and IVC between the renal hila and sacral promontory — demonstrable by CT (= muscle), US (hypoechoic) or MRI (low signal on T_1W, high signal on T_2W in the active stage, low signal on T_2W in the chronic stage). Contrast enhancement in the early, active sage.
6. Clinically — back pain, high ESR and elevated creatinine.

1. **Idiopathic** — >50% all cases. May be due to an immune reaction to artheromatous material in the aorta.
2. **Retroperitoneal malignancy** — lymphoma and metastases from colon and breast especially. The tumour initiates a fibrotic reaction around itself.
3. **Aortic aneurysm**
4. **Trauma**
5. **Surgery**

} fibrosis occurs secondary to blood in the retroperitoneal tissues.

6. **Inflammatory conditions** — Crohn's disease, diverticular disease, actinomycosis, pancreatitis and extravasation of urine from the pelvicalyceal system.
7. **Connective tissue diseases** — ankylosing spondylitis, systemic lupus erythematosus, Wegener's granulomatosis and polyarteritis nodosa.
8. **Drugs** — methysergide.

DIFFERENTIAL DIAGNOSIS OF MEDIALLY PLACED URETERS

1. **Normal variant** — 15% of individuals. Commoner in blacks, in whom bilateral displacement is also commoner.
2. **Pelvic lipomatosis** — other signs suggesting the diagnosis are: (a) elevation and elongation of the bladder; (b) elongation of the rectum and sigmoid with widening of the rectorectal space; and (c) increased lucency of the pelvic wall.
3. **Following abdominoperineal resection** — the ureters are medially placed inferiorly.

4. **Retrocaval ureter** — the right ureter passes behind the IVC at the level of LV4. The distal ureter lies medial to the dilated proximal portion.

Further Reading

Brooks A.P. (1990) Computed tomography of idiopathic retroperitoneal fibrosis ('periaortitis'): variants, variations, patterns and pitfalls. *Clin. Radiol.*, 42: 75–9.
Kottra J.J. & Dunnick N.R. (1996) Retroperitoneal fibrosis. *Radiol. Clin. North Am.*, 34(6): 1259–75.
Vivas I., Nicolas A.I., Velazquez P. *et al.* (2000) Retroperitoneal fibrosis: typical and atypical manifestations. *Br. J. Radiol.*, 73: 214–22.

8.33 FILLING DEFECT IN THE BLADDER (IN THE WALL OR IN THE LUMEN)

1. **Prostate.**
2. **Neoplasm** — especially transitional cell carcinoma in an adult and rhabdomyosarcoma in a child.
3. **Blood clot.**
4. **Instrument** — urethral or suprapubic catheter.
5. **Calculus.**
6. **Ureterocoele.**
7. **Schistosomiasis.**
8. **Endometriosis.**

8.34 BLADDER CALCIFICATION

IN THE LUMEN

1. **Calculus.**
2. **Foreign body** — encrustation of the balloon of a Foley catheter.

IN THE WALL

1. **Transitional and squamous cell carcinoma** — radiographic incidence about 0.5%. Usually surface calcification which may be linear, curvilinear or stippled. Punctate calcification of a villous tumour may suggest chronicity. No extravesical calcification.
2. **Schistosomiasis** — an infrequent cause in the Western hemisphere but the commonest cause of mural calcification worldwide. Thin curvilinear calcification outlines a bladder of normal size and shape. Calcification spreads proximally to involve the distal ureters (appearing as two parallel lines) in 15%.
3. **Tuberculosis** — rare and usually accompanied by calcification elsewhere in the urogenital tract. Unlike schistosomiasis, the disease begins in the kidney and spreads distally. Contracted bladder.
4. **Cyclophosphamide-induced cystitis.**

Further Reading

Pollack H.M., Banner M.P., Martinez L.O. *et al.* (1986) Diagnostic considerations in urinary bladder wall calcification. *Am. J. Roentgenol.,* 136: 791–7.

8.35 BLADDER FISTULA

CONGENITAL

1. **Ectopia vesicae.**
2. **Imperforate anus** — high type.
3. **Patent urachus.**

INFLAMMATORY

1. **Diverticular disease.**
2. **Crohn's disease*.**
3. **Appendix abscess** — and other pelvic sepsis.

NEOPLASTIC

1. **Carcinoma of the colon, bladder or reproductive organs.**
2. **Radiotherapy.**

TRAUMA

1. **Accidental.**
2. **Iatrogenic** — particularly in obstetrics and gynaecology.

8.36 BLADDER OUTFLOW OBSTRUCTION IN A CHILD

1. Distended bladder with incomplete emptying.
2. ± Bilateral upper tract dilatation.
3. ± Upper tract cystic disease.

CAUSES (FROM PROXIMAL TO DISTAL)

1. **Vesical diverticulum** — posteriorly behind the bladder base. It fills during micturition and compresses the bladder neck and proximal urethra. More common in males.
2. **(Bladder neck obstruction** — probably not a distinct entity and only occurs as part of other problems such as ectopic ureterocoele and rhabdomyosarcoma.)
3. **Ectopic ureterocoele** — 80% are associated with the upper moiety of a duplex kidney. 15% are bilateral. More common in

females. Opens into the urethra, bladder neck or vestibule. May be largely outside the bladder and the bladder base may be elevated. 'Drooping flower' appearance of lower moiety. May prolapse into the urethra.

4. **Posterior urethral valves** — posterior urethra is dilated and the distal urethra is small. Almost exclusively males.
5. **Urethral stricture** — post-traumatic strictures are most commonly at the penoscrotal junction and follow previous instrumentation or catheterization.
6. **Anterior urethral diverticulum** — a saccular wide-necked, ventral expansion of the anterior urethra, usually at the penoscrotal junction. The proximal lip of the diverticulum may show as an arcuate filling defect and during micturition the diverticulum expands with urine and obstructs the urethra.
7. **Prune-belly syndrome** — almost exclusively males. High mortality. Bilateral hydronephrosis and hydroureters with a distended bladder are associated with undescended testes, hypoplasia of the anterior abdominal wall and urethral obstruction.
8. **Calculus or foreign body.**
9. **Meatal stenosis** } clinical diagnosis.
10. **Phimosis** }

NB. The commonest cause in males is posterior urethral valves and in females is ectopic ureterocoele.

8.37 CALCIFICATION OF THE SEMINAL VESICLES OR VAS DEFERENS

1. **Diabetes mellitus** — the cause in the vast majority of cases.
2. **Chronic infection** — tuberculosis, schistosomiasis, chronic urinary tract infection and syphilis.
3. **Idiopathic.**

Further Reading

King J.C. & Rosenbaum H.D. (1971) Calcification of the vasa deferentia in non-diabetes. *Radiology*, 100: 603–6.

8.38 ULTRASOUND OF THE TESTES AND SCROTUM

TESTICULAR

Neoplastic

Colour Doppler does not accurately differentiate neoplasm from acute inflammation or benign from malignant tumours.

1. **Germ cell tumours** — 95% of primary testicular tumours. 40% are of mixed histology. 8% are bilateral.
   (a) *Seminoma* — most common testicular tumour in the adult. 40–50% of testicular germ cell tumours. 25% have metastases at presentation. Most common tumour in the undescended testis. A solid, homogeneous, hypoechoic, round or oval mass which is sharply delineated from normal testicular tissue.
   (b) *Embryonal carcinoma* — 20–25% of germ cell tumours. More aggressive than seminoma and more heterogeneous because of necrosis, haemorrhage, cysts and calcification.
   (c) *Choriocarcinoma* — rare.
   (d) *Teratoma* — 5–10% and most common in infants and children. Heterogeneous echo texture because of the different tissue elements present.
2. **Non-germ cell tumours** — usually benign. May secrete oestrogens (Sertoli cell) or testosterone (Leydig cell). Non-specific appearance but usually solid hypoechoic mass ± cystic areas.
3. **Metastases** — kidney, prostate, bronchus, pancreas. More common than germ cell tumours in the over 50-year age group. Patients with leukaemia or lymphoma may relapse in the testis and present as focal or diffuse decreased echogenicity in an enlarged testis.

Vascular

1. **Testicular torsion**
   (a) *Acute* — presentation within 24 hours.
   Enlarged hypoechoic or heterogeneous testis ± hydrocoele and enlargement of the epididymis. Colour Doppler: absent testicular flow; normal peritesticular flow.
   (b) *Subacute or missed* — presentation at 1–10 days.
   Colour Doppler: absent testicular flow; increased peritesticular flow.

(c) *Spontaneous detorsion*
Colour Doppler: normal or increased testicular flow; increased peritesticular flow.

Inflammatory

1. **Orchitis** — Generalized testicular swelling and hypoechogenicity, initially; progresses to patch focal low reflectivity. Hypoechoic areas are hypervascular. There may be swelling of the epididymis, hydrocoele and scrotal wall oedema. Complications occur in 50% — abscess formation, necrosis, haematoma and testicular atrophy.
2. **Abscess** — complicating epididymo-orchitis, often in a diabetic patient or those with mumps. Hypoechoic or mixed echogenic mass.

Idiopathic non-neoplastic cysts

1. **Tunica albuginea cyst** — 2–5 mm; typically in the upper anterior or lateral part of the testis; unilocular or multilocular.
2. **Simple cyst** — > 40 years of age; 2–20 mm; usually solitary and most are located near the mediastinum.

EXTRATESTICULAR

Inflammatory

1. **Epididymitis** — enlarged, hypoechoic, hypervascular epididymis with a hydrocoele and skin thickening. Normal testis in the absence of orchitis but frequently coexists with orchitis.

Idiopathic

1. **Hydrocoele** — fluid collection anterolaterally in the scrotum.
   (a) Congenital — due to persistence of the processus vaginalis.
   (b) Infantile — accumulation of fluid along the processus vaginalis but with no communication with the abdominal cavity.
   (c) Secondary to trauma, infection, torsion or neoplasm.

VASCULAR

1. **Varicocoele** — dilated pampiniform plexus of veins posterior to the testis. In 15% of adult males and virtually always on the left side. Important to exclude a compressive retroperitoneal aetiology if the varicocoele is right-sided or does not decompress in the erect position or with a Valsalva manoeuvre.

NEOPLASTIC

1. **Adenomatoid tumour of the epididymis** — a benign tumour which accounts for 30% of extratesticular tumours. Other tumours are varied and uncommon.

Further Reading

Atchley J.T. & Dewbury K.C. (2000) Ultrasound appearances of testicular epidermoid cysts. *Clin. Radiol.*, 55: 493–502.
Cook J.L. & Dewbury K. (2000) The changes seen on high-resolution ultrasound in orchitis. *Clin. Radiol.*, 55: 13–18.
Dogra V.S., Gottlieb R.H., Rubens D.J. *et al.* (2001) Benign intratesticular cystic lesions: US features. *RadioGraphics*, 21: S273–81.
Howlett D.C., Marchbank N.D. & Sallomi D.F. (2000) Ultrasound of the testis. *Clin. Radiol.*, 55: 595–601.
Sidhu P.S. (1999) Clinical and imaging features of testicular torsion: role of ultrasound. *Clin. Radiol.*, 54: 343–52.
Siegel M.J. (1997) The acute scrotum. *Radiol. Clin. North Am.*, 35(4): 959–76.
Strauss S., Gottlieb P., Kessler A. *et al.* (2000) Non-neoplastic intratesticular lesions mimicking tumour on ultrasound. *Eur. Radiol.*, 10: 1628–35.

9 Soft tissues

9.1 GYNAECOMASTIA

PHYSIOLOGICAL

1. **Neonatal** — due to high placental oestrogens.
2. **Pubertal** — due to an excess of oestradiol over testosterone.
3. **Senile** — due to falling androgen and rising oestrogen levels with age.

PHARMACOLOGICAL

1. **Oestrogen** — especially in the treatment of carcinoma of the prostate.
2. **Digitalis** — binds to oestrogen receptors.
3. **Anti-cancer drugs** — producing testicular damage.
4. **Anti-androgens** — spironolactone.
5. **Reserpine.**
6. **Phenothiazines.**
7. **Tricyclic antidepressants.**
8. **Methyldopa.**

PATHOLOGICAL

1. **Carcinoma of the bronchus** } secreting human
2. **Teratoma of the testis** } chorionic gonadotrophin.
3. **Cirrhosis** — due to increased conversion of androgens to oestrogens.
4. **Hypogonadism** — e.g. Klinefelter's syndrome and castration.
5. **Hypopituitarism** — including acromegaly.
6. **Testicular feminization** — androgen insensitivity.
7. **Adrenal tumours** } secreting
8. **Leydig cell tumours** } oestrogens.

9.2 LINEAR AND CURVILINEAR CALCIFICATION IN SOFT TISSUES

ARTERIAL

1. **Atheroma/aneurysm.**
2. **Diabetes.**
3. **Hyperparathyroidism*** — more common in secondary than primary.
4. **Werner's syndrome** — premature ageing in a Jewish diabetic (male or female).

NERVE

1. **Leprosy.**
2. **Neurofibromatosis*.**

LIGAMENT

1. **Tendonitis** — Pellegrini–Stieda syndrome, supraspinatus.
2. **Ankylosing spondylitis*.**
3. **Fluorosis.**
4. **Diabetes.**
5. **Alkaptonuria.**

BISMUTH INJECTION

In the buttocks. ± Neuropathic joints.

PARASITES

1. Cysticerci 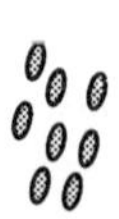 — oval with lucent centre. Often arranged in the direction of muscle fibres.
2. Guinea worm 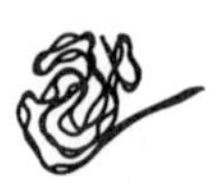 — irregular coiled appearance.

3. Loa loa 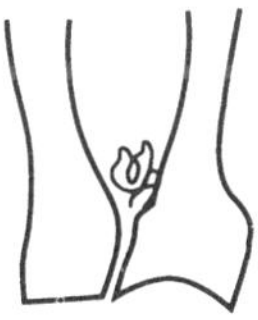 — thread-like coil. Particularly in the web spaces of the hand.

4. Armillifer 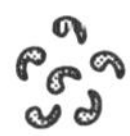 — 'comma'-shaped. Only in trunk muscles.

See also 9.4.

Further Reading

Rahalkar M.D., Shetty D.D., Kelkar A.B. *et al.* (2000) The many faces of cysticercosis. *Clin. Radiol.*, 55: 668–74.

9.3 CONGLOMERATE CALCIFICATION IN SOFT TISSUES

COLLAGENOSES

1. **Scleroderma*** — acrolysis and flexion contractures in the hands.
2. **Dermatomyositis.**
3. **Ehlers–Danlos syndrome.**

METABOLIC

1. **Hyperparathyroidism*** — more common in secondary hyperparathyroidism. Vascular calcification is common.
2. **Gout*** — calcified tophus.

TRAUMATIC

1. **Haematoma.**
2. **Burns.**
3. **Myositis ossificans** — outer part is more densely calcified than the centre.
4. **Calcifying myonecrosis.**

INFECTIVE

1. **Tuberculous abscess/node.**

NEOPLASTIC

1. **Benign**
   (a) Parosteal lipoma — lucent. ± Pressure erosion of adjacent bone.
   (b) Haemangioma — Suspect if phleboliths present in an unusual site. ± Soft-tissue mass with adjacent bone destruction.
2. **Malignant**
   (a) Parosteal osteosarcoma — age 20–40 years. Lobulated calcification around a metaphysis. Inner part is more densely calcified than the periphery. Early — a thin lucent line may separate it from underlying bone.
   (b) Extraskeletal osteosarcoma*.
   (c) Synovial sarcoma.

9.4 'SHEETS' OF CALCIFICATION/OSSIFICATION IN SOFT TISSUES

1. **Congenital myositis ossificans progressiva** — manifest in childhood. Initially neck and trunk muscles involved. Short first metacarpal and metatarsal.
2. **Dermatomyositis.**

9.5 PERIARTICULAR SOFT-TISSUE CALCIFICATION

INFLAMMATORY

1. **Scleroderma*** — ± Acro-osteolysis.
2. **Dermatomyositis.**
3. **Gout*** — calcified tophi. Punched-out erosions.
4. **Bursitis** — can be dense and lobulated.

DEGENERATIVE

1. **Calcific periarthritis (calcium hydroxyapatite deposition disease).**
2. **Calcium pyrophosphate deposition disease*.**

RENAL FAILURE

1. **Secondary hyperparathyroidism** — ± vascular calcification.
2. **Treatment with 1-α-OHD_3** — particularly shoulder, hip and metacarpophalangeal joints.

HYPERCALCAEMIA

1. **Sarcoidosis*** — rare. Affects hands and feet. ± Lace-like trabecular pattern in tubular bones.
2. **Hypervitaminosis D.**
3. **Milk-alkali syndrome.**

NEOPLASTIC

1. **Synovial osteochondromatosis** — age 20–50 years. Most commonly affects a large joint. Multiple calcified loose bodies. ± Secondary degenerative changes or pressure erosion of bone.
2. **Synovial sarcoma** — age 20–50 years. Soft-tissue mass with amorphous calcification, irregular bone destruction and osteoporosis.

IDIOPATHIC

1. **Tumoral calcinosis** — age 20–30 years. Adjacent to a major joint. Firm, non-tender, moveable mass which is well-defined, lobulated and calcified on X-ray. Osseous involvement is rare. ± Calcium fluid level.

9.6 SOFT-TISSUE OSSIFICATION

TRAUMATIC

1. **Myositis ossificans.**
2. **Burns.**
3. **Neurogenic** — paraplegia and post-comatose states.

NEOPLASTIC

1. **Synovial sarcoma.**
2. **Parosteal osteosarcoma.**
3. **Liposarcoma.**

IDIOPATHIC

1. **Fibrodysplasia ossificans progressiva.**

9.7 CT OF SWOLLEN LEGS

1. **Normal** — homogeneous subcutaneous fat containing superficial veins. Interstitial tissue not visible.
2. **Venous thrombosis and insufficiency** — increased cross-sectional areas of muscle and subcutaneous fat. Prominent interstitial tissues in the subcutaneous fat.
3. **Lymphoedema** — increased subcutaneous fat with visible interstitial tissue and skin thickening. When secondary to malignant pelvic lymphadenopathy, pelvic CT may give additional positive findings.
4. **Haematoma** — variable high attenuation dependent on the age of the haematoma.
5. **Popliteal cyst** — water density fluid collection between the medial head of gastrocnemius and soleus muscles.

Further Reading

Vaughan B.F. (1990) CT of swollen legs. *Clin. Radiol.*, 41: 24–30.

10 Breast disease and mammography

Michael Collins

10.1 INTRODUCTION

Modern mammography demands meticulously high standards in all its aspects. These include X-ray equipment, radiographic technique, film–screen combinations, processing, viewing conditions and interpretation. Shortcomings in any of these factors will lead to serious errors. Other factors that lead to difficulty include dense parenchymal background that may obscure malignancy, benign conditions that mimic malignancy, and malignant tumours with 'benign' appearances on mammography. The radiologist now has a central role in the management of breast disease and should have use of all facilities to ensure accurate diagnosis, including mammography, ultrasound and biopsy/localization techniques.

Close co-operation between radiologists, radiographers, surgeons and pathologists is essential.

Further Reading

Bassett L.W. (2000) Imaging of breast masses. *Radiol. Clin. North Am.*, 38(4) 669–91.

Orel S.G. & Schnall M.D. (2001) MR imaging of the breast for detection, diagnosis and staging of breast cancer. *Radiology,* 220:13–30.

Tabar L., Vitak B., Chen H.H. *et al.* (2000) The Swedish two county trial twenty years later. Updated mortality results and new insights from long term follow-up. *Radiol. Clin. North Am.*, 38(4): 625–51.

10.2 THE NORMAL BREAST

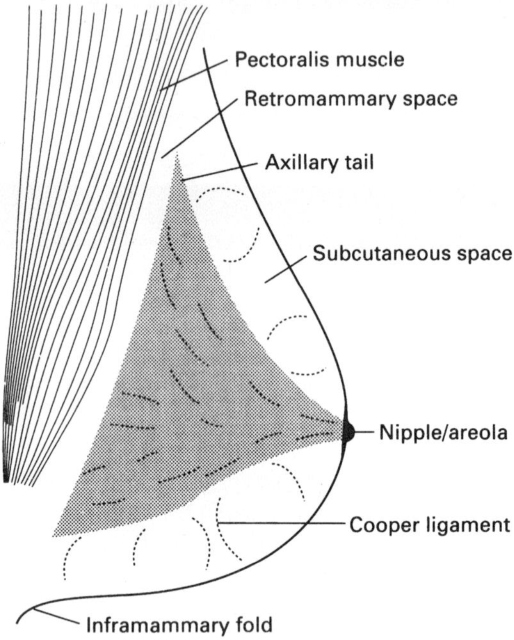

Normal lateral oblique projection

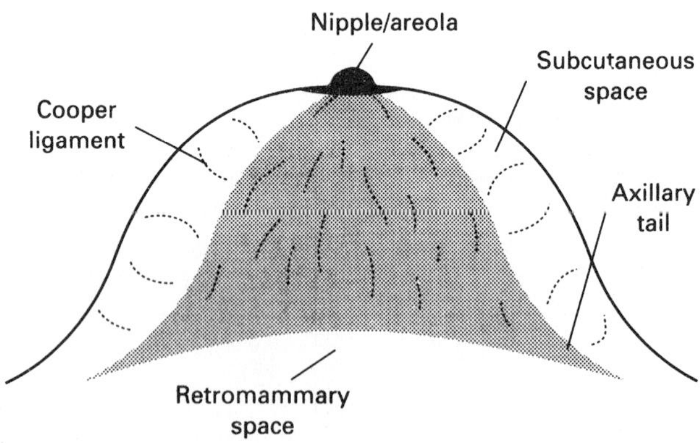

Normal craniocaudal projection

10.3 BENIGN v. MALIGNANT

1. **Opacity**	Smooth margin	Ill-defined margin — stellate, spiculated, comet tail.
	Low density	High density
	Homogeneous	Inhomogeneous
	Thin 'halo'	Wide 'halo'
2. **Calcification**		see 10.4
3. **Surrounding parenchyma**	Normal	Disrupted
4. **Nipple/areola**	± Retracted	± Retracted
5. **Skin**	Normal	Thickened
6. **Cooper ligaments**	Normal	Thickened, increased number
7. **Ducts**	Normal	Focal dilatation
8. **Subcutaneous/ retromammarty space**	Normal	Obliterated

NB. The above distinguishing features are not invariable and may be found in 'classic cases' only

10.4 CALCIFICATION

1. Microcalcification is defined as individual calcific opacities measuring < 0.5 mm in diameter.
2. Macrocalcification: opacities > 0.5 mm in diameter.
3. Microcalcification is not specific to carcinoma.
4. Microcalcification is seen in 30–40% of carcinomas on mammography.
5. Macrocalcification may be found in carcinoma.

DEFINITELY BENIGN (see figure, p. 367)

1. Arterial — tortuous, tramline.
2. Smooth, widely separated, some with radiolucent centre.
3. Linear thick, rod-like, widespread, some with radiolucent centre.
4. 'Egg-shell' curvilinear: margin of cyst, fat necrosis.
5. 'Pop-corn' in fibroadenoma.
6. Large individual calcific opacity > 2 mm, e.g. involutional fibroadenoma.
7. 'Floating' calcification — seen as calcific/fluid level on lateral oblique projection in 'milk of calcium' cysts.

PROBABLY BENIGN

1. Widespread — all one/both breasts.
2. Macrocalcification of one size.
3. Symmetrical distribution.
4. Widely separated opacities.
5. Superficial distribution.
6. Normal parenchyma.

POSSIBLY MALIGNANT – biopsy indicated – see microcalcification figure

1. Microcalcification — particularly segmental, cluster distribution (> 5 particles in 1.0 cm^3 space; of these 30% will be malignant).
2. Mixture of sizes and shapes — linear, branching, punctate.
3. Associated suspicious soft-tissue opacity.
4. Microcalcification eccentrically located in soft-tissue mass.
5. Deterioration on serial mammography.

Examples of definitely benign calcification

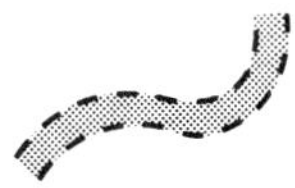

1. Arterial

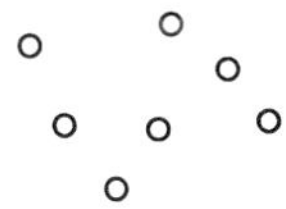

2. Smooth ± lucent centre widely separated

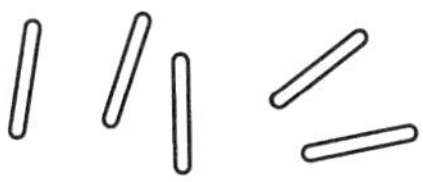

3. Linear, thick, rod-like ± lucent centres

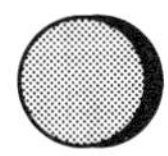

4 'Egg-shell'

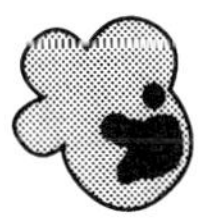

5. 'Pop-corn'

6. Large calcific opacity

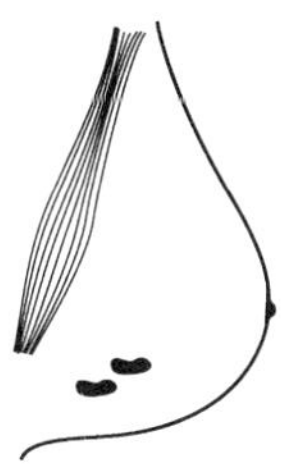

7. Floating calcification

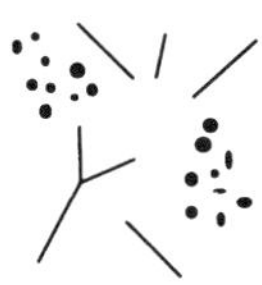

Microcalcification; mixture of sizes, shapes, cluster, haphazard arrangement, linear branching patterns

Further Reading

Hogge J.P., Robinson R.E., Magnant C.M. *et al.* (1995) The mammographic spectrum of fat necrosis of the breast. *RadioGraphics,* 15: 1347–56.

Monsees B.S. (1995) Evaluation of breast microcalcifications. *Radiol., Clin. North Am.,* 33(6): 1109–21.

Sickles E.A. (1986) Breast calcification: mammographic evaluation. *Radiology,* 160: 289–93.

10.5 DISAPPEARANCE OF CALCIFICATION

1. **Surgery.**
2. **Radiotherapy.**
3. **Chemotherapy.**
4. **Spontaneous.**

10.6 BENIGN LESIONS WITH TYPICAL APPEARANCES

1. **Lipoma** — large, rounded, radiolucent, well-defined with compression of adjacent parenchyma.
2. **Fibroadenoma** — rounded, lobulated, well-defined homogeneously dense soft-tissue opacity with eccentrically sited 'pop-corn' calcification.
3. **Intramammary lymph node** — well-defined, usually approximately 1.0 cm in diameter soft-tissue opacity, often with an eccentric radiolucency situated in the upper outer quadrant of the breast.
4. **Lipid cyst** — well-defined, multiplc, lucent, 'egg-shell' calcification.

10.7 SINGLE WELL-DEFINED SOFT-TISSUE OPACITY

BENIGN

1. **Cyst.**
2. **Fibroadenoma.**
3. **Intramammary lymph node.**
4. **Skin lesion.**
5. **Papilloma.**
6. **Nipple not in profile.**
7. **Galactocoele.**
8. **Hamartoma.**

MALIGNANT

1. **Cystosarcoma phylloides** — usually large, may be benign but have malignant potential.
2. **Carcinoma** — a small group of carcinomas look 'benign' on mammography, medullary, encephaloid, mucoid, papillary.

NB. Any well-defined opacity > 1.0 cm in diameter should be subjected to ultrasound; if solid, biopsy should be performed.

10.8 MULTIPLE WELL-DEFINED SOFT-TISSUE OPACITIES

1. **Cysts.**
2. **Fibroadenomas** — 10–20% are multiple.
3. **Skin lesions** — e.g. neurofibromas.
4. **Silicone injections** — usually dense.
5. **Intramammary lymph nodes.**
6. **Metastases** — lymphoma, lung, ovarian carcinoma and melanoma are common primary lesions.

10.9 LARGE (> 5 CM) WELL-DEFINED OPACITY

1. **Giant cyst.**
2. **Giant fibroadenoma.**
3. **Lipoma.**
4. **Sebaceous cyst.**
5. **Cystosarcoma phylloides.**

10.10 BENIGN CONDITIONS THAT MIMIC MALIGNANCY

1. **Microcalcification**
   (a) Sclerosing adenosis: one/both breasts, widely separated opacities.
2. **Suspicious soft-tissue opacity**
   (a) Fibroadenoma — when one margin ill-defined.
   (b) Fat necrosis — ill-defined, sometimes with radiolucent centre.
   (c) Post-biopsy scar.
   (d) Radial scar.
   (e) Plasma cell mastitis.
   (f) Haematoma.
   (g) Summation of normal tissues.
   (h) Irregular skin lesion, e.g. wart.

10.11 CARCINOMA

PRIMARY FEATURES

1. **Opacity** — ill-defined, spiculated outline, comet tail. Usually dense.
2. **Microcalcification** — mixture of sizes, shapes; linear, branching, punctate cluster arrangement. Eccentric to and/or outside soft-tissue opacity.

SECONDARY FEATURES

1. **Distortion** — adjacent tissues, obliteration subcutaneous, retromammary spaces.
2. **Skin, nipple retraction.**
3. **Oedema** — all or part of breast.
4. **Halo** — wide around primary opacity.
5. **Duct dilatation.**
6. **Venous engorgement.**

NB. Approximately 10% of palpable carcinomas in premenopausal women are not diagnosable on mammography.

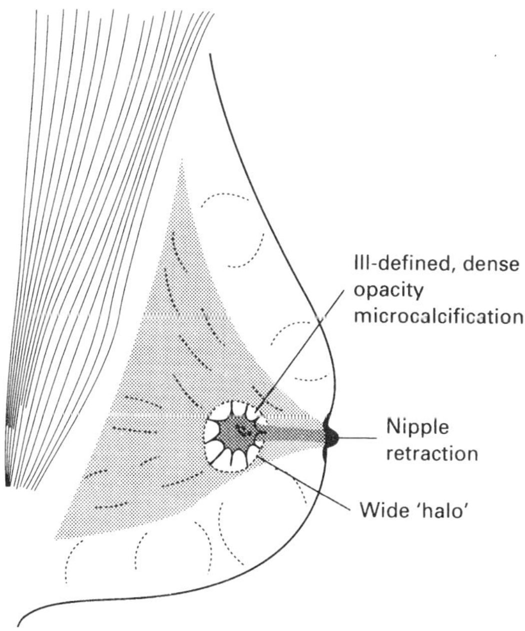

10.12 OEDEMATOUS BREAST

SIGNS ON MAMMOGRAPHY

1. Diffuse increased density.
2. Skin thickening (> 1.5 mm).
3. Coarse reticular pattern.
4. Prominent Cooper ligaments.

CAUSES

1. Inflammatory carcinoma.
2. Radiotherapy.
3. Lymphatic obstruction.
4. Venous obstruction.
5. Recent surgery.
6. Breast abscess.

10.13 ULTRASOUND IN BREAST DISEASE

USES AND INDICATIONS

1. Dense parenchyma in young women.
2. Breast tenderness (compression for mammography not possible).
3. Breast implant (mammography not useful).
4. Equivocal mammography, biopsy.
5. Biopsy, localization guidance.

TYPICAL APPEARANCES OF CARCINOMA

1. Poorly reflective mass.
2. Ill-defined mass.
3. Heterogeneous internal echo pattern.
4. Absent 'far wall' echoes.
5. Posterior acoustic shadowing.

TYPICAL APPEARANCES OF SIMPLE CYSTS

1. Round, oval in shape.
2. Well-defined.
3. Anechoic (echo-free).
4. Posterior wall enhancement.
5. Posterior acoustic enhancement.

TYPICAL APPEARANCES OF FIBROADENOMA

1. Rounded or oval (may be lobulated).
2. Poorly reflective.
3. Homogeneous echo pattern.
4. Variable posterior echo pattern.

Further Reading

Baker J.A., Soo M.S. & Rosen E.L. (2001) Artifacts and pitfalls in sonographic imaging of the breast. *Am. J. Roentgenol.*, 176: 1261–6.

Lister D., Evans A.J., Burrell H.C. *et al.* (1998) The accuracy of breast ultrasound in the evaluation of clinically benign, discrete symptomatic breast lumps. *Clin. Radiol.*, 53: 490–2.

Smith D.N. (2001) Breast ultrasound. *Radiol. Clin. North Am.*, 39(3): 485–97.

11 Face and neck

11.1 ORBITAL MASS LESIONS

Classify by site in relation to the muscle cone. Axial sections suffice in most cases, but coronal sections are useful for muscle cone lesions and abscesses. Most orbital lesions enhance following the administration of contrast medium so this is not a useful means of discrimination.

WITHIN OR INVOLVING THE GLOBE

1. **Retinoblastoma** — the most important ocular tumour of childhood. Incidence of 1:20 000 live births. Four types have been recognized:
   (a) Those that are non-inheritable.
   (b) Those that are inherited as an AD trait.
   (c) Those that are associated with a partial deletion of chromosome 13.
   (d) Bilateral retinoblastoma and pineal tumour — so-called trilateral retinoblastoma.

Most children present with leukokoria or white pupillary reflex. 20–40% of patients have bilateral tumours and this is most often the AD type. 5–10% of patients have a family history of retinoblastoma.

Over 90% of tumours show calcification on CT which may be small, large, single or multiple. Diffuse infiltrating tumours are less likely to show calcification. Intraocular calcification in children under 3 years of age is highly suggestive of retinoblastoma.

The non-calcified component of the tumour is moderately dense on CT, enhances poorly or not at all, and may be difficult to differentiate from the associated retinal detachment and subretinal effusion. The presence of enhancement excludes subretinal exudate and haemorrhage while marked enhancement suggests persistent hyperplastic primary vitreous (PHPV) (see 11.3).

On MRI, the tumour is slightly/moderately hyperintense on T_1W and moderately low intensity on T_2W. The tumour enhances following i.v. gadolinium.

Children with the hereditary form are at risk of developing second non-ocular malignancies, either within or out of the radiation field. Osteosarcoma is the commonest tumour.

2. **Melanoma** — increases in frequency after middle age. Lentiform mass related to the choroid. Contrast-enhancing. High signal on T_1W MRI if melanotic. May invade outside the globe.
3. **Detachment and choroidal effusion** — may mimic melanoma.

WITHIN THE MUSCLE CONE (INTRACONAL)

1. **Optic nerve glioma** — see 11.2 and 11.4. Visual loss and painless with preservation of eye movements because the lesion is intraconal. There may also be other soft-tissue neurofibromas visible on the images. It should be remembered that patients with neurofibromas may have other causes of proptosis such as sphenoid wing dysplasia.
2. **Optic nerve meningioma** — see 11.4.
3. **Haemangioma (usually cavernous) and arteriovenous malformation** — an enhancing mass but usually not seen on angiography, except for the relatively rare AVM.
4. **Inflammatory orbital pseudotumour** — an enhancing soft-tissue mass which may involve the muscle cone or optic nerve.
5. **Lymphoma and metastases.**
6. **Haematoma** — most are intraconal.
7. **Neurofibroma** — rare.

ARISING FROM THE MUSCLE CONE

1. **Inflammatory orbital pseudotumour.**
2. **Dysthyroid ophthalmopathy** — muscle tendons are spared.
3. **Rhabdomyosarcoma** — 10% arise in the orbit. The single most important cause of primary orbital malignancy in children. 50% are less than 7 years of age. Rapid onset of proptosis, usually with lateral deviation of the eye, as anteromedial or superomedial points of origin are most common. Vision is preserved. The tumour is closely related to the paranasal sinuses and, though extension out of the orbit anteriorly and medially is not uncommon, most tumours lie preseptally or extraconally and extension backwards into the brain is not common. It is important to differentiate between a primary orbital location and a parameningeal location (defined as a tumour close enough to the meninges to permit intracranial spread of tumour), because therapy differs.

OUTSIDE THE MUSCLE CONE (EXTRACONAL)

1. **Orbital cellulitis and abscess** — contrast-enhanced study may show the abscess cavity outlined by an enhancing wall; coronal sections should be performed if possible.
2. **Lymphoma and metastases.**
3. **Dermoid and teratoma** — mixed tissue densities on CT. Most common in the lateral aspect of the orbit. Majority associated with localized bone changes. Most cysts have a wall with no soft-tissue component outside the cyst.
4. **Lymphangioma, lymphohaemangioma** — tumours of childhood. See 11.2.
5. **Spread from lacrimal gland tumours.**

ARISING FROM THE ORBITAL WALL

1. **Metastases and lymphoma.**
2. **Langerhans cell histiocytosis*.**
3. **Invasion by ethmoidal or maxillary antral tumours.**
4. **Ethmoidal mucocoele.**
5. **Spread of ethmoidal or antral infection.**

Further Reading

Bilaniuk L.T. (1999) Orbital vascular lesions. Role of imaging. *Radiol. Clin. North Am.*, 37(1): 169–83.

Chawda S.J. & Moseley I.F. (1999) Computed tomography of orbital dermoids: a 20-year review. *Clin. Radiol.*, 54: 821–5.

Dobben G.D., Philip B., Mafee M.F. *et al.* (1998) Orbital subperiosteal hematoma, cholesterol granuloma, and infection. *Radiol. Clin. North Am.*, 36(6): 1185–1200.

Flanders A.E., Espinosa G.A., Markiewicz D.A. *et al.* (1987) Orbital lymphoma. Role of CT and MRI. *Radiol. Clin. North Am.*, 25 (3): 601–13.

Kaste S.C., Jenkins J.J. III, Pratt C.B. *et al.* (2000) Retinoblastoma: sonographic findings with pathologic correlation in paediatric patients. *Am. J. Roentgenol.*, 175: 495–501.

Kaufman L.M., Mafee M.F. & Song C.D. (1998) Retinoblastoma and simulating lesions. Role of CT, MR imaging and use of Gd-DTPA contrast enhancement. *Radiol. Clin. North Am.*, 36: 1101–17.

Mafee M.F., Pai E. & Philip B. (1998) Rhabdomyosarcoma of the orbit. Evaluation with MR imaging and CT. *Radiol. Clin. North Am.*, 36(6): 1215–27.

Price H. & Danziger A. (1979) The computerised tomographic findings in paediatric orbital tumours. *Clin. Radiol.*, 30: 435–40.

Sohaib S.A., Moseley I. & Wright J.E (1998) Orbital rhabdomyosarcoma — the radiological characteristics. *Clin. Radiol.*, 53: 357–62.

Weber A.L., Romo L.V. & Sabates N.R. (1999) Pseudotumour of the orbit. *Radiol. Clin. North Am.*, 37(1): 151–68.

112 FEATURES OF ORBITAL MASSES IN CHILDREN
CT CHARACTERISTICS OF ORBITAL MASSES IN CHILDREN

	Clinical features	*Age*	*Location*							*Extension*		*CT*		*MRI signal intensities*	
			Preseptal	Extraconal	Intraconal	Muscle only	Orbital expansion	Bone destruction	Calcification	Intracranial	Facial	Attenuation	Enhancement	T_1W	T_2W
Optic nerve glioma	Visual loss; painless proptopsis; occasionally bilateral, especially in neurofibromatosis	< 10 y; (50% < 5 y)	–	–	++	–	+	–	–	+	–	Isodense ± central lucencies	++	↓	↑
Rhabdomyo-sarcoma	Rapid unilateral proptosis ± lid swelling; vision is preserved; may be parameningeal spread	90% < 16 y	++	++	+	+	–	++	–	++	++	Isodense or increased	++	↓	↑
2° Neuro-blastoma	Proptosis and orbital ecchymosis. Diagnosis known in 90%	< 4 y	+	++	–	–	–	++	++	++	+	Isodense or increased	++	↓	↑
Leukaemia	Proptosis, lid oedema, pain, chemosis. May be bilateral. ± Haemorrhage. Chloroma describes focal tumour deposits, usually in AML	> 10 y	++	++	++	++	–	+	+	+	–	Increased	++	↓	↑
Lymphoma	Usually Burkitt type and bilateral	> 10 y	++	++	+	–	–	+	–	+	+	Increased	++	Homogeneous ↓	Homogeneous ↑

	Clinical features	Age	Location							Extension		CT		MRI signal intensities	
			Preseptal	Extraconal	Intraconal	Muscle only	Orbital expansion	Bone destruction	Calcification	Intracranial	Facial	Attenuation	Enhancement	T_1W	T_2W
Haemangioma	Increase in size followed by regression. 30% have cutaneous naevus	0–3 m	++	++	++	–	+	–	+	+	+	Mixed	++	Heterogeneous ↓	Heterogeneous ↑
Lymphangioma	Variable proptosis. Lids and conjunctiva. No spontaneous resolution. May haemorrhage	0–10 y	++	++	+	–	++	–	+	–	+	Mixed low	+	Heterogeneous ↓	Heterogeneous ↑
Dermoid	Usually upper, outer orbital margin but may be deep	Newborn	++	++	+	–	+	–	+	–	–	Low	–	↑	↑
Cellulitis	Pain; fever; sinus disease	Any age	++	++	+	–	–		–	+	++	Isodense or low	++	↓	↑
Pseudotumour	Painful proptosis; malaise; lid swelling; chemosis; may be recurrent	Any age	++	++	++	++	–	–	–	+	–	Isodense	++	↓	↓

Modified from Lallemand *et al.*

– not present; + uncommon; ++ common. ↑ increased; ↓ decreased.

Further Reading

Kaufman L.M., Villablanca J.P. & Mafee M.F (1998) Diagnostic imaging of cystic lesions in the child's orbit. *Radiol. Clin. North Am.,* 36(6): 1149–63.

Lallemand D.P., Brasch R.C., Char D.H. *et al.* (1984) Orbital tumours in children. Characterisation by computed tomography. *Radiology,* 151: 85–8.

Mafee M.F., Pai E. & Philip B. (1998) Rhabdomyosarcoma of the orbit — evaluation with MR imaging and CT. *Radiol. Clin. North Am.,* 36: 1215–27.

McHugh K. & Boothroyd A.E. (1999) The role of radiology in childhood rhabdomyosarcoma. *Clin. Radiol.,* 54: 2–10.

11.3 DIFFERENTIAL DIAGNOSIS OF RETINOBLASTOMA

More than 50% of children presenting with a clinical diagnosis of retinoblastoma may have another diagnosis. Ocular toxocariasis, PHPV and Coat's disease are the three commonest conditions confused with retinoblastoma. Under the age of 3 years, which is when retinoblastoma usually presents, none of the conditions shown in the table show calcification, but above that age some, e.g. retinal astrocytoma, retrolental fibroplasia and toxocariasis, may do so.

	Clinical features	*Age*	*Radiology*
Persistent hyperplastic primary vitreous	Unilateral leukokoria	At or soon after birth	Microphthalmia. Small irregular lens; shallow anterior chamber. No calcification. Increased attenuation of the vitreous. Enhancement of abnormal intravitreal tissue. Triangular retrolental density with its apex on the posterior lens and base on the posterior globe. Fluid level on decubitus scanning
Coat's disease	A vascular anomaly of telangiectatic vessels which leak proteinaceous material into the subretinal space. Usually boys; unilateral. Present at birth but usually asymptomatic until the retina detaches and vision deteriorates	4–8 y	Appearances of retinal detachment. Indistinguishable from non-calcified retinoblastoma on CT. High signal subretinal effusion on T_1W and T_2W MRI

	Clinical features	*Age*	*Radiology*
Retinopathy of prematurity	Uni- or bilateral leukokoria. Appropriate previous medical history of oxygen therapy and prematurity	7–10 weeks	No calcification (but may calcify in the older child). Microphthalmia
Toxocariasis	Close contact with dogs. No systemic symptoms. Positive ELISA test	Mean 6 y	Opaque vitreous or a localized, irregular retinal mass. No contrast enhancement
Chronic retinal detachment	Rare. Presentation late. More common in developmentally abnormal eyes and dysmorphic syndromes		No enhancement or calcification
Retinal astrocytoma (astrocytic hamartoma)	In 40% of patients with tuberous sclerosis or, less commonly, neurofibromatosis, retinitis pigmentosa or as an isolated abnormality		May be bilateral. Multiple, small retinal masses. May calcify in the older child
Retinal dysplasia	Bilateral leukokoria	At or soon after birth	Bilateral retrolental masses. No calcification

Further Reading

Edward D.P, Mafee M.F., Garcia-Valenzuela E. *et al.* (1998) Coat's disease and persistent hyperplastic primary vitreous. *Radiol. Clin. North Am.*, 36(6): 1119–31.

Kaufman L.M., Mafee M.F. & Song C.D. (1998) Retinoblastoma and simulating lesions. Role of CT, MR imaging and use of Gd-DTPA contrast enhancement. *Radiol. Clin. North Am.*, 36: 1101–17.

11.4 OPTIC NERVE GLIOMA V. OPTIC NERVE SHEATH MENINGIOMA. CLINICAL AND RADIOLOGICAL DIFFERENTIATION

Glioma	Meningioma
50% less than 5 years of age.	Usually middle-aged women.
± Bilateral.	Usually unilateral.
Slowly progressive, painless loss of vision; central scotoma. Childhood tumours may remain quiescent for years, particularly in the presence of NF. Adult tumours are aggressive.	Slowly progressive, painless loss of vision; proptosis.
Neurofibromatosis* NF1 in 25%; 15% of NF1 have optic nerve glioma; bilateral disease strongly suggests neurofibromatosis.	Neurofibromatosis (1 or 2) in 4–6%; bilateral disease may occur with or without NF.
No orbital hyperostosis.	Hyperostosis.
Widened optic canal in 90% but intracranial extension is unusual.	Widened optical canal in 10%.
Kinking and buckling of the optic nerve is common. Smooth outline.	Straight optic nerve, but tumour may be eccentric.
Well-defined margins.	More infiltrative. Localized or fusiform thickening.
Calcification rare without prior radiotherapy.	Calcification (linear, plaque-like or granular) are more common.
Isointense to brain on T_1W MRI; hyperintense on T_2W MRI.	Similar signal to optic nerve on most unenhanced MR pulse sequences.
Variable contrast enhancement with mottled lucencies due to mucinous degeneration.	Diffuse homogeneous enhancement ± serrated margins.
	Negative image of optic nerve within the tumour (tram-track sign).

Further Reading

Hollander M.D., FitzPatrick M., O'Connor S.G. *et al.* (1999) Optic gliomas. *Radiol. Clin. North Am.*, 37(1): 59–71.

Mafee M.F., Goodwin J. & Dorodi S. (1999) Optic nerve sheath meningiomas. *Radiol. Clin. North Am.*, 37(1): 37–58.

11.5 ENLARGED ORBIT

Exclude small contralateral orbit, e.g. enucleation as a child.

1. **Neurofibromatosis*** — ± 'bare' orbit due to elevation of the lesser wing of the sphenoid and associated dysplasia.
2. **Congenital glaucoma (buphthalmos)** — asymmetrical enlargement.
3. **Any space-occupying lesion** — if present long enough. The enlargement in children occurs much faster. (See 11.1.)

11.6 'BARE' ORBIT

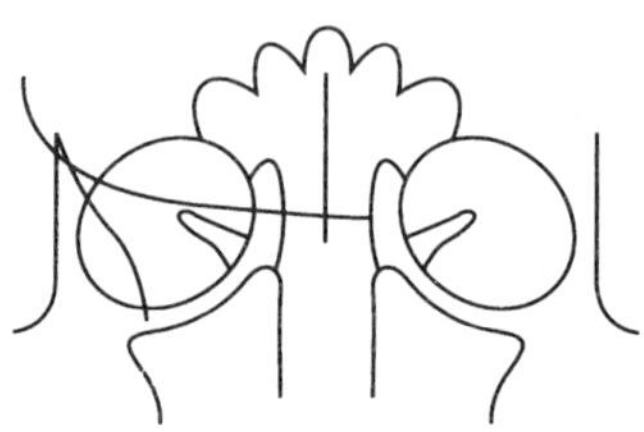

1. **Neurofibromatosis*** — dysplasia of the sphenoid.
2. **Metastasis** — bone destruction.
3. **Meningioma** — adjacent bone sclerosis.

Further Reading

Burrows E.H. (1963) Bone changes in orbital neurofibromatosis. *Br. J. Radiol.*, 36: 549–61.

11.7 ENLARGED OPTIC FORAMEN

Diameter greater than 7 mm (normal range of 4.4–6 mm is reached by the age of 4 years). However, the final arbiter is always comparison with the asymptomatic side. A difference in diameter of 1 mm is abnormal.

CONCENTRIC ENLARGEMENT

1. **Optic nerve glioma** — child/young adult. 25% associated with neurofibromatosis. Bone margins intact.
2. **Neurofibroma** — may occur without any associated glioma.
3. **Extension of retinoblastoma.**
4. **Vascular** — ophthalmic artery aneurysm, arteriovenous malformation.
5. **Granuloma** — very rarely in sarcoidosis or pseudotumour.

LOCAL DEFECT

Roof

1. **Adjacent neoplasm** — meningioma, metastases, glioma.
2. **Raised intracranial pressure** — due to thinning of the floor of the anterior and cranial fossa.

Medial wall

1. **Adjacent neoplasm** — carcinoma of the ethmoid/sphenoid.
2. **Sphenoid mucocoele.**

Inferolateral wall

1. **Same conditions as cause enlarged superior orbital fissure** (q.v.).

11.8 ENLARGED SUPERIOR ORBITAL FISSURE

1. **Normal variant.**
2. **Neurofibromatosis*.**
3. **Extension of intracranial lesion**
   (a) Meningioma — adjacent sclerosis.
   (b) Infraclinoid aneurysm — occurs in 75%. Usually accompanied by erosion of the inferior surface of the anterior clinoid.
   (c) Parasellar chordoma.
4. **Metastasis to wing of sphenoid.**
5. **Extension of orbital lesion (anterior clinoids not eroded)**
   (a) Arteriovenous malformation.
   (b) Haemangioma.
   (c) Orbital meningioma.
   (d) Lymphoma.

11.9 INTRAORBITAL CALCIFICATION

IN THE GLOBE

1. **Cataract.**
2. **Retinoblastoma** — see 11.1 and 11.3.
3. **Old trauma/infection** — of the vitreous humour.

OUTSIDE THE GLOBE

1. **Phleboliths**
   (a) Arteriovenous malformation — enlarged orbit and proptosis. ± Prominent vascular markings. Can also occur in an arteriovenous shunt (e.g. secondary to a traumatic carotico-cavernous fistula).
   (b) Haemangioma — only rarely have calcified phleboliths.
2. **Orbital meningioma** — 12% calcify (more common in extradural location). 10% show enlargement of the optic foramen. Sclerosis of the orbital apex may be present if extradural in location.
3. **Others** — rarely in neurofibroma, intraorbital dermoid and adenocarcinoma of the lacrimal gland.

11.10 HYPEROSTOSIS IN THE ORBIT

1. **Meningioma.**
2. **Sclerotic metastases.**
3. **Fibrous dysplasia*** — bone expansion may cause some reduction in size of the orbit.
4. **Paget's disease*** — usually widespread changes in the calvarium.
5. **Osteopetrosis*** — and other sclerosing bone dysplasias. See 12.5.
6. **Chronic osteomyelitis** — adjacent to a chronically infected frontal sinus.
7. **Lacrimal gland malignancy.**
8. **Langerhans cell histiocytosis*.**
9. **Radiotherapy.**

11.11 SMALL OR ABSENT SINUSES

CONGENITAL

1. **Congenital absence** — absence of the frontal sinuses occurs in 5% of the normal population.
2. **Cretinism*.**
3. **Down's syndrome*** — 90% have absent frontal sinuses.
4. **Kartagener's syndrome** — dextrocardia, bronchiectasis and absent frontal sinuses.

OVERGROWTH OF BONY WALL

1. **Paget's disease*.**
2. **Fibrous dysplasia*.**
3. **Haemolytic anaemia*.**
4. **Post Caldwell–Luc operation.**

11.12 OPAQUE MAXILLARY ANTRUM

TRAUMATIC

1. **Fracture** — blood in the antrum.
2. **Overlying soft-tissue swelling** — gives apparent opacification of the antrum.
3. **Postoperative** — washout/Caldwell–Luc.
4. **Epistaxis.**
5. **Barotrauma.**

INFLAMMATORY/INFECTIVE

1. **Infection.**
2. **Allergy.**
3. **Pyocoele** — infected mucocoele (rare in the antrum). Severe systemic symptoms.

NEOPLASTIC

1. **Carcinoma** — ± bone destruction and extension of the soft-tissue mass.
2. **Lymphoma*.**

OTHERS

1. **Fibrous dysplasia*** — ± bone expansion.
2. **Cysts** — dentigerous and mucous retention cysts may be large enough to fill the antrum.
3. **Wegener's granulomatosis.**
4. **Technical** — overtilted view.
5. **Anatomical** — thick skull vault, sloping antral wall.

Further Reading

Kronemer K.A. & McAlister W.H. (1997) Sinusitis and its imaging in the pediatric population. *Pediatr. Radiol.*, 27: 837–46.

11.13 MASS IN THE MAXILLARY ANTRUM

1. **Cysts**
   (a) Mucous retention cyst — complication of sinusitis. Maxillary antrum is a common site, and it often arises from the floor. Commoner than a polyp, but hard to differentiate between them.
   (b) Dentigerous cyst — expands upwards into the floor of the antrum. The involved tooth may be displaced into the antrum.
2. **Trauma** — due to 'tear-drop' of prolapsed muscle through the roof of the antrum in an orbital blow-out fracture.
3. **Neoplasms**
   (a) Polyp — complication of sinusitis.
   (b) Carcinoma — ± bone destruction and soft-tissue mass extending beyond the boundary of the antrum.
4. **Wegener's granulomatosis** — age usually 40–50 years. Early mucosal thickening progresses to a mass with bone destruction.

11.14 CYSTIC LESIONS IN THE JAW

DENTAL

1. **Periodontal/radicular/periapical cyst** — develops in a carious tooth, often in an asymptomatic patient. Well-defined lucency with a thin sclerotic margin at the apex of a tooth. If large may erode the inner cortex of the mandible, displace adjacent teeth and/or extend into the maxillary antrum.
2. **Dentigerous cyst** — adjacent to the crown of an unerupted tooth (usually a wisdom tooth or canine). Well-defined, unilocular or multilocular. If large, may displace adjacent teeth. Maxillary cysts may extend into the maxillary antra or nose. Multiple cysts occur in Gorlin's syndrome (multiple basal cell naevi, rib anomalies and lamellar falx calcification; AD).

NON-DENTAL

1. **Developmental/fissural cysts**
   (a) Nasopalatine duct cyst/incisive canal cyst — usually between fourth and sixth decades. A small asymptomatic cyst near the anterior palatine papilla.
   (b) Globulomaxillary cyst — between the lateral incisor and canine.
   (c) Nasolabial cyst — in the soft tissues between the nose and the upper lip. There may be resorption of the adjacent maxilla.
2. **Hyperparathyroidism** — a common site for a brown tumour.
3. **Neoplasms**
   (a) Ameloblastoma — 80% in mandible, 20% in maxilla. Most mandibular lesions are near the angle. Slow-growing, painless mass which can reach a considerable size. Unilocular or multilocular, well-defined, bony expansion ± extension through the cortex to form an extra-bony soft-tissue mass.
   (b) Langerhans cell histiocytosis*.
   (c) Aneurysmal bone cyst*.
   (d) Giant cell tumour*.
   (e) Haemangioma.
   (f) Metastases.
4. **Fibrous dysplasia*** — rare site.
5. **Bone cyst** — possibly following an injury. Usually second decade of life. Asymptomatic. Unilocular, indistinct borders and most commonly in the marrow space of the mandibular body.

Further Reading

Gupta M., Kaste S.C. & Hopkins K.P. (2002) Radiologic appearance of primary jaw lesions in children. *Pediatr. Radiol.*, 153–68.

Scholl R.J., Kellett H.M., Neumann D.P. *et al.* (1999) Cysts and cystic lesions of the mandible: clinical and radiologic–histopathologic review. *RadioGraphics*, 19: 1107–24.

Weber A.L. (1993) Imaging of cysts and odontogenic tumours of the jaw. *Radiol. Clin. North Am.*, 31(1): 101–20.

11.15 'FLOATING' TEETH

No obvious supporting bone for the teeth.

1. **Severe periodontal disease.**
2. **Langerhans cell histiocytosis*.**
3. **Hyperparathyroidism*.**
4. **Metastases.**
5. **Multiple myeloma*.**

11.16 LOSS OF LAMINA DURA OF TEETH

GENERALIZED

1. **Endocrine/metabolic**
   (a) Osteoporosis (q.v.).
   (b) Hyperparathyroidism*.
   (c) Cushing's syndrome*.
   (d) Osteomalacia (q.v.).
2. **Paget's disease*.**
3. **Scleroderma*** — thickened periodontal membrane.

LOCALIZED

1. **Infection.**
2. **Neoplasms** — leukaemia, multiple myeloma, metastases, Burkitt's lymphoma, Langerhans cell histiocytosis.

11.17 MASS IN THE NASOPHARYNX

1. **Adenoids** — enlargement is normal between 1 and 7 years of age.
2. **Trauma** — fracture of the base of the skull or upper cervical spine with associated haematoma.
3. **Infection** — abscess may be confined above C2 by strong attachment of the prevertebral fascia. ± Speckled gas in the mass.
4. **Neoplasms, benign**
   (a) Adolescent angiofibroma — very vascular. Young male: ± spontaneous regression after adolescence. Can cause pressure erosion of the sphenoid and opacification of the antra.
   (b) Antro-choanal polyp.
5. **Neoplasms, malignant**
   (a) Nasopharyngeal carcinoma.
   (b) Lymphoma*.
   (c) Rhabdomyosarcoma.
   (d) Plasmacytoma*.
   (e) Extension — carcinoma of the sphenoid/ethmoid, and chordoma.
6. **Encephalocoele** — midline defect in the base of the skull.

Further Reading

Chong V.F. & Fan Y.F. (2000) Radiology of the retropharyngeal space. *Clin Radiol.,* 55: 740–8.

McHugh K. & Boothroyd A.E. (1999) The role of radiology in childhood rhabdomyosarcoma. *Clin. Radiol.,* 54: 2–10.

11.18 PREVERTEBRAL SOFT-TISSUE MASS ON THE LATERAL CERVICAL X-RAY

CHILD

NB. Anterior bucking of the trachea with an increase in the thickness of the retropharyngeal tissues may occur as a normal phenomenon in expiration during the first 2 years of life and is due to laxity of the retropharyngeal tissues. These soft tissues may contain a small collection of air, trapped in the inferior recess of the laryngeal pharynx above the contracted upper oesophageal sphincter. An ear lobe may also mimic a prevertebral mass.

1. **Trauma/haematoma** — ± an associated fracture.
2. **Abscess** — ± gas lucencies within it. Unlike the normal variant described above these lucencies are constant and persist during deep inspiration.
3. **Neoplasms**
   (a) Cystic hygroma.
   (b) Lymphoma*.
   (c) Nasopharyngeal rhabdomyosarcoma.
   (d) Neuroblastoma.

ADULT

1. **Trauma**
2. **Abscess.**
3. **Neoplasms**
   (a) Post-cricoid carcinoma.
   (b) Lymphoma*.
   (c) Chordoma.
4. **Pharyngeal pouch** — ± air/fluid level within it.
5. **Retropharyngeal goitre.**

See also 11.17.

Further Reading

Brenner G.H. (1964) Variations in the depth of the cervical prevertebral tissues in normal infants studied by cine fluorography. *Am. J. Roentgenol.*, 91: 573–7.

Currarino G. & Williams B. (1993) Air collection in the retropharyngeal soft tissues observed in lateral expiratory films of the neck in 9 infants. *Pediatr. Radiol.*, 23: 186–8.

11.19 NECK MASSES IN INFANTS AND CHILDREN

Ultrasound is a valuable first imaging modality. MRI is generally preferred to CT.

SOFT

1. **Lipoma** — may be firm. Solid and usually well-defined homogeneously echo bright. Fat shows characteristic signal on MRI.
2. **Haemangioma** — solid and of variable echo texture. Capillary haemangiomas have tiny vessels and appear hyperechoic. Cavernous haemangiomas may have visible vessels within. All are usually bright on heavily T_2W MRI.
3. **Lymphangioma (cystic hygroma)** — predominantly cystic and may be haemorrhagic. Locally infiltrative and may extend into the chest. MRI shows medium signal (T_1W) and high signal (T_2W).

FIRM

1. **Cyst**
   (a) Thyroglossal — midline position. Unless they are haemorrhagic or infected they are fluid-filled and thin-walled.
   (b) Branchial cleft — lateral position. Unless they are haemorrhagic or infected they are fluid-filled and thin-walled.
   (c) Lingual.
   (d) Thymic.
2. **Abscess** — lateral X-ray may show gas lucencies within it.
3. **Haematoma.**
4. **Inflammatory lymphadenopathy** — round or oval masses becoming confluent. Central low echoes suggest suppuration.
5. **Neoplastic lymphadenopathy** — e.g. leukaemia, lymphoma.
6. **Neoplasia**
   (a) Benign — e.g. fibroma (commonly seen as an oval, hyperechoic lesion in the sternocleidomastoid muscle in an infant), ectopic thymus.
   (b) Malignant — rare, e.g. neuroblastoma, rhabdomyosarcoma. On US they are often hyperechoic and may show areas of

necrosis. Intermediate signal on T_1W and increased signal on T_2W MRI.

7. **Thyroid**
   (a) Diffuse enlargement — Graves' disease, multinodular goitre, thyroiditis.
   (b) Focal mass — cyst, benign adenoma. Malignancy is rare.

Further Reading

Swischuk L.E. & John S.D. (1997) Neck masses in infants and children. *Radiol. Clin. North Am.*, 35(6): 1329–40.

11.20 WHOLE BODY IODINE SCAN FOR LOCALIZING METASTASES

1. **Metastases** visualization depends on the amount of ^{131}I given. A low activity gives false negative results.
2. **Thyroid bed** — a small amount of uptake is normal.
3. **Normal thyroid tissue**
   (a) Ectopic, retrosternal, sublingual.
   (b) Aberrant — liver, thyroid lymph nodes (unless an ablative dose of iodine has already been given).
4. **Normal uptake** — genitourinary tract, nasopharynx, salivary glands, stomach, breasts.

Further Reading

Shapiro B., Rufini V., Jarwan A. *et al.* (2000) Artifacts, anatomical and physiologic variants, and unrelated diseases that might cause false-positive whole-body 131-I scans in patients with thyroid cancer. *Semin. Nucl. Med.*, 30(2): 115–32.

11.21 PHOTOPENIC (COLD) AREAS IN RADIONUCLIDE THYROID IMAGING

LOCALIZED

1. **Colloid cyst.**
2. **Adenoma** — non-functioning.
3. **Carcinoma** — medullary may be bilateral.
4. **Multinodular goitre.**
5. **Local thyroiditis** — may be increased uptake also
   (a) Acute.
   (b) De Quervain's.
   (c) Hashimito's.
   (d) Riedel's.
6. **Vascular** — haemorrhage or infarct.
7. **Artefacts.**
8. **Abscesses.**

GENERALIZED REDUCTION IN UPTAKE

1. **Medication** — thyroxine, glucocorticoids, phenylbutazone sulphonylureas.
2. **Hypothyroidism** — primary or secondary.
3. **Ectopic hormone production.**
4. **De Quervain's thyroiditis.**
5. **Ectopic thyroid** — lingual or retrosternal.

Further Reading

Cases J.A. & Surks M.I. (2000) The changing role of scintigraphy in the evaluation of thyroid nodules. *Semin. Nucl. Med.,* 30(2): 81–7.

Fogelman I. & Maisey M. (1988) *An Atlas of Clinical Nuclear Medicine.* London: Martin Dunitz, pp. 160–216.

12 Skull and brain

Stuart Coley

12.1 ACUTE ARTERIAL INFARCT – CT APPEARANCES

1. **Normal** — the conspicuity of an acute infarct depends upon the size and location of the insult, duration of ischaemia and scan quality. Large strokes involving the middle cerebral artery (MCA) territory often show some abnormality by 4–6 hours, but the changes are usually subtle at this stage.
2. **Low-density region** — the typical appearance of a cortical infarct is a bland wedge-shaped area of low attenuation involving both grey and white matter. Loss of grey–white matter differentiation is a feature of acute infarction and is the earliest radiological abnormality. The 'insular ribbon sign' is a finding of early MCA infarction caused by loss of the normal anatomical boundaries formed by the alternating grey and white matter structures of the peri-insular region. The normal 'striated' appearance of this area is replaced by a swollen homogeneous area of low attenuation. Alternatively, the basal ganglia may 'disappear' as the infarcted grey matter acquires the same CT attenuation as the surrounding white matter.
3. **Mass effect** — local effacement of the cerebral sulci and fissures may be followed by more diffuse brain swelling. Maximal swelling usually occurs after 3–5 days. Infarcts that do not have a typical appearance must be differentiated from other solitary intracranial masses (see 12.24).
4. **Hyperdense artery** — represents acute thrombus within the vessel. Most commonly recognized with basilar and proximal MCA thrombosis. False positives can occur if a vessel is partially calcified or if the haematocrit is raised (i.e. polycythaemia).
5. **Haemorrhage** — frank haemorrhage into an arterial infarct typically occurs a few days after the initial stroke. If there is haemorrhage within an infarct from the outset, a venous stroke or arterial embolus should be considered.

6. **Contrast enhancement** — usually occurs by 4 days and reflects impairment of the blood–brain barrier. Typically gyriform (following the cerebral cortex), but may appear ring-enhancing or confluent. Subsides by 4–8 weeks.
7. **Arterial occlusion** — CT angiography may demonstrate stenosis or complete arterial occlusion prior to spontaneous recanalization.
8. **Perfusion defect** — CT can demonstrate the extent and degree of cerebral ischaemia with the use of iodinated contrast medium or xenon.

Further Reading

Beauchamp N.J. & Bryan R.N. (1998) Acute cerebral ischemic infarction: a pathophysiologic review and radiologic perspective. *Am. J. Roentgenol.*, 171: 73–84.

12.2 ACUTE ARTERIAL INFARCT – MRI APPEARANCES

1. **Diffusion abnormality** — abnormalities may be seen within minutes of arterial occlusion with diffusion-weighted MRI. This early indicator of brain ischaemia is associated with low signal on apparent diffusion coefficient (ADC) images, whilst old infarcts and areas of vasogenic oedema are associated with increased ADC values. Although early diffusion changes are potentially reversible (by prompt revascularization), they normally indicate brain that will subsequently infarct.
2. **Absent arterial flow void** — an immediate sign of vessel occlusion best seen on T_2W and FLAIR imaging. An occluded vessel returns high signal on these sequences.

3. **Increased T_2W signal** — T_2W signal change represents cytotoxic oedema and typically becomes visible by 3–6 hours. The earliest changes are identified within the grey matter structures. Accompanied by a reduction in T_1W signal.
4. **Mass effect** — local effacement of the cerebral sulci and fissures may be followed by more diffuse brain swelling. Maximal swelling usually occurs after 3–5 days. Infarcts that do not have a typical appearance must be differentiated from other solitary intracranial masses (see 12.24).
5. **Intravascular stasis of contrast medium** — prolonged transit of contrast medium through distal/collateral vessels causes high arterial signal on post-gadolinium T_1W images.
6. **Reduced perfusion** — contrast-based MRI techniques show a qualitative fall in brain perfusion within the relevant vascular territory. A mismatch between perfusion and diffusion abnormalities may indicate brain that is potentially salvageable if prompt revascularization occurs (the ischaemic penumbra).
7. **Arterial occlusion** — MR angiography may demonstrate vessel stenosis or occlusion. Spontaneous recanalization is a feature of thromboembolic stroke, but may not occur until after a period of irreversible ischaemia.
8. **Meningeal enhancement** — observed at 24 hours in the meninges adjacent to an infarct. Parenchymal enhancement is maximal at 4–7 days and is usually gyriform or patchy in appearance.
9. **Haemorrhage** — high T_1W signal within the cortex of infarcted brain represents 'petechial haemorrhage' and should not be considered a contraindication to the use of antiplatelet agents.

Further Reading

Beauchamp N.J. & Bryan R.N. (1998) Acute cerebral ischemic infarction: a pathophysiologic review and radiologic perspective. *Am. J. Roentgenol.*, 171: 73–84.

12.3 ACUTE VENOUS INFARCT

It is important to distinguish between venous and arterial infarcts since the conditions are managed differently. The following radiological features are suggestive of venous infarction.

1. **Venous occlusion** — the vast majority of venous infarcts are caused by venous thrombosis. Acute thrombus is hyperdense on pre-contrast CT and expands the occluded sinus/vein. Clot within the cortical and deep venous systems may present as a hyperdense linear structure. Thrombus is visualized on MRI as loss of the normal venous flow void on T_2W-weighted sequences. Diagnostic difficulties arise with congenital variations of the venous system (i.e. normal hypoplasia of the transverse sinuses), arachnoid granulations and normal slow turbulent flow. Acute thrombus may be hypointense on T_2W MRI and should not be mistaken for the normal flow void.
2. **Bilateral infarcts** — occlusion of the midline veins (deep veins, straight sinus, superior sagittal sinus) may result in bilateral areas of low attenuation on CT and increased T_2W signal on MRI. Thrombosis of the deep cerebral veins may involve the basal ganglia, thalami, midbrain and mesial temporal lobes in a relatively symmetrical fashion.
3. **Unilateral infarct** — thrombosis of the transverse sinus and/or vein of Labbé may result in an infarct involving the grey and white matter of the temporal lobe in a non-arterial distribution. Midline venous occlusion may also present with unilateral infarcts.
4. **Haemorrhage** — haemorrhage is common within an acute venous infarct and is seen as an area of high attenuation on CT. MR signal intensity depends on the age of the haemorrhage (see 12.8).
5. **Mass effect** — marked brain swelling is often seen with venous infarction, even on day 1. Arterial infarcts usually show maximal swelling at 3–5 days.
6. **Dural thickening** — the 'empty delta' sign of peripheral enhancement around a central 'core' of acute thrombus represents hypervascularity and engorgement of the dura, not a patent peripheral channel. Persistent dural thickening is a feature of subacute/chronic venous thrombosis.

Further Reading

Provenzale J.M., Joseph G.J. & Barboriak D.P. (1998) Dural sinus thrombosis: findings on CT and MR imaging and diagnostic pitfalls. *Am. J. Roentgenol.*, 170: 777–83.

12.4 INDICATIONS FOR MRI IN STROKE

1. **Investigation of arterial dissection** — spin-echo sequences (T_1W/T_2W) can demonstrate a crescentic haematoma within the wall of the dissected vessel. The overall diameter of the vessel may be enlarged by the intramural haematoma, but the patent lumen is usually much reduced. MR angiography demonstrates vessel occlusion or long segment stenosis/irregularity. The angiography source data should always be reviewed as an intramural clot and/or an intimal flap may be shown, even if the maximum intensity projections appear normal.
2. **Investigation of venous thrombosis** — loss of the normal 'flow void' within a dural sinus or cerebral vein may indicate thrombosis. MR venography is also helpful in the diagnosis of venous thrombosis (see 12.3).
3. **Posterior circulation stroke** — MRI is vastly superior to CT in the evaluation of the posterior fossa and can demonstrate even small brainstem strokes. MR angiography can demonstrate arterial thrombosis and dissection.
4. **Children and young adults** — since the incidence of atherosclerotic stroke is relatively low in these groups, MRI should be considered. (See 12.6).
5. **Normal CT** — MRI is more sensitive than CT for the diagnosis of early ischaemic stroke and small vascular insults.
6. **Detection of reversible ischaemia** — current belief is that MRI can delineate areas of ischaemic brain amenable to salvage using the combination of perfusion and diffusion MRI. Any mismatch in size between the diffusion abnormality and a larger perfusion defect may depict an area of reversible ischaemia. MR angiography shows the presence and extent of arterial occlusion.
7. **Non-invasive assessment of the vascular tree** — MR angiography can demonstrate the intracranial circulation as well as the extracranial vertebral and carotid vessels.

12.5 DIFFERENTIATING BETWEEN INFARCT AND TUMOUR

It is usually straightforward to differentiate a brain tumour from an infarct, especially if the clinical history is known. The following features may be helpful in difficult cases, but in rare circumstances the diagnosis will not be clear cut and biopsy cannot be prevented.

1. **Clinical history** — the abrupt onset of a focal neurological deficit suggests infarct. Seizures, gradual onset and progressive deficit suggest tumour.
2. **Grey matter changes** — cortical infarcts often simultaneously involve the cerebral cortex and juxtacortical white matter. An acute infarct may also involve (radiologically) just the cerebral cortex on MRI and should not be mistaken for an area of encephalitis. The majority of metastases and 'high-grade' gliomas are centred upon the cerebral white matter and spare the overlying grey matter. Certain tumours, however, often appear to involve the cerebral cortex (e.g. dysembryoplastic neuroepithelial tumour and other 'low-grade' gliomas).
3. **Shape** — the typical cortical infarct is wedge- or box-shaped with its base towards the brain surface. Most tumours are spherical or ovoid. Difficulties arise if the tumour is infiltrative with little or no mass effect.
4. **Distribution** — tumours are not confined to vascular territories.
5. **Contrast enhancement** — gyriform enhancement is not specific to brain infarction, but is rarely encountered with tumour unless seizures have occurred, or if there is meningeal disease.
6. **Arterial flow void** — absence of an arterial flow void implies vascular occlusion.
7. **Diffusion weighted imaging** — an acute arterial infarct will usually demonstrate restricted diffusion (low apparent diffusion coefficient) for at least 4 days.
8. **MR spectroscopy** — infarcts and tumours can often be differentiated by virtue of their spectroscopic signatures.
9. **Natural history** — ageing infarcts involute and result in an area of focal atrophy. Tumours remain static or progress. Repeat imaging after 4–6 weeks may therefore be of help.

12.6 CAUSES OF STROKE IN CHILDREN AND YOUNG ADULTS

1. **Emboli** — cyanotic heart disease (secondary to right-to-left intracardiac shunt), cardiomyopathies, mitral valve prolapse, Osler–Weber–Rendu (secondary to pulmonary arteriovenous malformations).
2. **Arterial dissection** — trauma, spontaneous, fibromuscular dysplasia (also vessel stenoses and saccular dilatations, intracranial aneurysms), Marfan's syndrome, Ehlers–Danlos syndrome and homocystinuria (see 12.4).
3. **Venous thrombosis** — pregnancy, postpartum, oral contraceptive pill, skull base/intracranial sepsis, inflammatory bowel disease, systemic lupus erythematosus*, Behcet's disease and malignancy (see 12.3).
4. **Infection** — purulent meningitis may cause arterial and venous strokes. Viral infection is a well-recognized cause of arterial stroke due to a 'vasculitis' that usually involves the proximal MCA (infarction of basal ganglia with sparing of the cortical territories).
5. **Trauma** — arterial dissection and hypoxia.
6. **Drugs** — cocaine, amphetamines.
7. **Blood disorders** — sickle-cell anaemia*, polycythaemia, protein C and S deficiency.
8. **Migraine** — usually posterior circulation.
9. **Vasculopathy, vasculitis** — neurofibromatosis*, fibromuscular dysplasia, Kawasaki's, systemic lupus erythematosus*, sarcoidosis*.
10. **Idiopathic** — in many cases, a cause is not found.

Further Reading

Ball W.S. (1994) Cerebrovascular occlusive disease in childhood. *Neuroimaging Clin. North Am.*, 4: 393–421.

Provenzale J.M. & Barboriak D.P. (1997) Brain infarction in young adults: etiology and imaging. *Am. J. Roentgenol.*, 169: 1161–8.

12.7 ACUTE INTRACEREBRAL HAEMATOMA – CT APPEARANCES

0–2 hours — freshly extravasated blood has a mixed density (40–60 HU). Some components of the haematoma may be the same density as normal grey matter.
3–48 hours — the density (60–80 HU) of the haematoma increases as the clot 'retracts' and the haematocrit increases. Large haematomas may show fluid/fluid levels comprising a hypodense supernatant of serum overlying a dependent aggregation of blood cells.
Days 3–7 — as the haematoma matures an ill-defined hyperdense core is surrounded by a low-density halo (serum extrusion and reactive vasogenic oedema). Mass effect and pathological contrast enhancement is usually maximal at this time.
Weeks 2–4 — density of haematoma decreases from periphery to centre. Peripheral enhancement (disruption of the blood–brain barrier) around an isodense mass may at this time be mistaken for tumour.
Months 2 onwards — slit-like low density cavity.

Further Reading

Parizel P.M., Makkat S., Van Miert E. *et al.* (2001) Intracranial haemorrhage: principles of CT and MRI interpretation. *Eur. Radiol.* 11: 1770–83.

12.8 ACUTE INTRACEREBRAL HAEMATOMA – MRI APPEARANCES

	Hyperacute <12 hours	Acute 12–72 hours	Early subacute 4–7 days	Late subacute 8–30 days	Chronic 1 month plus
T_1W	⇔	⇔	⇑	⇑⇑ (From periphery to centre)	⇓
	Oxyhaemoglobin	Deoxyhaemoglobin	Intracellular methaemoglobin	Extracellular methaemoglobin	Haemosiderin Ferritin
T_2W	⇑	⇓⇓	⇓ ⇓	⇑⇑	⇓⇓

Further Reading

Parizel P.M., Makkat S., Van Miert E. *et al.* (2001) Intracranial haemorrhage: principles of CT and MRI interpretation. *Eur. Radiol.*, 11: 1770–83.

12.9 INTRACRANIAL ANEURYSMS

PRESENTATION

1. **Haemorrhage**
   (a) Subarachnoid haemorrhage — see 12.10.
   (b) Parenchymal haemorrhage — the compartments of the brain into which blood enters during rupture depend on the site and orientation of the aneurysm. Blood may appear to lie exclusively within the substance of the brain but there is usually at least a small amount of blood in the subarachnoid space.
   (c) Subdural haemorrhage — seen in aneurysms that are located near to the dural covering, e.g. rupture of a posterior communicating artery aneurysm pointing laterally and inferiorly may produce a subdural haemorrhage (SDH) within the middle cranial fossa.
   (d) Intraventricular haemorrhage — aneurysms (e.g. anterior communicating region) may rupture directly into the ventricular system. Blood may also migrate into the ventricular system from the subarachnoid space.
   (e) Epistaxis — large petrocavernous aneurysms can rupture directly into the sphenoid sinus and present with torrential bleeding. These aneurysms are often the result of skull base fracture.
2. **Mass effect**
   (a) Cranial nerve palsy — classic example is a third nerve palsy caused by a posterior communicating or superior cerebellar aneurysm. Hearing loss, facial pain, facial palsy and ophthalmoplegia are associated with large aneurysms of the petrous and cavernous segments of the inferior cerebellar artery (ICA). Compression of the anterior optic pathways by large ICA, anterior cerebral and posterior circulation aneurysms can produce visual field deficits and reduced acuity. Lower cranial nerves may be compromised by large posterior fossa aneurysms (e.g. posterior inferior cerebellar artery (PICA).
   (b) Brainstem compression — pyramidal tracts and lower cranial nerves may be compromised by posterior circulation aneurysms.
   (c) Supratentorial dysfunction — giant frontal aneurysms may present with dementia, epilepsy, visual disturbance and hydrocephalus. MCA lesions can present with progressive hemiparesis and speech disturbance.

   (d) Horner's syndrome — constricted pupil and ptosis due to involvement of the sympathetic fibres surrounding the ICA.
   (e) Localized pain/generalized headache — especially if the aneurysm is in contact with the dura.
   (f) Pulsatile tinnitus — petrous aneurysm.
3. **Incidental finding** — approximately 2–3% of the general population harbour an asymptomatic unruptured aneurysm. The cumulative risk of haemorrhage is currently estimated to be in the order of 0.5–1.5% per annum. Aneurysm size and location, cigarette smoking, female gender and age (inversely) have some influence on the risk of rupture.
4. **Thromboembolism** — aneurysms may present as a result of intra-aneurysmal thrombosis and/or distal embolism.

NON-INVASIVE IMAGING

CT: high-attenuation extra-axial mass within the subarachnoid space. Large aneurysms may invaginate the brain and appear intra-axial. Large/giant lesions may show peripheral calcification and internal thrombosis. The patent lumen enhances strongly with contrast medium. CT angiography is becoming more sophisticated with the advent of multislice spiral scanners.

MRI: small aneurysms are usually visible on T_2W sequences as areas of flow void contiguous with the parent vessel. Large/giant aneurysms tend to experience turbulent intra-aneurysmal flow resulting in a complex pattern of mixed signal return on each sequence. Partially thrombosed aneurysms may reveal multilaminated clot that varies in signal. Phase-encoding artefact can corrupt the image and help differentiate a large aneurysm from a tumour. MR angiography continues to evolve and is a non-invasive, but inferior, alternative to catheter angiography.

Further Reading

Byrne J.V. & Guglielmi G. (1998) *Endovascular Treatment of Intracranial Aneurysms*. Berlin, Springer-Verlag.

Weir B. (2002) Unruptured intracranial aneurysms: a review. *J. Neurosurgery,* 96: 3–42.

12.10 SUBARACHNOID HAEMORRHAGE

CAUSES

1. **Ruptured intracranial aneurysm.**
2. **Perimesencephalic venous haemorrhage** — diagnosis of exclusion in patients with blood in the pontine cistern and normal cerebral angiography. Good prognosis.
3. **Trauma.**
4. **Parenchymal haematoma** — any haematoma that extends up to the surface of the brain and dissects into the subarachnoid space.
5. **Brain arteriovenous malformation/fistula.**
6. **Spinal arteriovenous malformation.**
7. **Cervical ependymoma.**
8. **No cause found.**

DIAGNOSIS

1. **CT** — acute subarachnoid haemorrhage (SAH) presents as high-density material within the basal cisterns and cerebral fissures. Blood may also be identified within the ventricles, brain parenchyma and subdural space (see 12.9). Blood disappears from the subarachnoid space after only a few days and therefore only 50% of scans are still positive at 7 days. Important 'review areas' for blood include the basal cisterns (including the interpeduncular fossa), Sylvian fissures, occipital horns and interhemispheric fissure. See 'Complications of SAH' below. A mild communicating hydrocephalus may be the only abnormality if the patient is imaged late (e.g. after 7 days).
2. **Lumbar puncture** — all CT-negative patients investigated for SAH must have a lumbar puncture for xanthochromia.
3. **MRI** — MRI is potentially superior to CT in the delayed diagnosis of SAH (i.e. after 7 days). Gradient echo, proton density and FLAIR sequences are the most sensitive MRI sequences for the detection of blood.
4. **Angiography** — once a diagnosis of SAH is made, the search for a vascular malformation begins. In the case of multiple aneurysms (20% of patients) the largest, most irregular lesion is usually, but not invariably, the source. A rupture point (false aneurysm) may be seen on the relevant aneurysm. Catheter angiography remains the gold standard at this time, but considerable advances in CT and MR angiography are being made.

COMPLICATIONS OF SAH

1. **Hydrocephalus** — either post-haemorrhagic communicating hydrocephalus, or an obstructive hydrocephalus if the ventricular system becomes blocked (e.g. occlusion of the cerebral aqueduct).
2. **Vasospasm** — low-attenuation (CT) within a vascular territory is suggestive of 'vasospasm' in the acute phase of SAH, but may be reversible and does not therefore indicate irreversible brain injury. Often maximal several days after the initial bleed.
3. **Infarct** — severe or prolonged vasospasm causes permanent injury.
4. **Rebleeding** — usually recognizable on clinical grounds.
5. **Diffuse cerebral swelling and cerebral herniation** — bilateral posterior cerebral infarcts can occur during transtentorial herniation because of compression of the vessels against the free edge of the tentorium.

Further Reading

Mitchell P., Wilkinson I.D., Hoggard N. *et al.* (2001) Detection of subarachnoid haemorrhage with magnetic resonance imaging. *J. Neurol. Neurosurg. Psychiatry,* 70: 205–11.

12.11 VASCULAR MALFORMATIONS

ARTERIOVENOUS SHUNTING

1. **Brain arteriovenous malformation** — brain AVMs typically present in 20–40-year olds with haemorrhage, seizures, headache or neurological deficit. AVM consists of single or multiple arterial pedicles, a nidus through which arteriovenous shunting occurs and enlarged draining veins. The annual cumulative risk of rupture is estimated at 3% per year. Multiple AVMs occur in Osler–Weber–Rendu and Wyburn–Mason syndromes.

CT: hyperdense serpiginous, enlarged feeding and draining vessels with strongly enhancing nidus. Nidal calcification (speckled or solid) is common. Local atrophy may occur.
MRI: AVMs are most obvious on T_2W and PD sequences as a nidus of flow voids with enlarged feeding and draining vessels. The surrounding brain may show evidence of gliosis (increased T_2W signal) or old haemorrhage (low T_2W signal).
Catheter angiography: gold standard for detailed evaluation of nidal architecture, related aneurysms (arterial, nidal and venous), stenoses, varices and direct arteriovenous fistulae.

2. **Dural arteriovenous fistula (DAVF)** — DAVFs are acquired lesions that present in an older population (50–70 years) than brain AVMs. They can result from damage to the venous structures as a result of thrombosis or surgery. Symptoms and complications result from arterialization of the venous system and can be predicted by the pattern of venous drainage. Lesions that involve the dural sinuses often present with a bruit, pulsatile tinnitus (transverse sinus) or intracranial hypertension, whilst those that directly involve the cortical veins, or do so indirectly by reflux from the diseased sinus, are at greatest risk of severe neurological complications (haemorrhage, seizures, focal neurological deficits, myelopathy and dementia).
CT: usually normal unless complications such as haemorrhage have occurred. A carotid–cavernous fistula may show enlargement of the cavernous sinus and ophthalmic veins with signs of venous hypertension within the orbit (proptosis, chemosis).
MRI: conventional spin-echo and static angiography techniques are insensitive to DAVF. MRI may be entirely normal unless there is occlusion of the venous sinus (loss of T_2W flow void), enlarged arterial pedicles (e.g. occipital artery), engorged cortical veins or established intracranial complications such as venous ischaemia and haemorrhage. Conventional MR venography may be normal or show non-specific abnormalities of flow. Dynamic MR subtraction angiography shows great promise for non-invasive diagnosis.
Catheter angiography: gold standard for the diagnosis and classification of DAVF.

NO ARTERIOVENOUS SHUNTING

1. **Cavernous angioma (cavernoma)** — may present with seizures, haemorrhage and progressive neurological deficit, although many are incidental findings. Cavernomas are endothelial-lined sinusoidal spaces most commonly occurring in the pons, but can arise anywhere within the brain. They are frequently multiple and may be found in combination with a venous angioma. Familial cases are well recognized.
   CT: isodense/hyperdense focus ± minor contrast enhancement. Speckled calcification common.
   MRI: central 'pop-corn' core of high T_1W and T_2W signal with surrounding rim of haemosiderin (very low T_2W signal). Smaller lesions present as uniform foci of low signal on T_2W and gradient echo sequences. Multiple lesions are common, especially if the brain is imaged with gradient echo sequences. No surrounding oedema unless there has been recent haemorrhage.
   Catheter angiography: faint vascular stain, or normal.
2. **Developmental venous anomaly (venous angioma)** — probably represents embryonic veins that persist because of abnormal venous maturation. They are not thought to have an increased risk of haemorrhage.
   CT: contrast-enhanced study shows enhancing linear structure draining towards the cerebral cortex or ventricular system.
   MRI: most easily seen on post-contrast studies but larger anomalies can be seen as a linear structure with flow void (T_2W) or flow-related enhancement (T_1W/GE sequences).
   Catheter angiography: caput medusae of smaller draining veins feed a single transcerebral vein that enters either a superficial cortical or subependymal vein.
3. **Telangiectasia** — dilated capillary beds that are almost invariably asymptomatic. Usually found only at post-mortem within the posterior fossa. Visible on MRI as very hypointense areas of haemosiderin staining. Patients with Osler–Weber–Rendu may have telangiectasia, cavernomas, DAVFs and brain AVMs.

Further Reading

Osborn A.G. (1994) *Diagnostic Neuroradiology,* Ch. 10. St Louis: Mosby, pp. 284–329.

12.12 ACUTE BACTERIAL MENINGITIS

1. **Normal** — most common finding in early bacterial meningitis.
2. **Diffuse brain swelling** — effacement of the cerebral sulci and basal cisterns. The ventricles may be reduced or totally effaced by diffuse swelling.
3. **Meningeal enhancement** — absence of contrast enhancement does not exclude meningitis. CT is relatively insensitive in detecting meningeal enhancement and is performed primarily to exclude other complications (e.g. abscess and empyema).
4. **Ventriculitis** — linear enhancement of the ependymal lining. May progress to a chronic adhesive arachnoiditis.
5. **Hydrocephalus** — a purulent exudate can produce an intraventricular obstruction, but more typically results in a communicating hydrocephalus because of impairment of CSF resorption by the arachnoid granulations.
6. **Subdural empyema** — CT reveals a low density/isodense extrinsic collection that may or may not enhance avidly with contrast medium. Often located in the interhemispheric fissure and secondary to frontal sinus infection. Subtemporal empyema secondary to temporal bone pathology is best evaluated with MRI. Subdural empyema is a neurosurgical emergency.
7. **Sterile collections** — sterile subdural effusions are commonly encountered in young children. The fluid is similar to CSF on both CT and MRI. The majority will resolve spontaneously, but a small number may become secondarily infected.
8. **Focus of sepsis within temporal bone, paranasal sinus or skull vault** — skull base/sinus infection, cranial surgery and penetrating head injury are potential causes of intracranial sepsis.
9. **Arterial infarct** — vessels passing through the subarachnoid space may be compromised by a purulent CSF (e.g. tuberculosis).
10. **Venous infarct** — cortical thrombophlebitis and dural sinus occlusion may occur, particularly in the context of an empyema.
11. **Cerebritis/cerebral abscess** — ill-defined infection within the parenchyma may progress to frank abscess formation. An abscess is usually low density on CT with a thin enhancing rim surrounded by extensive white matter oedema.
12. **Atrophy/encephalomalacia** — late features of infection.

Further Reading

Osborn A.G. (1994) *Diagnostic Neuroradiology*, Ch. 16. St Louis: Mosby, pp. 680–94.

12.13 VIRAL ENCEPHALITIS

Herpes simplex (HSV) is the most common viral encephalitis in the developed world. It causes a haemorrhagic necrotizing encephalitis with a predilection for the limbic system, medial temporal lobes and inferior frontal lobes. MRI is often highly suggestive of the diagnosis and is an important diagnostic tool that can prevent a biopsy. Early treatment with antiviral drugs can be life-saving.

1. **Herpes simplex**

CT:

(a) Normal — early changes may not be evident on CT.
(b) Low-attenuation temporal lobe(s) — sparing of the putamen helps to differentiate SV from MCA infarct in atypical clinical presentations. Beam-hardening artefact may seriously limit the study and therefore MRI should be performed if the diagnosis of HSV is strongly considered.
(c) Temporal lobe swelling — unilateral or, less commonly, bilateral.
(d) Haemorrhage — macroscopic haemorrhage is a feature of fulminant encephalitis.
(e) Contrast enhancement — patchy parenchymal and gyral uptake of contrast medium.

MRI:

(a) T_2W signal change — predominantly involves the cerebral cortex and adjacent white matter of the temporal lobe (especially the hippocampus and parahippocampal gyrus), insula and cingulate gyrus. Changes are often bilateral but usually asymmetrical, and are not always limited to the limbic system.
(b) Gyral enhancement — uptake of gadolinium may be seen in the cortex, producing a 'gyral' pattern of enhancement.
(c) Haemorrhage — small foci of haemorrhage will be most conspicuous on MRI and present as high signal areas on the pre-contrast T_1W.
(d) Atrophy and encephalomalacia — local atrophy and T_2W signal change may result.

2. **HIV** — see 12.14.
3. **Sporadic Creutzfeldt–Jakob disease** — rapidly progressive dementia associated with myoclonus, ataxia, pyramidal and extrapyramidal signs, and cortical blindness. High T_2W signal

lesions within the corpus striatum (i.e. putamen and caudate head) and less commonly within the thalamus, globus pallidus and periaqueductal grey matter. Cortical signal change best detected with FLAIR.

4. **Variant Creutzfeldt–Jakob disease** — clinical features include sensory disturbance, withdrawal, depression, abnormal eye movements and involuntary movements. Causal link with bovine spongiform encephalopathy (BSE). High T_2W/FLAIR signal lesions with the posterior thalamic nuclei (pulvinar). Changes also reported in the tectal plate, periaqueductal grey matter and cerebral cortex. Atrophy is unusual.
5. **Progressive multifocal leukoencephalopathy** — see 12.14.
6. **Subacute sclerosing panencephalitis** — progressive encephalitis that occurs several years after measles infection. MRI shows gross atrophy and non-specific foci of T_2W signal change in the cerebral and cerebellar white matter.
7. **Rasmussen's encephalitis** — progressive neurological deficits and intractable seizures in children. MRI reveals atrophy and non-specific signal change localized to one cerebral hemisphere.
8. **Polio** — increased T_2W signal in the ventral horns of spinal grey matter ± brainstem encephalitis (bulbar polio).
9. **Acute cerebellitis** — viral syndrome characterized by symmetrical grey/white matter changes plus swelling of the cerebellar hemispheres. May result in obstructive hydrocephalus.

Further Reading

Collie D.A., Sellar R.J., Zeidler M. *et al.* (2001) MRI of Creutzfeldt–Jakob disease: imaging features and recommended MRI protocol. *Clin. Radiol.*, 56: 726–39.

Leonard J.R., Moran C.J. & Cross D.T. III (2000) MR imaging of herpes simplex type 1 encephalitis in infants and young children: a separate pattern of findings. *Am. J. Roentgenol.*, 174: 1651–5.

12.14 HIV AND THE BRAIN

HIV is a neurotropic virus that can directly involve the central nervous system. The most common opportunistic infections to involve the brain are toxoplasmosis, cryptococcosis and progressive multifocal leukoencephalopathy.

A. INFECTIONS

Viral

1. **HIV** — HIV produces a subacute encephalitis that results in progressive dementia and generalized neurological decline. The most usual appearance on CT is diffuse low-attenuation change within the white matter plus cerebral atrophy. MRI shows ill-defined patchy/diffuse bilateral signal change within the white matter and/or basal ganglia. Mass effect and contrast enhancement is usually absent. Other abnormalities include cerebral/cerebellar atrophy and infarcts secondary to vasculitis.
2. **Cytomegalovirus** — patchy/diffuse periventricular signal change (MRI) ± ependymitis. May present with cranial nerve neuropathies.
3. **Progressive multifocal leukoencephalopathy** — caused by papovaviruses (JC virus). Destruction of oligodendroglia results in myelin and axon loss. Imaging shows multifocal or extensive confluent involvement of the cerebral white matter with relative sparing of the cerebral cortex. Mass effect is usually minimal and typically there is little or no enhancement with contrast media. Involvement of the deep grey nuclei is unusual. The abnormalities are not usually symmetrical and there is no atrophy; these features are more typical of HIV encephalopathy.
4. **Herpes simplex and zoster** — non-specific signal change within the cerebral white matter ± grey matter involvement.

Fungal

1. **Cryptococcus** — a meningitis that can be complicated by invasive seeding of the brain along the perivascular spaces. Produces multiple punctate foci of increased T_2W signal within the basal ganglia and pons.
2. **Aspergillus** — rare in AIDS. More commonly seen in other forms of immunocompromise such as bone marrow transplantation. Can present as an invasive paranasal sinusitis with extension into orbit and brain. Also presents as cerebral

abscess and infarct, the latter secondary to fungal occlusion of the cerebral vessels.

3. ***Candida*** — rare. May produce meningitis, meningoencephalitis, abscess, microabscesses and granulomas.

Protozoal

1. **Toxoplasma** — imaging reveals solitary/multiple, small nodules/ring-enhancing lesions with a predilection for the basal ganglia, thalami and corticomedullary junction. Surrounding oedema is variable. The appearances may mimic lymphoma (see below), but multiple abnormalities are more suggestive of toxoplasmosis.

Bacterial

1. **Tuberculosis** — leptomeningeal thickening/enhancement, cerebritis, abscess, hydrocephalus and infarcts.
2. **Nocardia** — multiple abscesses.
3. **Syphilis** — acute meningitis with leptomeningeal enhancement, hydrocephalus, cranial nerve neuropathies ± parenchymal gummas (nodular or ring-enhancing). Also meningovascular with meningeal thickening and brain infarcts.
4. **Listeria.**
5. **Pyogenic.**

B. TUMOUR

1. **Lymphoma*** — a periventricular location with subependymal spread suggests lymphoma instead of toxoplasmosis. In HIV, lymphoma may present with solitary or multiple ring-enhancing mass(es), as well as the appearances encountered in the immunocompetent (see 12.34).

Further Reading

Donovan Post M.J. (1997) Neuroimaging of AIDS 1 & 2. *Neuroimaging Clin. North Am.*

12.15 CONGENITAL CNS INFECTIONS

1. **Cytomegalovirus** — CMV 'targets' the developing germinal matrix and produces multiple foci of calcification, predominantly in a periventricular distribution. Other features are microcephaly, deafness, chorioretinitis and polymicrogyria. Lissencephaly, hypoplastic cerebellum and marked ventriculomegaly occur with early *in-utero* infection.
2. **Toxoplasma** — the foci of calcification encountered with congenital toxoplasmosis are more scattered than those seen with CMV infection and tend to involve the basal ganglia, periventricular region and cerebral cortex. Hydrocephalus occurs secondary to aqueduct stenosis caused by ependymitis. Microcephaly, porencephaly and chorioretinitis are other manifestations.
3. **Rubella** — deafness, cataracts, chorioretinitis, microphthalmia, microcephaly, atrophy and parenchymal calcification.
4. **Herpes simplex** — acute neonatal encephalitis produces diffuse or focal white matter oedema (± haemorrhage) that accentuates the cerebral cortex on CT. The infection is not localized to the limbic system as it is in older children and adults. Meningeal enhancement occurs in the acute phase. Subsequent atrophy and cystic encephalomalacia.
5. **HIV** — diffuse cerebral atrophy. Calcification of the basal ganglia after the first year of life.

Further Reading

Barkovich A.J. (2000) *Pediatric Neuroimaging,* Ch. 11, 3rd edn. Philadelphia: Lippincott Williams & Wilkins, pp. 715–23.

12.16 HEAD INJURY

PRIMARY BRAIN INJURY

Extra-axial

1. **Extradural haemorrhage** — high-attenuation, lentiform, extra-axial haematoma usually caused by laceration of the middle meningeal artery and seen in combination with a skull fracture. Venous extradural haemorrhages (EDHs) are less common and result from injury to the dural sinuses (e.g. torcula).
2. **Subdural haemorrhage** — crescentic extra-axial haematoma crossing suture lines.
3. **Subarachnoid haemorrhage.**
4. **Intraventricular/choroid plexus haemorrhage.**
5. **Skull fracture** — high-density fluid (blood) in the sphenoid sinus or temporal bone is suggestive of a basal fracture.
6. **CSF leak** — usually associated with fracture of the anterior cranial fossa floor in the region of the cribriform plate.
7. **Pneumocephalus** — skull base fracture with dural tear may lead to pneumocephalus if there is communication with an air-containing structure (i.e. paranasal sinus or temporal bone).
8. **Cranial nerve palsy** — VII nerve palsy secondary to temporal bone fracture.

Intra-axial

1. **Diffuse axonal injury** — shearing injuries caused by sudden rotational or accelerating/decelerating forces. High-attenuation lesions (CT) located at the corticomedullary junction, corpus callosum, internal capsule and brainstem. Small petechial haematomas are most conspicuous on GE MRI. Late atrophy.
2. **Haemorrhagic contusions** — occur as brain impacts adjacent skull or dura. Usually subfrontal, anterior temporal and cerebral convexities. High-attenuation on CT ± surrounding brain swelling.
3. **Deep grey matter and brainstem lesions** — shearing forces disrupt small perforating vessels and cause focal injuries. The midbrain may also strike the tentorium.
4. **Hypoxia** — see 12.29.

SECONDARY BRAIN INJURY

1. **Intracerebral herniation** — subfalcine herniation, when severe, may cause anterior cerebral artery infarction if the free inferior edge of the falx impinges on the displaced vessels. Unilateral hydrocephalus occurs if the foramen of Monro is obstructed by the mass effect. Descending transtentorial herniation causes posterior cerebral artery infarction as the vessel is compromised by the free edge of the tentorium.
2. **Diffuse cerebral oedema and ischaemia.**
3. **Embolic complications** — secondary to arterial damage (i.e. dissection).
4. **Meningitis** — and its complications.
5. **Hypoxia** — see 12.29.

DELAYED

1. **Atrophy** — focal (cortical contusion) or diffuse.
2. **CSF leak** — frontal sinus, anterior cranial fossa floor or temporal bone.
3. **Arterial pseudoaneurysm** — following arterial laceration.
4. **Arteriovenous fistula** — direct carotid–cavernous fistula.
5. **Leptomeningeal cyst** — usually due to the dura being trapped in the fracture line. Continuing CSF pulsation prevents fracture repair and may produce a ‘growing fracture’.

Further Reading

Osborn AG (1994) *Diagnostic Neuroradiology,* Ch. 8. St Louis: Mosby, pp. 199–247.

12.17 NON-ACCIDENTAL INJURY*

In cases of suspected NAI, head CT should be performed as soon as the child is stabilized. Plain skull radiographs should also be performed to confirm the presence and extent of skull fractures. If the initial brain CT is abnormal, or if a child has neurological symptoms despite a normal or equivocal CT, brain MRI should be performed and interpreted by a neuroradiologist. Delayed CT at days 8–10 may clarify the presence and extent of any abnormality seen on the initial CT. MRI at 3 months documents the extent of permanent damage.

1. **Subdural haematoma** — haematomas of different ages are highly suspicious of NAI. Posterior interhemispheric and occipital SDHs are common and occur following laceration of bridging veins. Chronic SDHs with CSF signal must be differentiated from benign enlargement of the subarachnoid space. The latter is most often seen overlying the anterior frontal lobes. MRI may aid diagnosis in difficult cases since haematomas should not be isointense with CSF on PD and FLAIR sequences.
2. **Skull fracture** — complex, bilateral, depressed, multiple and non-parietal fractures are suggestive of NAI.
3. **Cortical contusions/shearing injuries** — see 12.16.
4. **Cerebral oedema** — effacement of the cerebral sulci and basal cisterns plus loss of normal grey–white matter differentiation.
5. **Hypoxia** — The cerebellum and thalami appear relatively hyperdense in comparison with the low-density cerebral hemispheres as a result of asphyxia (reversal sign).
6. **Subarachnoid and intraventricular haemorrhage.**
7. **Subdural hygromas** — tears in the arachnoid may allow CSF to collect within the subdural space.
8. **Cerebral laceration** — best identified by ultrasound and MRI. Virtually pathognomonic of shaking injury in the first 6 months.
9. **Vascular injuries** — dissection of intracranial or cervical vessels. May lead to pseudoaneurysm formation.
10. **Late sequelae** — hydrocephalus, atrophy, gliosis and growing fractures.
11. **Coexistent non-CNS injuries** — retinal haemorrhages, skeletal fractures, visceral injuries.

Further Reading

Harwood-Nash D.C. (1992) Abuse to the pediatric central nervous system. *Am. J. Neuroradiol.*, 13: 569–75.

Jaspan T., Griffiths P.D., McConachie N.S. *et al* (2002) Neuroimaging for non-accidental head injury in childhood: a proposed protocol. *Clin. Radiol.* (in press).

Kleinman P.K. (1998) *Diagnostic Imaging of Child Abuse,* Ch. 15, 2nd edn. St Louis: Mosby.

12.18 LARGE HEAD IN INFANCY

1. **Hydrocephalus.**
2. **Chronic subdural haematoma.**
3. **Neurofibromatosis*.**
4. **Mucopolysaccharidoses.**
5. **Megalencephaly.**
6. **Alexander's disease** — leukodystrophy that typically involves the frontal lobes early in its course.
7. **Canavan's disease** — leukodystrophy that typically affects the subcortical arcuate fibres, but often involves the entire cerebral white matter.
8. **Hydranencephaly.**

12.19 WIDE CRANIAL SUTURES

> 10 mm at birth; > 3 mm at 2 years; > 2 mm at 3 years.

NORMAL

Raised intracranial pressure

Only seen in children < 10 years.

1. **Intracranial tumour.**
2. **Subdural haematoma.**
3. **Hydrocephalus.**

Infiltration of sutures

1. **Neuroblastoma** — ± skull vault lucencies and 'sunray' spiculation (a reaction to subpericranial deposits).
2. **Leukaemia.**
3. **Lymphoma*.**

Metabolic disease

1. **Rickets*.**
2. **Hypoparathyroidism.**
3. **Lead intoxication.**
4. **Bone dysplasias with defective mineralization.**

Recovery from illness

Rapid rebound growth of the brain following:

1. **Deprivational dwarfism.**
2. **Chronic illness.**
3. **Prematurity.**
4. **Hypothyroidism.**

Trauma

Traumatic diastasis of the sutures.

12.20 HYDROCEPHALUS

Hydrocephalus can be classified in terms of 'communicating' and 'non-communicating' (obstructive) pathologies. These conditions must be differentiated from disorders producing ventricular enlargement secondary to cerebral atrophy. The more reliable radiological features favouring 'hydrocephalus' rather than atrophy include:

1. Commensurate enlargement of the temporal horns.
2. Ventricular enlargement disproportionate to the degree of sulcal widening.
3. Periventricular fluid secondary to transependymal flow of CSF.
4. Enlarged third ventricle with large suprapineal and chiasmatic recesses.
5. In children < 2 years head circumference is often the best distinguishing feature between hydrocephalus and atrophy.

NON-COMMUNICATING HYDROCEPHALUS (INTRAVENTRICULAR OBSTRUCTION)

Ventricular dilatation caused by intraventricular obstruction at, or above, the outlet foramina of the fourth ventricle.

1. **Lateral ventricles**
   (a) Intrinsic tumour — solid or ependymal. (See 12.52 and 12.53.)
   (b) Ventriculitis — following infection intraventricular adhesions may produce 'encysted' CSF collections which fail to drain (e.g. 'trapped' temporal horn).
   (c) Extraventricular tumour — mass effect from large parenchymal mass may also produce an 'encysted' temporal horn.
2. **Foramen of Monro**
   (a) Tumour — colloid cyst, subependymal giant cell astrocytoma.
   (b) Ventriculitis — adhesive arachnoiditis.
   (c) Haemorrhage — fresh clot or delayed adhesive arachnoiditis.
   (d) Cerebral swelling — severe mass effect with subfalcine herniation (e.g. SDH).
3. **Third ventricle**
   (a) Intraventricular tumour — see 12.52 and 12.53.
   (b) Extraventricular tumour — pituitary adenoma, craniopharyngioma, arachnoid cyst.

4. **Cerebral aqueduct**
   (a) Intraventricular tumour — ependymal seeding.
   (b) Extraventricular tumour — pineal, mesencephalic, tentorial mass lesions.
   (c) Developmental aqueduct stenosis.
   (d) Ventriculitis.
   (e) Haemorrhage.
5. **Fourth ventricle**
   (a) Intraventricular tumours — ependymoma, metastasis.
   (b) Extraventricular tumour — medulloblastoma, metastasis, haemangioblastoma, large posterior extrinsic masses (e.g. meningioma, vestibular schwannoma).
   (c) Outflow obstruction — infection (TB), haemorrhage (SAH), leptomeningeal malignancy

COMMUNICATING HYDROCEPHALUS (EXTRAVENTRICULAR 'OBSTRUCTION')

There is free flow of CSF throughout the ventricular system. Impaired resorption of CSF by the arachnoid granulations accounts for the majority of cases.

1. **Subarachnoid haemorrhage.**
2. **Infectious meningitis.**
3. **Malignant meningitis** — e.g. lung, breast, medulloblastoma.
4. **Granulomatous meningitis** — sarcoidosis, tuberculosis.
5. **Altered venous dynamics** — vein of Galen malformation, multisutural craniosynostosis, venous obstruction.

OTHERS

1. **'External' hydrocephalus** — misleading term used to describe the benign enlargement of the subarachnoid space seen in young children. Caused by disproportionate growth between the skull and intracranial contents. Must not be mistaken for subdural haematomas.
2. **Overproduction hydrocephalus** — choroid plexus papilloma is often quoted as a cause of hydrocephalus produced by excessive CSF production. It is more likely that the highly proteinaceous tumour exudate impairs CSF uptake at the arachnoid granulations.
3. **Normal pressure hydrocephalus** — clinical syndrome of memory loss, gait disturbance and urinary incontinence. Imaging

demonstrates ventricular enlargement disproportionate to the degree of sulcal widening, but has limited ability to select those patients that will benefit from CSF shunting. Underlying aetiology and mechanism of neural dysfunction remains contentious.

4. **Hydrocephalus *ex vacuo*** — misleading term that should be discontinued in favour of atrophy.

Further Reading

Boaz J.C. & Edwards-Brown M.K. (1999) Hydrocephalus in children. *Neuroimaging Clin. North Am.*, 9(1): 73–91.

Bradley W.G. (2001) Normal pressure hydrocephalus and deep white matter ischemia: which is the chicken and which is the egg? *Am. J. Neuroradiol.*, 22: 1638–9.

12.21 CONGENITAL SYNDROMES ASSOCIATED WITH ENLARGED VENTRICLES

COMMON

1. **Achondroplasia*.**
2. **X-linked hydrocephalus syndrome.**
3. **Soto's syndrome** — cerebral gigantism. Advanced skeletal maturity.
4. **Acrocephalosyndactyly** — types Apert and Pfeiffer.
5. **Crouzon's syndrome.**
6. **Fetal alcohol syndrome.**
7. **Lissencephaly.**
8. **Osteopetrosis*** — AR.

UNCOMMON

1. **Metachromatic leukodystrophy.**
2. **Mucopolysaccharidoses IH and VI.**
3. **Thanatophoric dysplasia.**

Further Reading

Jones K.L. (1988) *Smith's Recognizable Patterns of Human Malformation*, 5th edn. Philadelphia: WB Saunders.

Taybi H. & Lachman R.S. (1996) *Radiology of Syndromes, Metabolic Disorders and Skeletal Dysplasias*, 4th edn. St Louis: Mosby, p. 1017.

12.22 PNEUMOCEPHALUS

1. **Trauma** — major compound fractures of the skull vault allow entry of air. Fractures involving the frontal, ethmoidal or sphenoidal sinuses may allow air to enter the cranial cavity and fluid to collect in the sinuses (horizontal ray film essential for detection). CSF rhinorrhoea may occur (fluid tests positive for glucose).
2. **Iatrogenic** — postoperative.
3. **Osteoma of ethmoid sinus** — may erode the ethmoid roof, penetrating the dura to allow air to enter the cranial cavity.
4. **Tumours eroding the skull base arising in sinuses or nasopharynx.**
5. **Empty sella** — occasionally empty sella is complicated by the development of a spontaneous communication between the sella and the sphenoid sinus.

12.23 CT ATTENUATION OF CEREBRAL MASSES

(Relative to normal brain.)

HYPERDENSE

1. Neoplasms
   (a) Meningioma — 95%.
   (b) Lymphoma.
   (c) Metastases — 30%.
   (d) Glioma — 10% (most glioblastomas show mixed attenuation).
   (e) Ependymoma.
   (f) Papilloma.
   (g) Medulloblastoma — 80%.
   (h) Pituitary adenoma — 25%.
   (i) Craniopharyngioma — if solid.
   (j) Acoustic neuroma — 5%.
2. **Haematoma** — if ≤ 2 weeks old.
3. **Giant aneurysm.**
4. **Colloid cyst** — 50%.

ISODENSE

1. **Neoplasms**
   (a) Acoustic neuroma — 95%.
   (b) Pituitary adenoma — 65%.
   (c) Glioma — 10%.
   (d) Metastases — 10%.
   (e) Chordoma.
   (f) Pinealoma.
2. **Haematoma** — if 2–4 weeks old.
3. **Tuberculoma.**
4. **Colloid cyst** — 50%.

HYPODENSE

1. **Tumours**
   (a) Craniopharyngioma.
   (b) Glioma.
   (c) Metastases.
   (d) Prolactinoma.
   (e) Haemangioblastoma.
   (f) Lipoma.
   (g) Epidermoid.
   (h) Dermoid.
2. **Haematoma** — ± if >4 weeks old.
3. **Abscess** — pyogenic.
4. **Tuberculoma.**
5. **Cyst**
   (a) Arachnoid.
   (b) Porencephalic.
   (c) Hydatid.

12.24 DIFFERENTIAL DIAGNOSIS OF A SOLITARY INTRACEREBRAL MASS

1. **Glioblastoma multiforme** — heterogeneous irregular supratentorial mass. Usually large and located within the cerebral white matter. Composed of solid and cystic components; the former enhances avidly with contrast medium. Surrounding 'oedema' and overall mass effect is often considerable. Rarely GBM may appear multifocal. Calcification is rare.
2. **Metastasis** — homogeneous or heterogeneous lesion, either supratentorial or infratentorial. CT attenuation and MRI signal is highly variable and depends upon the primary lesion. Metastases vary from solid nodules to cystic lesions and are often multiple. Avid contrast enhancement (solid or ring) is usually accompanied by considerable white matter oedema. Usually smaller than GBM and often located near the grey–white matter junction.
3. **Arterial infarct** — homogeneous low-attenuation wedge-shaped lesion (CT) involving grey and white matter. Mass effect is variable and is maximal after 3–5 days. Contrast enhancement is often absent, but may be gyriform, 'ring-like' or solid. Size and location depends on the site of vessel occlusion and the collateral circulation. Increased signal on T_2W MRI, low signal on T_1W MRI. (See 12.1 and 12.2.)
4. **Abscess** — homogeneous low-attenuation lesion with thin enhancing rim and marked surrounding oedema. Often small and multiple if caused by haematogenous dissemination. Usually located at the grey–white matter junction and other small vessel territories. May lie next to a site of extradural sepsis (paranasal sinus or temporal bone).
5. **Demyelination** — an acute plaque of demyelination may present as a relatively large area of low attenuation on CT, with variable mass effect and contrast enhancement. High signal on T_2W MRI, sometimes with a 'target' appearance. Usually, but not invariably located within the white matter structures. Other lesions may also be identified.
6. **Haematoma** — high attenuation on CT with mass effect depending on the size of the lesion and the degree of surrounding oedema (see 12.7). Ageing haematomas become isodense with brain by approximately 14 days and may produce diagnostic difficulties, especially if there is ring enhancement. The characteristic progression of signal change on MRI aids diagnosis (see 12.8).

7. **Encephalitis** — ill-defined confluent or patchy low attenuation with variable mass effect on CT. Haemorrhage is a feature of fulminant herpes encephalitis. Increased T_2W signal on MRI characteristically involves grey matter structures and adjacent white matter. Contrast medium uptake is gyriform. (See 12.13.)
8. **Aneurysm** — CT reveals a high-density extrinsic mass that, if large, invaginates the adjacent brain. There is often incomplete peripheral calcification and avid enhancement with contrast unless the lesion is partially thrombosed. Mass effect depends on the size of the lesion and the presence of any surrounding oedema. Turbulent flow and internal thrombus causes heterogeneous signal return on MRI. Phase-encoding artefact may indicate that a large mixed signal mass is indeed an aneurysm.

12.25 INTRACRANIAL CALCIFICATION

NORMAL

1. **Pineal gland** — after 10 years of age on plain radiographs, earlier on CT.
2. **Choroid plexus** — atria of lateral ventricles, unusual in third and fourth ventricles.
3. **Dura** — falx and tentorium.
4. **Basal ganglia** — usually in the globus pallidus. Symmetrical speckled calcification. Sometimes unilateral.
5. **Habenular commissure** — C-shaped calcification within the tela choroidea of the third ventricle.
6. **Dentate nuclei** — posterolateral to the fourth ventricle.
7. **Parasellar ligaments** — petroclinoid and interclinoid ligaments.
8. **Arachnoid granulations** — related to the dural venous sinuses.

VASCULAR

1. **Atherosclerosis** — vertebrobasilar and carotid siphon.
2. **Aneurysms** — mural calcification in large/giant aneurysms.
3. **AVM** — see 12.11.
4. **Cavernous angioma** — see 12.11.
5. **Chronic SDH.**
6. **Old infarct/haemorrhage** — rare. Calcification may appear relatively early in paediatric infarcts, but may not be permanent.

TUMOURS

1. **Meningioma** — intratumoral calcification and bony hyperostosis.
2. **Glioma** — less than 10% of astrocytomas calcify. Usually feature of low-grade tumour.
3. **Oligodendroglioma** — approximately 50% calcify. Slow-growing heterogeneous mass typically located in the frontal lobe.
4. **Craniopharyngioma** — see 12.48.
5. **Dermoid** — fat containing partially calcified mass usually located in the parasellar region. May rupture and cause chemical meningitis with fat droplets in the subarachnoid space. High signal on T_1W MRI.
6. **Ependymoma** — see 12.41.
7. **Chordoma and chondrosarcoma** — see 12.57.
8. **Choroid plexus papilloma** — see 12.41.
9. **Dysembryoplastic neuroepithelial tumour (DNT)** — see 12.41.
10. **Central neurocytoma** — low-grade tumour related to the septum pellucidum. Cyst formation, necrosis and calcification common.
11. **Metastases** — adenocarcinoma (breast, gastrointestinal).
12. **Pineal tumours** — teratoma and germinoma. See 12.50.
13. **Lipoma** — crescentic calcification in midline malformation (corpus callosum).

INFECTIONS

1. **TORCH** — see 12.15.
2. **Cysticercosis** — periventricular, cisternal and corticomedullary nodules.
3. **Tuberculosis** — within basal cisterns, ventricles and parenchyma.

BASAL GANGLIA CALCIFICATION

1. **Normal.**
2. **Endocrine** — hypoparathyroidism, pseudohypoparathyroidism, hypothyroidism.
3. **Metabolic** — mitochondrial disorders, Fahr's disease, Cockayne's syndrome.
4. **Infection** — see above.
5. **Toxic** — hypoxia, carbon monoxide, lead.
6. **Chemotherapy/radiation** — mineralizing angiopathy most prominent in the basal ganglia, dentate nuclei and corticomedullary junction.

NEUROCUTANEOUS

1. **Sturge–Weber syndrome** — dystrophic calcification of the cerebral cortex. See 12.38.
2. **Tuberous sclerosis*** — periventricular and parenchymal. (See 12.38.)
3. **Neurofibromatosis*** — choroid plexus (premature and excessive), subependymal and basal ganglia, neoplastic.

12.26 ENHANCEMENT OF THE MENINGES ON CT AND MRI

NORMAL

1. **Dura** — falx, tentorium and cavernous sinus wall.
2. **Leptomeninges** — thin smooth discontinuous uptake of contrast is normal on MRI.
3. **Vessels** — large and medium calibre intracranial arteries and veins.

LEPTOMENINGEAL

1. **Infection** — bacterial, tuberculosis, fungal, syphilis, viral and Lyme's disease.
2. **Tumour** — metastases (breast and lung), glioblastoma multiforme, leukaemia, lymphoma, germinoma, pineoblastoma, ependymoma, medulloblastoma, Langerhans cell histiocytosis.
3. **Sarcoidosis*** — see 12.47.
4. **Subarachnoid haemorrhage** — subacute.
5. **Infarct** — modest enhancement overlying subacute infarcts.
6. **Neurocutaneous** — Sturge–Weber syndrome (pial angioma).
7. **Rheumatoid arthritis.**

DURAL

1. **Infection** — skull base osteomyelitis, paranasal infection.
2. **Tumour** — meningioma, metastasis, lymphoma.
3. **Intracranial hypotension** — other features include subdural effusions (especially infratentorial), engorgement of the dural sinuses and brainstem descent. Uniform dural thickening may be seen following lumbar puncture.
4. **Postoperative** — craniotomy, shunt insertion.
5. **Idiopathic pachymeningitis.**
6. **Venous thrombosis.**
7. **Sarcoidosis*.**
8. **Extramedullary haematopoiesis** — e.g. myelofibrosis.
9. **Rheumatoid arthritis.**

Further Reading

Collie D.A., Brush J.P., Lammie G.A. *et al.* (1999) Imaging features of leptomeningeal metastases. *Clin. Radiol.*, 54: 765–71.

Ginsberg L.E. (1994) Contrast enhancement in meningeal and extra-axial disease. *Neuroimaging Clin. North Am.*, 4: 133–52.

12.27 ENHANCEMENT OF THE EPENDYMA AND SUBARACHNOID SPACE ON CT AND MRI

EPENDYMA

1. **Infection** — bacterial, tuberculosis, fungal, syphilis or viral ventriculitis (e.g. cytomegalovirus).
2. **Tumour** — metastases (breast and lung), glioblastoma multiforme, leukaemia, lymphoma, germinoma, pineoblastoma, ependymoma, medulloblastoma, Langerhans cell histiocytosis.
3. **Sarcoidosis*.**
4. **Enlarged ependymal veins** — AVM, venous angioma, and centripetal venous drainage due to dural venous occlusion or Sturge–Weber syndrome.
5. **'Inflammatory'** — intrathecal chemotherapy/post-shunt insertion.

SUBARACHNOID SPACE

1. **Meningitis** — contrast may leak into the CSF in the presence of a malignant or infective meningitis (e.g. Lyme disease).
2. **Neoplasm.**
3. **Post-angiography.**

12.28 MULTIPLE RING-ENHANCING LESIONS ON CT AND MRI

1. **Metastases** — ring-enhancing or solid nodules most commonly at the corticomedullary junction. Commonest primaries are lung, breast, kidney, colon and melanoma. Multiple in approximately 80% of cases. May be simultaneous involvement of the meninges, subarachnoid space and skull. Most common infratentorial mass in adults. Contrast-enhanced MRI superior to CT.
2. **Abscesses** — abscesses differ from metastases in that they tend to have a thin uniform wall, homogeneous centre and florid surrounding oedema. Tuberculosis has several radiological manifestations, including basal meningitis, communicating hydrocephalus and calcifying parenchymal granulomas. Other infections producing multiple small lesions include toxoplasmosis, cryptococcosis and cysticercosis.
3. **Demyelination** — enhancing lesions (solid or ring) are indicative of acute inflammation with breakdown of the blood–brain barrier. (See 12.34.)
4. **Lymphoma*** — lymphoma in immunocompetent individuals usually presents as solid enhancing periventricular tumour with ependymal spread. In AIDS, however, lymphoma is often ring-enhancing and must be differentiated from toxoplasmosis.
5. **Multicentric glioma** — although glioma may appear multicentric on imaging studies these lesions are usually diffusely infiltrating and confluent histologically.
6. **Infarcts** — multiple infarcts suggest an embolic source. Enhancement may be gyriform, ring-like or solid.
7. **Contusions/haematomas** — peripheral enhancement occurs as a result of injury to the blood–brain barrier. A subacute isodense haematoma on CT with peripheral ring enhancement must not be mistaken for a neoplasm.

12.29 BASAL GANGLIA – BILATERAL ABNORMALITIES

The functional unit of the basal ganglia includes the caudate nucleus (CN), putamen (P), globus pallidus (GP), substantia nigra, subthalamic nucleus and ventral tegmentum. The corpus striatum (S) describes the head of the CN and P.

NORMAL

1. **Age-related change** — light, speckled calcification is commonly seen within the GP with advancing age. This may cause a slight increase in signal on T_1W MRI. Increased iron deposition in the GP and P reduces signal on T_2W sequences.
2. **Perivascular spaces** — sharply defined CSF-containing structures that surround small arteries as they penetrate the brain. (See 12.34.)

VASCULAR

1. **Lacunar infarcts** — punctate well-defined foci of low attenuation ± lesions within the white matter and brainstem. May be unilateral.
2. **Hypoxia** — following severe acute asphyxia in the neonatal period, abnormalities are seen in the posterior putamina, lateral thalami, hippocampi, corticospinal tracts and perirolandic/ calcarine cortices. Bilateral lesions in the GP/P are seen following heroin overdose, cardiac arrest and drowning.
3. **Venous infarction** — thrombosis of the deep cerebral veins may result in bilateral infarcts that involve the basal ganglia, mesial temporal lobes and thalami.

NEURODEGENERATIVE DISEASE

1. **Parkinson's disease** — see 12.35.
2. **Huntington's disease** — see 12.35.
3. **Other extrapyramidal disorders** — e.g. multisystem atrophy, supranuclear palsy (see 12.35).

TOXIC

1. **Exogenous** — methanol, cyanide (P), carbon monoxide and hydrogen sulphide. Manganese in total parenteral nutrition can cause increased T_1W signal on MRI.
2. **Endogenous** — acquired hepatocellular degeneration also causes increased signal on T_1W MRI within the basal ganglia. Kernicterus (bilirubin encephalopathy) causes lesions in the GP.

ACQUIRED METABOLIC DISEASE

1. **Hypoglycaemia** — putamina, cerebral cortex/adjacent white matter (parietal and occipital lobes).
2. **Osmotic myelinolysis** — see 12.34.
3. **Haemolytic–uraemic syndrome.**

INHERITED METABOLIC DISEASE

1. **Wilson's disease (S) and Kearns–Sayre disease (GP).**
2. **Mitochondrial cytopathies** — e.g. Leigh's disease (S, GP ± thalami, brainstem, cerebral cortex).
3. **Leukodystrophies** — e.g. Krabbe's disease(thalami and periventricular white matter).
4. **Amino acid disorders** — e.g. methylmalonic acidaemia (GP).
5. **Lipidoses** — e.g. Tay–Sachs disease (S and thalami). Cerebral atrophy.
6. **Hallervorden–Spatz** — low signal on T_2W MRI (excess iron deposition) in GP ± 'eye of the tiger' appearance (surrounding gliosis).

OTHERS

1. **Basal ganglia calcification** — see 12.25.
2. **Neurofibromatosis 1*** — non-neoplastic 'neurofibromatous bright objects'.
3. **Viral encephalitides** — e.g. sporadic Creutzfeld–Jakob disease. (See 12.13.)
4. **Microabscesses** — e.g. cryptococcosis, toxoplasmosis.
5. **Acute disseminated encephalomyelitis** — further lesions within the white matter.

Further Reading

Barkovich A.J. (2000) *Pediatric Neuroimaging,* Ch. 3, 3rd edn. Philadelphia: Lippincott Williams & Wilkins, pp. 71–156.

Lai P.H., Chen C., Liang H.L. *et al.* (1999) Hyperintense basal ganglia on T-1 weighted MR imaging. *Am. J. Roentgenol.,* 172: 1109–15.

12.30 HYPERECHOIC LESIONS IN THE BASAL GANGLIA OF NEONATES AND INFANTS

Single punctate, multiple punctate or stripe-like densities.

1. **Congenital infections** — CMV, toxoplasmosis, rubella, HIV and syphilis.
2. **Asphyxia/hypoxia.**
3. **Cardiac disease** — particularly hypoplastic left heart syndrome.
4. **Chromosome disorders.**
5. **Fetal alcohol and drug exposure.**
6. **Twin–twin transfusion.**
7. **Idiopathic.**

Further Reading

Coley B.D., Rusin J.A. & Boue D.R. (2000) Importance of hypoxic/ischemic conditions in the development of cerebral lenticulostriate vasculopathy. *Pediatr. Radiol.*, 30: 846–55.
Teele R.L., Hernanz-Schulman M. & Sorel A. (1988) Echogenic vasculature in the basal ganglia of neonates: a sonographic sign of vasculopathy. *Radiology*, 169: 423.

12.31 HYPERINTENSE BASAL GANGLIA ON T_1W MRI

DUE TO PARAMAGNETIC SUBSTANCES

1. **Intracranial haemorrhage.**
2. **Haemorrhagic infarction.**
3. **Wilson's disease.**
4. **Japanese encephalitis.**
5. **Long-term total parenteral nutrition** — due to manganese deposition.

CALCIFICATION

Calcification is usually iso-intense or hypointense on T_1W and T_2W sequences, but may, occasionally, be hyperintense on T_1W images because of the crystalline structure of the calcification. (See 12.25.)

HAMARTOMA

1. **Neurofibromatosis type I*** — most common sites are the globus pallidus, internal capsule, brainstem and dentate nucleus. No perilesional oedema or enhancement. Lesions tend to resolve by adulthood.

INDETERMINATE CAUSES

1. **Profound hypoxia/ischaemia** — with involvement of the perirolandic region.
2. **Chronic liver disease with a portocaval shunt** — CT and T_2W images are normal.

Further Reading

Lai P.H., Chen C., Liang H.L. *et al.* (1999) Hyperintense basal ganglia on T1-weighted MR imaging. *Am. J. Roentgenol.*, 172: 1109–15.

12.32 THALAMUS – BILATERAL ABNORMALITIES

VASCULAR

1. **Lacunar infarcts** — small, well-defined, non-cortical infarcts that are similar to CSF in terms of attenuation/signal. May be unilateral or bilateral. Also occur within the basal ganglia, pons and corona radiata.
2. **Arterial infarct** — perforating arteries from the tip of the basilar artery may simultaneously supply both thalami. Occlusion causes symmetrical infarction of both thalami.
3. **Venous infarct** — thrombotic occlusion of the vein of Galen and/or straight sinus. High-attenuation thrombus within the veins on pre-contrast CT and loss of the normal venous flow void on MRI. Lesions within the mesial temporal lobes indicate occlusion of the basal veins.
4. **Severe anoxia** — infants surviving severe abrupt anoxia or profound circulatory arrest suffer injury to the ventrolateral thalami, lateral putamina, hippocampi and eloquent cortices since these are all metabolically active areas.

INFECTION

1. **Variant CJD** — the 'pulvinar' sign of symmetrical high T_2W signal within the posterior thalamic nuclei.
2. **Japanese encephalitis** — involvement of the substantia nigra also occurs.

METABOLIC

1. **Carbon monoxide poisoning** — low-attenuation CT and high T_2W signal on MRI. Lesions also within the basal ganglia.
2. **Wernicke's encephalopathy** — thiamine deficiency in chronic alcoholics presents with confusion, ataxia and ophthalmoplegia. The mesial thalamic nuclei, mammillary bodies, midbrain and floor of the third ventricle may show increased T_2W signal change and/or pathological enhancement with contrast. Atrophy may follow.
3. **Inherited metabolic diseases** — e.g. mitochondrial cytopathies (e.g. Leigh's disease) and certain leukodystrophies (e.g. Krabbe's disease).

OTHERS

1. **Acute disseminated encephalomyelitis** — there are usually more lesions within the white matter or other grey matter structures. (See 12.34.)

Further Reading

Antunez E., Estruch R. & Cardenal C. (1998) Usefulness of CT and MR imaging in the diagnosis of acute Wernicke's encephalopathy. *Am. J. Roentgenol.*, 171: 1131–7.

Zeidler M., Sellar R.J., Ironside J. *et al.* (2000) The pulvinar sign on magnetic resonance imaging in variant Creutzfeldt–Jakob disease. *Lancet*, 355: 1412–8.

12.33 INHERITED METABOLIC WHITE MATTER DISEASE

White matter diseases show low density on CT, low signal on T_1W and high signal on T_2W MRI. T_2W MRI is the most sensitive method for detection. The early echo on multiple echo sequences shows periventricular lesions in greater relief against lower signal ventricular CSF. Acute lesions may show focal contrast uptake due to blood–brain barrier damage. Conditions can be considered under two main categories: dysmyelinating diseases (primary abnormalities of formation of myelin) and demyelinating diseases (which are the result of myelin loss after its normal formation).
(See also 12.34.)

DYSMYELINATION (LEUKODYSTROPHIES)

Enzyme deficiencies prevent the normal formation or maintenance of myelin. They are disorders of children and present with variable mental retardation.

Lysosomal disorders

1. **Metachromatic leukodystrophy** — arylsulphatase-A deficiency. AR. Usually presents at 2–3 years but may be later. Rapidly progressive. Diffuse symmetrical abnormalities but with sparing of the subcortical arcuate fibres. Cerebellar lesions may be present. Cerebral atrophy.
2. **Krabbe's (globoid) leukodystrophy** — galactosylceramide β-galactosidase deficiency. AR. Presentation in the first 6 months of life with death in early childhood. Symmetrical abnormalities in the posterior white matter of the optic radiations, centrum semiovale, thalami and caudate nuclei. Severe atrophy is common late in the disease.

Peroxisomal disorders

1. **Adrenoleukodystrophy (ALD)** — different phenotypes include cerebral ALD (40%), adrenomyeloneuropathy (46%; progressive spastic diplegia in adults), and primary adrenocortical insufficiency without CNS involvement. ALD is further divided into childhood, adolescent and adult forms. X-linked recessive trait (i.e. boys only). Childhood cerebral ALD presents between 5 and 10 years and there are three patterns of involvement on MRI:
   (a) (80%) Deep parieto-occipital white matter, splenium and posterior body of corpus callosum, visual and auditory pathways, and corticospinal tracts.
   (b) (15%) Deep anterior frontal white matter, genu and anterior body of corpus callosum, and cerebellar deep white matter.
   (c) (5%) Projectional white matter fibres. Enhancement may be evident at the leading edges of the lesions, indicating demyelination. Calcification rarely seen in the parieto-occipital regions.
2. **Zellweger's (cerebrohepatorenal) syndrome** — presentation in the newborn. Hepatomegaly, polycystic kidneys and stippled calcification, particularly of the patellae. Extensive white matter changes with pachygyria and, in some cases, vermian hypoplasia.

Mitochondrial dysfunction

Defects of respiratory chain enzymes which are expressed as myopathic diseases or multisystem disorders with encephalopathy. Among the latter group are:

1. **Leigh's disease** — mostly AR. Lesions in the grey and white matter but predominantly the former. CT and MRI abnormalities in the midbrain, pons, periaqueductal grey matter, substantia nigra, floor of fourth ventricle and dentate nuclei. Lesions in the caudate nucleus and putamen are common and may show cavitation.
2. **MELAS (mitochondrial myopathy, encephalopathy, lactic acidosis and stroke-like episodes)** — focal cortical and brainstem white matter changes with basal ganglia calcification ± cerebral and cerebellar atrophy.
3. **MERFF (myoclonus epilepsy with ragged red fibres).**
4. **Alper's disease** — primarily affects cerebral grey matter.

5. **Kearns–Sayre syndrome** — onset in childhood or adolescence of progressive external ophthalmoplegia and pigmentary retinal degeneration, and at least one of the following: heart block, elevated CSF protein and cerebellar dysfunction. White matter disease is associated with cortical and/or cerebellar atrophy and calcification in the basal ganglia or deep white matter.

Amino acid and organic acid metabolic disorders

1. **Canavan's disease** — AR. Found predominantly in children of Ashkenazi Jewish descent. Manifests in the first few months of life; progressive increase in head size, hypotonia, seizures, progressing to spasticity and death by 2 years of age. Increased urine and plasma N-acetylaspartic acid. Bilaterally symmetrical changes, most severe in the subcortical white matter and globus pallidus with relative sparing of the brainstem and internal capsule. Cerebral atrophy is late.
2. **Maple syrup urine disease.**

Others

1. **Pelizaeus–Merzbacher disease** — rare. X-linked recessive. Onset in infancy with nystagmus, ataxia and spasticity. Death in adolescence. Generalized white matter disease.
2. **Alexander's disease** — Presentation in the first year with developmental delay, macrocephaly, spasticity and seizures. Death in early childhood. Frontal involvement occurs earliest and is most severe. Enhancement may occur in the caudate nuclei, periventricular white matter and optic radiations. Megalencephaly and ventricular dilatation.

NB. A useful mnemonic for the differential diagnosis of the common dysmyelinating leukodystrophies is **'LACK P**roper **M**yelin' (Hatten, 1991).

L	=	Leigh's disease
A	=	Alexander's disease
		Adrenoleukodystrophy
C	=	Canavan's disease
K	=	Krabbe's disease
P	=	Pelizaeus–Merzbacher disease
M	=	Metachromatic leukodystrophy.

Further Reading

Barkovich A.J., Lyon G. & Evrard P. (1992) Formation, maturation and disorders of white matter. *Am. J. Neuroradiol.*, 13: 447–61.

Greenberg S.B., Faerber E.N., Riviello J.J. *et al.* (1990) Subacute necrotizing encephalomyelopathy (Leigh disease): CT and MRI appearances. *Pediatr. Radiol.*, 21: 5–8.

Hatten H.P. Jr (1991) Dysmyelinating leukodystrophies: 'LACK Proper Myelin'. *Pediatr. Radiol.*, 21: 477–82.

Kendall B.E. (1992) Disorders of lysosomes, peroxisomes and mitochondria. *Am. J. Neuroradiol.*, 13: 621–53.

Melhem E.R., Barker P.B., Raymond G.V. *et al.* (1999) X-linked adrenoleukodystrophy in children: review of genetic, clinical, and MR imaging characteristics. *Am. J. Roentgenol.*, 173: 1575–81.

12.34 MULTIPLE SCLEROSIS AND ITS DIFFERENTIAL DIAGNOSIS

Multiple sclerosis is the most common demyelinating disorder to affect the brain and spinal cord. MRI is far superior to CT and typically demonstrates ovoid high T_2W signal lesions within the corpus callosum and periventricular white matter that typically lie perpendicular to the ventricular margin. Other characteristic sites include the optic radiation, brainstem (dorsal), cerebellar peduncles and optic nerves. Abnormalities in the cerebral cortex, deep grey nuclei and 'peripheral' white matter are less common, but are by no means rare. Acute lesions are usually ill-defined and may display surrounding oedema. The latter contributes to the 'target' appearance that is sometimes seen with acute plaques. Solid and 'ring-like' contrast uptake is a feature of acute demyelination, regardless of the cause. Large acute lesions may be mistaken for tumours if there is considerable mass effect. As lesions age they shrink, become more circumscribed and fail to enhance with contrast medium. Sagittal T_2W, proton density and FLAIR sequences are recommended for routine diagnostic purposes.

DIFFERENTIAL DIAGNOSIS

Normal

1. **Virchow–Robin spaces** — sharply defined CSF-containing structures that surround small arteries as they penetrate the brain. Most commonly seen in the centrum semiovale, basal ganglia and upper brainstem. May appear slightly hyperdense to CSF on CT because of partial volume effects. V–R spaces are isointense with CSF signal on all MRI sequences (proton density and FLAIR sequences are helpful). May be very large, especially in the lentiform nuclei.
2. **Age-related white matter lesions** — small peripheral white matter lesions are commonly seen in the normal ageing brain. Periventricular lesions are best seen on FLAIR MRI and may present as a thin uniform rim, frontal 'caps' or more patchy areas of signal change. The loose term 'small vessel ischaemia' is a convenient, but inaccurate, description of most age-related white matter change.

Vascular

1. **'Small vessel disease'** — premature cerebrovascular disease in hypertensive and diabetic patients presents as either confluent or highly discrete white matter abnormalities. Ischaemic white matter lesions are located more peripherally than typical MS plaques and only very rarely do they involve the corpus callosum, dorsal brainstem or cerebellar peduncles. Discrete abnormalities within the ventral pons, basal ganglia and thalami that have low T_1W and high T_2W signal on MRI are consistent with small vessel infarcts.
2. **Infarct** — a solitary abnormality with modest mass effect, little or no contrast uptake that involves white matter and adjacent cortex can cause diagnostic uncertainty. A reduced apparent diffusion coefficient on diffusion imaging suggests an acute infarct. Loss of the arterial flow void indicates vessel occlusion.
3. **Vasculitis** — imaging appearances are entirely non-specific and range from extensive confluent abnormalities to focal white matter lesions. Catheter angiography may demonstrate segmental irregularity and/or occlusion.

Demyelination

1. **Acute disseminated encephalomyelitis (ADEM)** — monophasic autoimmune demyelinating disorder following viral infection or immunization. When compared to MS, ADEM is associated with fewer, but larger lesions. Involvement of grey matter and juxtacortical white matter is also more in keeping with ADEM. Mass effect is not a predominant feature. Lesions enhance in the acute phase.
2. **Osmotic myelinolysis** — changes are usually seen in the pons following correction of chronic hyponatraemia in alcoholic and malnourished individuals. The pons is swollen and returns low T_1W and high T_2W signal. Extrapontine lesions may be symmetrical and occur in either grey or white matter structures. The diagnosis is rarely confused with MS if the clinical history is well documented.
3. **Chemotherapy/radiotherapy** — the use of cytotoxics such as methotrexate can result in an acute necrotizing leukoencephalopathy with multifocal white matter abnormalities. Concurrent brain irradiation increases the risk of neurotoxicity. Late features include calcification in the basal ganglia, corticomedullary junction and dentate nuclei, plus diffuse cerebral atrophy.
4. **Miscellaneous toxins** — solvents and alcohol (e.g. Marchiafava–Bignami).

Infection

1. **Encephalitis** — viral encephalitides, including HIV and progressive multifocal leukoencephalopathy, may present with multiple white matter lesions. (See 12.13 and 12.14.)
2. **Lyme disease** — multisystem disease caused by the spirochaete *Borrelia*. White matter lesions may resemble MS plaques. Abnormalities also appear within the basal ganglia and brainstem, and there may be associated parenchymal and meningeal enhancement.

Tumour

1. **Lymphoma*** — primary CNS lymphoma presents as a solitary/multiple enhancing periventricular mass(es). These tumours are typically iso/hyperdense on pre-contrast CT and isointense with grey matter on T_2W sequences. They may also be located within the corpus callosum, basal ganglia and thalami. Ependymal spread is common.
2. **Glioma** — a large solitary plaque of demyelination in the acute phase can be mistaken for a primary brain tumour.
3. **Multicentric glioma** — although glioma may appear multicentric on imaging studies these lesions are usually diffusely infiltrating and confluent histologically.

Other

1. **Sarcoidosis*** — although sarcoidosis may present with multiple white matter abnormalities, the presence of meningeal enhancement means that the diagnosis is not normally confused with MS.

Further Reading

Brant-Zawadzki M. (1992) Multiple sclerosis and its imitators. In: Huckman M.S. (ed.) *ARRS Neuroradiology Categorical Course Syllabus*. American Roentgen Ray Society, pp. 229–32.

Erdag N., Bhorade R.M. & Alberico R.A. (2001) Primary lymphoma of the CNS: typical and atypical CT and MR imaging appearances. *Am. J. Roentgenol.*, 176: 1319–26.

Fuller G.N. & Bone I. (2001) Neurology in practice: multiple sclerosis. *J. Neurol. Neurosurg. Psyhiatry*, 71 (Suppl II): ii1–27.

Singh S., Alexander M. & Korah I.P. (1999) Acute disseminated encephalomyelitis: MR imaging features. *Am. J. Roentgenol.*, 173: 1101–8.

12.35 CEREBRAL ATROPHY

DIFFUSE

1. **Normal ageing.**
2. **Excessive alcohol intake.**
3. **Severe head injury.**
4. **Multiple sclerosis.**
5. **Cerebrovascular disease** — hypoxic–ischaemic insult, 'small vessel disease' and multifocal cortical infarcts.
6. **Drugs** — e.g. corticosteroids.
7. **Encephalitis/meningitis.**
8. **Radiation and chemotherapy.**
9. **Neurodegenerative disease** — see below.
10. **Human immunodeficiency virus** — see 12.14.
11. **Pregnancy.**

FOCAL

1. **Infarct** — infarcted brain involutes and may be associated with antegrade degeneration (atrophy ± signal change) of associated tracts (Wallerian degeneration).
2. **Haemorrhage** — large haematomas typically evolve into collapsed slit-like cavities.
3. **Encephalitis/meningitis** — focal or diffuse.
4. **Trauma** — focal brain contusions.
5. **Alzheimer's disease** — most common dementia. Atrophy may be diffuse but the changes in the mesial temporal lobes (hippocampus) are usually the most severe.
6. **Frontotemporal dementia** — anterior frontal and/or temporal atrophy.
7. **Parkinson's disease** — generalized cerebral atrophy plus atrophy of the substantia nigra (with reduced iron deposition). Increased iron deposition within the putamen leads to reduced T_2W signal.
8. **Progressive supranuclear palsy** — atrophy of the midbrain (tectum), globus pallidus and frontal lobes.
9. **Pick's disease** — typically produces severe frontal and anterior temporal atrophy.
10. **Huntington's disease** — focal atrophy of the caudate nuclei (and putamena).
11. **Corticobasal degeneration** — posterior parietal and/or frontal lobes.

Further Reading

Miller B.L. (2002) Past glory and future promise: maximising and improving understanding of atrophy patterns in the diagnosis of degenerative dementias. *Am. J. Neuroradiol.*, 23: 33–4.

12.36 DIFFUSE CEREBELLAR ATROPHY

1. **Normal ageing.**
2. **Excessive alcohol intake.**
3. **Drugs** — e.g. phenytoin.
4. **Paraneoplastic** — e.g. oat cell carcinoma, ovary.
5. **Radiation** — e.g. posterior fossa tumours in children.
6. **Ataxia telangiectasia** — hereditary oculocutaneous telangiectasia and cerebellar ataxia. Increased incidence of infection and malignant tumours (mainly lymphoma and leukaemias).
7. **Neurodegenerative diseases** — e.g. olivopontocerebellar degeneration is characterized by small medullary olives, a flattened pons and atrophic cerebellar peduncles and vermis. Multisystem atrophy may present with cerebral and cerebellar atrophy, a 'hot-cross bun sign' of high T_2W signal within the pons and linear signal change in the lateral putamina.
8. **Hereditary spinocerebellar ataxias** — e.g. Friedreich's ataxia.
9. **Idiopathic cerebellar ataxias.**
10. **Gluten sensitivity** — associated with sporadic cerebellar ataxia.

Further Reading

Hadjivassilou M., Grunewald R.A., Chattopadhyay A.K. *et al.* (1998) Clinical, radiological, neurophysiological and neuropathological characteristics of gluten ataxia. *Lancet*, 352: 1582–5.

Macia F., Yekhlef F., Ballon G. *et al.* (2001) T2-hyperintense lateral rim and hypointense putamina are typical but not exclusive of multisystem atrophy. *Arch. Neurol.*, 58: 1024–6.

12.37 DISORDERS OF NEURONAL MIGRATION

The neuronal population of the normal cerebral cortex arrives by a process of outward migration from the periventricular germinal matrix between the 8th and 16th weeks of gestation. This complex process of cell migration can be interfered with by many causes, sporadic and unknown, chromosomal or genetic.

1. **Agyria–pachygyria** — poorly formed gyri and sulci, the former being more severe. Focal pachygyria may be the cause of focal epilepsy. Polymicrogyria (see below) may coexist with pachygyria. Extreme cases with a smooth brain may be termed lissencephaly. Complete lissencephaly ≡ agyria. Several distinct forms are recognized.
   Type I lissencephaly — small brain with few gyri; smooth, thickened four-layer cortex resembling that of a 13-week fetus with diminished white matter and shallow vertical sylvian fissures ('figure-of-eight' appearance on axial images). ± agenesis of the corpus callosum. Severe mental retardation, diplegia, seizures, microcephaly and limited survival. Some infants have specific dysmorphic features: Miller–Dieker syndrome and Norman–Roberts syndrome. Pachygyria may also be observed in Zellweger syndrome and prenatal CMV infection.
   Type II lissencephaly (Walker–Warburg syndrome) — smooth cortex, cerebellar hypoplasia and vermian aplasia and hydrocephalus (in 75%) due to cisternal obstruction by abnormal meninges or aqueduct stenosis.
2. **Polymicrogyria** — the neurons reach the cortex but are distributed abnormally. Macroscopically the surface of the brain appears as multiple small bumps. Localized abnormalities are more common than generalized and often involve arterial territories, especially the middle cerebral artery. The most common location is around the sylvian fissure. The cortex is isointense to grey matter but in 20% of cases the underlying white matter has high signal on T_2W. Linear flow voids due to anomalous venous drainage may be present. Polymicrogyrias may be present in the vicinity of a porencephalic cyst, be associated with heterotopic grey matter or agenesis of the corpus callosum or with evidence of fetal infection such as intracranial calcification. Symptoms and signs depend on the size, site and

presence of associated abnormalities. The majority have mental retardation, seizures and neurological signs.

3. **Schizencephaly** — clefts which extend through the full thickness of the cerebral mantle from ventricle to subarachnoid space. The cleft is lined by heterotopic grey matter and microgyrias, indicating that it existed prior to the end of neuronal migration. Unilateral or bilateral (usually asymmetrical) and usually near the sylvian fissure. May be associated with absence of the septum pellucidum or, less commonly, dysgenesis of the corpus callosum. There are variable clinical manifestations, from profound retardation to isolated partial seizures.
4. **Heterotopic grey matter** — collections of neurons in a subependymal location, i.e. at the site of the germinal matrix or arrested within the white matter on their way to the cortex. Isointense to normal grey matter on all imaging sequences. Nodules or bands and may have mass effect. Frequently a part of complex malformation syndromes or, when isolated, may be responsible for focal seizures which are amenable to surgical treatment. Small heterotopias are probably asymptomatic.
5. **Cortical dysplasia** — focal disorganization of the cerebral cortex. A single enlarged gyrus resembling focal pachygyria. Usual presentation is with partial epilepsy.

Further Reading

Aicardi J. (1992) *Clinics in Developmental Medicine. Diseases of the Nervous System in Childhood*, Ch. 3, 2nd edn. London: MacKeith Press, pp. 69–130.

Barkovich A.J. (2000) *Pediatric Neuroimaging*, 3rd edn.. Philadelphia: Lippincott Williams & Wilkins, pp. 281–318.

12.38 INTRACRANIAL MANIFESTATIONS OF WELL-KNOWN NEUROCUTANEOUS DISORDERS

NEUROFIBROMATOSIS 1*

1. **Optic pathway glioma.**
2. **Non-optic glioma** — tectum, brainstem.
3. **Plexiform neurofibroma.**
4. **Neurofibromatous bright objects.**
5. **Vascular abnormalities** — aneurysm, ectasia, progressive arterial occlusion, moya moya, arteriovenous fistula.
6. **Skull** — sphenoid wing dysplasia, calvarial defects, dural ectasia.
7. **Orbit** — Lisch nodules, retinal phakomas, buphthalmos and pulsatile exophthalmos, 'harlequin orbit'.

NEUROFIBROMATOSIS 2*

1. **Cranial nerve schwannomas.**
2. **Meningiomas.**
3. **Non-neoplastic choroid plexus lesions.**
4. **Ependymomas.**

TUBEROUS SCLEROSIS*

1. **Cortical 'tubers'.**
2. **Subependymal nodules.**
3. **Giant cell astrocytoma.**
4. **White matter lesions** — disorganized collections of dysplastic cells. On MRI appear as well-defined foci of increased T_2W signal.
5. **Orbit** — retinal phakomas.
6. **Vascular abnormalities** — aneurysm, vessel stenosis.

STURGE–WEBER SYNDROME (SWS)

1. **Cerebral atrophy** — with compensatory thickening of the skull vault/enlargement of the frontal sinus.
2. **Cortical calcification** — 'tram track' gyriform calcification underlying the pial angioma.
3. **Surface enhancement** — corresponds to the embryonic pial angioma that persists in SWS because of hypoplasia of the cortical veins. Bilateral in 20%.

4. **Enlarged choroid plexus.**
5. **Enlarged medullary/subependymal veins** — centripetal shunting, often by anomalous venous structures, in response to an inadequate cortical venous system.
6. **Orbit** — buphthalmos, scleral/choroid angiomas, glaucoma.

VON HIPPEL–LINDAU

1. **Haemangioblastoma** — commonest lesion is a cystic tumour with an enhancing mural nodule in one of the cerebellar hemispheres. Smaller lesions are often solid and hypervascular.
2. **Orbit** — retinal angioma, microphthalmia ± dystrophic calcification.
3. **Non-CNS** — visceral cysts, phaeochromocytoma, renal cell carcinoma.

OSLER–WEBER–RENDU (HEREDITARY HAEMORRHAGIC TELANGIECTASIA)

1. **Cerebral abscess** — caused by septic emboli passing through pulmonary arteriovenous malformations.
2. **Embolic infarcts** — as above.
3. **Vascular abnormalities** — telangiectasia, cavernoma, AVM, AVF, aneurysm and epistaxis.
4. **Non-CNS** — mucocutaneous (skin, gut) and visceral (pulmonary, hepatic) telangiectasia.

Further Reading

Barkovich A.J. (2000) *Pediatric Neuroimaging,* Ch. 6, 3rd edn. Philadelphia: Lippincott Williams & Wilkins, pp. 383–441.

Griffiths P.D. (1996) Sturge–Weber revisited: the role of neuroradiology. *Neuropediatrics,* 11: 417–9.

Griffiths P.D. & Martland T.R. (1997) Tuberous sclerosis complex: the role of neuroradiology. *Neuropediatrics,* 28: 1–9.

Mukonoweshuro W., Blaser S. & Griffiths P.D. (1999) Neurofibromatosis type 1: the role of neuroradiology. *Neuropediatrics,* 30: 111–9.

12.39 HIGH SIGNAL ON T_1W MRI

NORMAL

1. **Posterior lobe of pituitary** — the pituitary gland is uniformly high signal up to 6 months.
2. **Moving structures** — flow-related 'enhancement', particularly in dural venous sinuses and other vascular structures. Moving CSF may also produce the same effect.
3. **Ossification of the falx.**
4. **Calcification within the basal ganglia.**
5. **Rathke's cleft cyst.**
6. **Fat.**

PATHOLOGICAL

1. **Haemorrhage** — methaemoglobin in 'subacute' haematomas causes markedly increased T_1W signal (see 12.8). Also haemorrhagic metastases. 'Petechial haemorrhage' is also seen as high T_1W signal within the cerebral cortex of subacute infarcts.
2. **Thrombus** — partially thrombosed large/giant aneurysms may have a substantial high T_1W signal component. Intraluminal thrombus associated with venous thrombosis and arterial stroke is often readily visualized.
3. **Fat** — lipoma of the corpus callosum, perimesencephalic and chiasmatic cisterns. Dermoids may also have a large fat component.
4. **Proteinaceous fluid** — e.g. craniopharyngioma, colloid cyst.
5. **Melanin** — melanoma, neurocutaneous melanosis.
6. **Heavy metals** — e.g. manganese in total parenteral nutrition and Wilson's disease.

12.40 SIGNAL VOID ON T_2W MRI

NORMAL

1. **Normal arterial and venous flow** — loss of a normal vascular flow void on a T_2W sequence implies reduced flow or occlusion. Loss of a T_2W flow void is therefore an important feature of venous sinus thrombosis and acute arterial stroke. A potential pitfall in the diagnosis of venous sinus thrombosis is the presence of very acute thrombus that may return profoundly low T_2W signal (deoxyhaemoglobin). Other problems with interpretation arise because of normal variations in the venous structures (asymmetry of the lateral sinuses), arachnoid granulations within the sinus (focal areas of CSF signal) and normal slow or turbulent flow.
2. **Densely packed bone** — because the temporal bone is composed of dense bone and air cells it normally has no T_2W signal return. As a result, the CSF-filled membranous labyrinth is highlighted.
3. **Dural calcification** — dense calcification of the falx may present as an area of T_2W void.
4. **Air.**
5. **CSF flow** — movement of CSF within the ventricles may lead to T_2W signal voids (e.g. cerebral aqueduct).

PATHOLOGICAL

1. **Aneurysms** — may appear as saccular or fusiform signal voids related to the arterial circulation. Large or giant aneurysms with complex turbulent flow ± internal thrombus more commonly display mixed patterns of signal return on spin-echo sequences. Aneurysms must not be mistaken for temporal bone, parasellar or sellar neoplasms since surgery may be fatal. Large aneurysms arising from peripheral divisions of the cerebral vessels have been mistaken for hemisphere tumours.
2. **Arteriovenous malformations** — the enlarged feeding and draining vessels of parenchymal/ependymal AVMs present as serpiginous flow voids. The AVM nidus may also appear as an area of flow void and is sometimes associated with haemorrhage and gliosis.
3. **Acute haemorrhage** — deoxyhaemoglobin is a product of blood cell degradation and is seen in acute intracerebral haematomas (days 1–3).

4. **Chronic haemorrhage** — haemosiderin deposition is a feature of chronic haemorrhage and is seen to surround old haematoma cavities, and to coat the brain and cranial nerves following repeated subarachnoid bleeds (superficial siderosis).

12.41 SUPRATENTORIAL TUMOURS IN CHILDREN

Primary CNS tumours are the second most common malignancy in children (leukaemia is the commonest). Overall, supratentorial and infratentorial tumours occur with equal incidence.

1. **Hemispheric astrocytoma** — solid, solid with a necrotic centre, or cystic with a mural nodule. Usually large at presentation and can involve the basal ganglia and thalami. Most are low grade. Enhancement with contrast medium does not correlate with histological grade. Associated with NF1.
2. **Craniopharyngioma** — more than half of all craniopharyngiomas occur in children (8–14 years). Cystic/solid partially calcified suprasellar mass presenting with headache, visual disturbance and endocrine abnormalities. (See 12.48.)
3. **Optic pathway glioma** — low grade, but infiltrating pilocytic astrocytomas associated with NF1. Solid enhancing tumours that extend along the length of the anterior optic pathways and may invade adjacent structures (e.g. hypothalamus) and extend posteriorly into the optic tracts and radiations.
4. **Giant cell subependymal astrocytoma** — slow-growing partially cystic, partially calcified tumour occurring in tuberous sclerosis. Located at the foramen of Monro and presents with obstructive hydrocephalus.

5. **Germ cell tumours** — germinomas, teratoma. (See 12.50.)
6. **Primitive neuroectodermal tumour (PNET)** — large heterogeneous hemispheric mass presenting in neonates and small infants. Necrosis, haemorrhage and enhancement are common.
7. **Dysembryoplastic neuroepithelial tumour (DNT)** — benign cortical tumour often presenting with seizures. Cortical (temporal) mass, usually small, that may demonstrate internal cyst formation and calcification.
8. **Ganglioglioma** — well-circumscribed peripheral tumour that often presents with seizures. Cystic tumour with mural nodule ± calcification.
9. **Choroid plexus papilloma** — presents in young children with hydrocephalus. Most occur in the atrium of the lateral ventricle (fourth ventricle in adults) and appear as a well-circumscribed multilobulated avidly enhancing intraventricular mass ± calcification. Invasion of brain suggests choroid plexus carcinoma.
10. **Ependymoma** — often in the frontal lobe adjacent to the frontal horn, but not usually within the ventricular system.

Further Reading

Barkovich A.J. (2000) *Pediatric Neuroimaging,* 3rd edn.. Philadelphia: Lippincott Williams & Wilkins, pp. 487–545.

Edwards-Brown M.K. (1994) Supratentorial brain tumors. *Neuroimaging Clin. North Am.,* 4: 437–55.

Griffiths P.D. (1999) A neuroimaging protocol for imaging children with brain tumours. *Clin. Radiol.,* 54: 558–62.

12.42 INFRATENTORIAL TUMOURS IN CHILDREN

These comprise 50% of paediatric cerebral tumours. The majority arise from the cerebellar parenchyma. Cerebellar astrocytomas, medulloblastomas and ependymomas present with symptoms of raised intracranial pressure and ataxia. Brainstem gliomas involve the cranial nerve nuclei and long tracts at an early stage.

1. **Cerebellar astrocytoma** — 20–25% of posterior fossa tumours. Vermis (50%) or hemispheres (20%) or both sites (30%) ± extension into the cavity of the fourth ventricle. Calcification in 20%.
   CT/MRI: Large lesion displacing the fourth ventricle → obstructive hydrocephalus. 80% are juvenile pilocytic astrocytomas with an excellent prognosis. Tumour can be cystic, solid or solid with central necrosis. 50% of all tumours are a cyst with an isodense enhancing mural nodule. The cyst contents have slightly > CSF attenuation on CT. 40–45% are solid with central necrosis. The solid component is isodense to hypodense to white matter on CT, low signal on T_1W MRI and high signal on T_2W MRI. The solid component enhances on CT and MRI. Larger tumour at diagnosis than the solid type. The solid type accounts for 10%.
2. **Medulloblastoma** — 30–40% of posterior fossa tumours. Short history. 80% located in the vermis; 30% extend into the brainstem.
   CT: Moderately well-defined, ovoid or spherical mass; slightly > surrounding cerebellum; rim of oedema. Usually uniform enhancement; non-enhancement rarely. Calcification (in 10%) is usually small, homogeneous and eccentric. Dystrophic calcification occurs after radiotherapy. Small cystic or necrotic areas are unusual.
   MRI: Low signal on T_1W; heterogeneous iso- to low signal on T_2W. Variable enhancement.
   Dissemination of tumour by: (a) seeding of the subarachnoid space; (b) retrograde ventricular extension; or (c) extracranial metastases to bone, lymph nodes or soft tissues. Recurrence of tumour is demonstrated by: (a) enhancement at the site of the lesion; (b) enhancement of the subarachnoid space (basal cisterns, sylvian, fissures, sulci and ependymal surfaces of ventricles; or (c) progressive ventricular enlargement.

3. **Ependymoma** — most commonly in the floor of the fourth ventricle. 8–15% of posterior fossa tumours. Usually a long clinical history.
   CT: Typically, an isodense to hyperdense fourth ventricular mass with punctate calcifications, small cysts and heterogeneous or homogeneous enhancement. Calcification within a fourth ventricular mass or adjacent to the fourth ventricle ≡ ependymoma.
   MRI: Homogeneous or heterogeneous. Slightly hypointense on T_1W and isointense to grey matter on T_2W. Tumour extension through the foramen of Magendie, foramen magnum (behind the spinal cord) and foramen of Luschka (into the cerebellopontine angle) are important clues to the diagnosis.
4. **Brainstem glioma** — 20–30% of posterior fossa tumours. Insidious onset because of the location and tendency to infiltrate cranial nerve nuclei and long tracts without producing CSF obstruction until late. Four subgroups: (a) medullary, (b) pontine, (c) mesencephalic and (d) those associated with NF1. Tumours may also be diffuse (> 50–75% of the brainstem in the axial plane) or focal (< 50%). Calcification rare.
   (a) Medullary — least common. Young children. May be differentiated into focal dorsally exophytic and diffuse forms (with significantly worse prognosis). Low attenuation (CT), low signal (T_1W) and high signal (T_2W).
   (b) Pontine — most common. Diffuse tumours are low attenuation (CT), low signal (T_1W) and high signal (T_2W). Flattening of the floor of the fourth ventricle. Contrast enhancement is rare. Focal tumours are very uncommon but do exhibit heterogeneous enhancement.
   (c) Mesencephalic — focal tumours are more common than diffuse. Symptoms depend on the exact location of the mass.
   (d) Associated with NF1 — most commonly in the medulla. Similar imaging appearances to those without NF1, but patients may be asymptomatic and progression is slower.

Further Reading

Barkovich A.J. (2000) *Pediatric Neuroimaging*, 3rd edn.. Philadelphia: Lippincott Williams & Wilkins, pp. 446–68.

Griffiths P.D. (1999) A neuroimaging protocol for imaging children with brain tumours. *Clin. Radiol.*, 54: 558–62.

Vezina L.-G. & Packer R.J. (1994) Infratentorial brain tumors of childhood. *Neuroimaging Clin. North Am.*, 4: 423–36.

12.43 SMALL PITUITARY FOSSA

1. **Normal variant.**
2. **Dystrophia myotonica** — hereditary. Usually starts in early adult life. Cataracts, frontal baldness, testicular atrophy, thick skull and large frontal sinus.
3. **Radiotherapy as child.**
4. **Hypopituitarism.**

12.44 EXPANDED PITUITARY FOSSA

1. **Size** — normal range is: height 6.5–11 mm
length 9–16 mm
breadth 9–19 mm.
2. **Double floor** — can be a normal variant (asymmetrical development) but a tumour should be suspected.
3. **Elevation/destruction of clinoid processes.**
4. **Loss of lamina dura.**

1. **Para/intrasellar mass.**
2. **Raised intracranial pressure** — due to dilated third ventricle.
3. **Empty sella.**
4. **Nelson's syndrome** — post-adrenalectomy for Cushing's syndrome.

12.45 J-SHAPED SELLA

Flattened tuberculum sellae with a prominent sulcus chiasmaticus.

1. **Normal** — 5% of normal children.
2. **Optic chiasm glioma** — if the chiasmatic sulcus is markedly depressed (W- or omega-shaped sella), the tumour may be bilateral.
3. **Neurofibromatosis*.**
4. **Achondroplasia*.**
5. **Mucopolysaccharidoses.**
6. **Chronic hydrocephalus** — bone erosion occurs due to the downward pressure of an enlarged third ventricle.

12.46 INTRASELLAR MASS

NEOPLASTIC

1. **Pituitary microadenoma** — adenomas < 10 mm. Enhance more slowly than surrounding normal pituitary and are therefore seen as areas of reduced contrast uptake on gadolinium studies. Frequently seen on pre-contrast T_1W and T_2W sequences. May cause visible asymmetry of the gland, infundibulum or sella.
2. **Pituitary macroadenoma** — adenomas > 10 mm. Solid or mixed solid/cystic enhancing midline pituitary mass. Often evidence of asymptomatic haemorrhage (high T_1W). Imaging important for the assessment of tumour extension (optic pathway compression, cavernous sinus/sphenoid/clivus invasion and vessel encasement).
3. **Meningioma** — tuberculum or diaphragma sellae meningiomas may extend into the sella. Purely intrasellar tumour rare.
4. **Craniopharyngioma** — see 12.48.
5. **Chordoma** — Expansile lytic mass arising from the central skull base (clivus). Locally aggressive with foci of calcification (50%).
6. **Pituitary metastasis** — rare (breast most common). May appear identical to pituitary adenomas.

NON-NEOPLASTIC

1. **Pituitary 'cyst'** — all focal intraglandular abnormalities are not adenomas. Pars intermedia cysts may be seen as central well-defined cystic structures.
2. **Pituitary hyperplasia** — normal menstruating females and pregnancy. Nelson's syndrome. Generalized homogeneous enlargement of the gland.
3. **Internal carotid artery aneurysm** — must not be mistaken for intrasellar tumour. (See 12.9.)
4. **Ectatic carotid artery** — medially positioned ICAs may be bilateral and produce 'kissing carotids'.
5. **Rathke's cleft cyst** — intrasellar, suprasellar or both. Cystic or solid. Hyperdense on CT with rim enhancement. High T_1W signal on MRI.
6. **Lymphocytic hypophysitis** — lymphocytic infiltration of the anterior pituitary occurring in pregnancy/postpartum period. Enlarged enhancing gland and infundibulum.
7. **Langerhans cell histiocytosis*** — more commonly the pituitary infundibulum is thickened and enhances with gadolinium.
8. **Pituitary abscess** — rare.

Further Reading

FitzPatrick M., Tartaglino L.M., Hollander M.D. *et al.* (1999) Imaging of sellar and parasellar pathology. *Radiol. Clin. North Am.*, 37(1): 101–21.
Osborn A.G. (1994) *Diagnostic Neuroradiology*, Ch. 12. St Louis: Mosby, pp. 461–71.

12.47 INFUNDIBULAR MASS

NEOPLASTIC

1. **Germinoma** — usually involves the infundibulum, anterior recesses of the third ventricle and hypothalamus. MRI shows an avidly enhanced infiltrating homogeneous mass. Synchronous involvement of the pineal region in 10%. Meningeal/ependymal dissemination is relatively common.
2. **Lymphoma*** — may involve the pituitary gland, infundibulum and hypothalamus. Isointense on T_1W with strong uniform enhancement. Coexistent disease may be visible in the paranasal sinuses or orbit.
3. **Leukaemia.**
4. **Glioma.**
5. **Metastasis** — haematogenous (breast) and leptomeningeal (medulloblastoma).

NON-NEOPLASTIC

1. **Sarcoidosis*** — sarcoidosis has numerous intracranial manifestations, including nodular or diffuse thickening and enhancement of the dura, leptomeninges and cranial nerves. Enhancement involving the optic apparatus/floor of the third ventricle and pituitary infundibulum is particularly suggestive of sarcoidosis. Non-specific white matter lesions may be associated with enhancing parenchymal nodules. Strokes occur in microvascular territories due to vessel obliteration by granulomata.
2. **Lymphocytic hypophysitis** — lymphocytic infiltration of the anterior pituitary occurring in pregnancy/postpartum period. Enlarged enhancing gland and infundibulum.
3. **Langerhans cell histiocytosis*** — commonest radiological presentation is a thickened, enhancing infundibulum with loss of the normal posterior pituitary 'bright spot'. Parenchymal, cranial nerve, meningeal and skull lesions also occur.

Further Reading

Osborn A.G. (1994) *Diagnostic Neuroradiology*, Ch. 12. St Louis: Mosby, p. 482.

12.48 SUPRASELLAR MASS

NEOPLASTIC

1. **Pituitary macroadenoma** — large tumours extend into the chiasmatic cistern where they can compress the optic apparatus. Macroadenomas typically have a 'cottage loaf' or 'figure-of-eight' appearance. Haemorrhage, cyst formation and midline origin is suggestive of macroadenoma rather than meningioma.
2. **Meningioma** — arises from the anterior cranial fossa, sphenoid wing or diaphragma sellae. Meningiomas are almost invariably homogeneous with T_2W signal similar to that of grey matter. Enhancement is uniform. The pituitary gland should be identified separately.
3. **Craniopharyngioma** — usually has sellar and suprasellar components but may occupy either compartment alone or sit in the anterior third ventricle. CT demonstrates a midline solid/cystic mass with calcification that extends superiorly and posteriorly. The solid component enhances with contrast medium. The cyst fluid may be high signal on T_1W MRI. Children 8–14 years, second peak in middle age.
4. **Chiasmatic glioma** — see 12.41.
5. **Infundibular tumour** — see 12.47.
6. **Germinoma** — see 12.47.
7. **Hypothalamic hamartoma** — sessile or pedunculated tumour lying between the pituitary stalk and mamillary bodies. Patients present with either precocious puberty or gelastic seizures (paroxysms of inappropriate emotional outbursts, usually laughing).

NON-NEOPLASTIC

1. **Aneurysm or ectatic carotid artery.**
2. **Arachnoid cyst** — CSF signal on all MRI sequences. Can cause local mass effect and obstructive hydrocephalus.
3. **Epidermoid** — lobulated non-enhancing parasellar mass. Low density on CT. Signal on MRI is similar to that of CSF but usually T_1W and PD signal is slightly brighter (this allows differentiation from arachnoid cyst). Epidermoids will also show increased signal on diffusion-weighted imaging when compared to CSF.

4. **Dermoid** — occurs in suprasellar region as midline mass with fat and calcification. May rupture and cause chemical meningitis with fat droplets in the subarachnoid space.
5. **Rathke's cleft cyst** — usually intrasellar as well. (See 12.46.)
6. **Lymphocytic hypophysitis** — see 12.46.
7. **Sarcoidosis*** — see 12.47.
8. **Langerhans cell histiocytosis*** — see 12.47.

Further Reading

Felsberg G.J. & Tien R.D. (1994) Sellar and parasellar lesions involving the skull base. *Neuroimaging Clin North Am.*, 4: 543–60.

Osborn A.G. (1994) *Diagnostic Neuroradiology*, Ch. 12. St Louis: Mosby, pp. 472–82.

12.49 CAVERNOUS SINUS/PARASELLAR MASS

NEOPLASTIC

1. **Schwannoma** — large trigeminal schwannomas can simultaneously involve the cerebellopontine angle (CPA), Meckel's cave, cavernous sinus, skull base and pterygomaxillary fissure. Extension of the tumour from the cavernous sinus through the foramen ovale into the gasserian ganglion helps differentiate a schwannoma from a meningioma.
2. **Meningioma** — enhancing homogenous mass.
3. **Pituitary adenoma** — direct local invasion from the sella.
4. **Metastasis.**
5. **Lymphoma*** — unilateral or bilateral, ± leptomeningeal, extradural or orbital disease.
6. **Invasion by skull base tumour** — e.g. chordoma, chondrosarcoma.
7. **Nasopharyngeal carcinoma** — direct superior extension.

NON-NEOPLASTIC

1. **Aneurysm or ectatic carotid artery.**
2. **Cavernous sinus thrombosis** — usually a result of orbital sepsis. The cavernous sinus may be expanded and return abnormal signal.
3. **Carotid–cavernous fistula** — a direct (from internal carotid artery) or indirect (dural) fistula results in enlargement of the sinus and its venous tributaries. An enlarged superior ophthalmic vein with retrograde flow is the most readily identified abnormality and may be associated with ophthalmoplegia, proptosis, chemosis and visual deterioration. A carotid–cavernous fistula does not always drain through the orbit and may use alternative venous routes (e.g. petrosal sinuses, pterygoid plexus). Therefore a normal orbital study does not exclude a fistula.
4. **Invasive sinusitis** — in immunocompromised patients, *Aspergillus* can invade the orbit and intracranial compartment by direct spread from the paranasal sinuses. Involvement of the cavernous sinus is well recognized.
5. **Dermoid/epidermoid** — see 12.48.
6. **Sarcoidosis*** — see 12.47.
7. **Lymphocytic hypophysitis** — see 12.46.
8. **Tolosa–Hunt syndrome** — painful, steroid-responsive, ophthalmoplegia caused by a non-specific granulomatous infiltration of the cavernous sinus and superior orbital fissure.

Further Reading

FitzPatrick M., Tartaglino L.M., Hollander M.D. *et al.* (1999) Imaging of sellar and parasellar pathology. *Radiol. Clin. North Am.*, 37(1): 101–21.

12.50 PINEAL REGION MASS

Accurate localization of the mass is crucial in the differential diagnosis of pineal tumours, but is not always easy, especially if the lesion is very large.

PINEAL GLAND

1. **Benign cyst** — simple cystic structure within the gland measuring < 1.5 cm. Slightly higher signal than CSF on all sequences. A common incidental finding on MRI studies. Unlikely to be significant when no mass effect and when there are no relevant symptoms.
2. **Germinoma** — most common pineal germ cell tumour. Males predominate (10:1). 10% have synchronous infundibular/suprasellar germinoma. Well-defined hyperdense calcified mass with avid uniform enhancement (CT). MRI helps delineate local and distant seeding of the subarachnoid space (spinal imaging also required). Serum markers (alpha-fetoprotein) may also be positive.
3. **Teratoma** — second most common pineal germ cell tumour. Heterogeneous mass with fat, calcification and cyst formation. Little or no enhancement. There is a spectrum of malignant potential.
4. **Parenchymal cell tumour** — whilst germinomas occur in the first two decades of life, pineal parenchymal tumours may present in later life. Pineocytomas tend to be slow-growing and present as non-specific enlargement of the pineal gland. Pineoblastoma is usually larger, more heterogeneous with much greater propensity for local invasion and CNS dissemination.

POSTERIOR BRAINSTEM

1. **Glioma** — usually low-grade tectal tumour causing aqueduct stenosis.
2. **Metastasis.**
3. **Demyelination** — rarely, an acute demyelinating disorder can present as a brainstem mass.
4. **Infarct** — arterial and venous infarcts may mimic a tumour mass.
5. **Haemorrhagic contusion.**
6. **Cavernoma** — may present with acute brainstem syndrome ± hydrocephalus following haemorrhage.

POSTERIOR THIRD VENTRICLE

1. **Glioma.**
2. **Metastasis.**
3. **Choroid plexus papilloma** — see 12.41.

PERIMESENCEPHALIC CISTERN

1. **Arachnoid cyst** — CSF density/signal on all imaging sequences.
2. **Dermoid** — see 12.48.
3. **Lipoma** — fat density/signal on imaging.
4. **Meningioma** — arising from the tentorium.
5. **Metastasis.**
6. **Arteriovenous malformation** — including vein of Galen malformation.
7. **Aneurysm** — of the posterior cerebral artery.

Further Reading

Barboriak D.P., Lee L. & Provenzale J.M. (2001) Serial MR imaging of pineal cysts: implications for natural history and follow-up. *Am. J. Roentgenol.*, 176: 737–43.

Osborn A.G. (1994) *Diagnostic Neuroradiology*, Ch. 14. St Louis: Mosby, pp. 607–13.

12.51 HYPERDENSE CHOROID PLEXUS ON CT IN A CHILD

1. **Calcification** — normal in an adult. Unusual < 10 years and, when bilateral, consider neurofibromatosis*.
2. **Haemorrhage** — in the neonate the incidence is inversely proportional to the gestational age.
3. **Haemangioma.**
4. **Choroid plexus neoplasm.**
5. **Aortic obstruction in the newborn** — upper extremity hypertension results in increased cerebral blood flow.

Further Reading

Doe F.D., Shuangsoti S. & Netsky M.G. (1972) Cryptic hemangioma of the choroid plexus: a cause of intraventricular hemorrhage. *Neurology*, 22: 1232–9.

Modic M.T., Weinstein M.A., Rothner A.D. *et al.* (1980) Calcification of the choroid plexus visualized by computed tomography. *Radiology*, 135: 369–72.

Rand J.C., Burton E.M., Tonkin I.L. *et al.* (1990) The hyperdense choroid plexus: a CT finding associated with aortic arch obstruction in the newborn. *Pediatr. Radiol.*, 21: 2–4.

Reeder J.D., Kaude J.V. & Setzer E.S. (1982) Choroid plexus hemorrhage in premature neonates; recognition by sonography. *Am. J. Neuroradiol.*, 3: 619–22.

12.52 INTRAVENTRICULAR MASS IN CHILDREN

LATERAL VENTRICLES

1. **Glioma.**
2. **Primitive neuroectodermal tumour** see 12.41.
3. **Choroid plexus papilloma** — see 12.41.
4. **Choroid plexus cyst.**
5. **Choroid plexus enlargement** — neurofibromatosis, Sturge–Weber.
6. **Subependymoma.**
7. **Meningioma.**
8. **Arteriovenous malformation** — enlarged draining veins.
9. **Subependymal heterotopia** — nodules of ectopic grey matter.
10. **Metastatic seeding** — e.g. medulloblastoma, ependymoma.

FORAMEN OF MONRO

1. **Subependymal giant cell astrocytoma** — see 12.41.

THIRD VENTRICLE

1. **Craniopharyngioma** — see 12.48.
2. **Glioma** — hypothalamic, chiasmatic. See 12.41.
3. **Langerhans cell histiocytosis*** — see 12.47.
4. **Germinoma** — see 12.50.
5. **Choroid plexus papilloma** — see 12.41.
6. **Metastatic seeding.**

FOURTH VENTRICLE

1. **Medulloblastoma** — see 12.42.
2. **Ependymoma** — see 12.42.
3. **Choroid plexus papilloma** — see 12.42.
4. **Exophytic brainstem glioma** — see 12.42.

12.53 INTRAVENTRICULAR MASS IN ADULTS

LATERAL VENTRICLES

1. **Glioblastoma multiforme.**
2. **Oligodendroglioma.**
3. **Central neurocytoma** — low-grade heterogeneous tumour typically applied to the septum pellucidum.
4. **Lymphoma*** — see 12.34.
5. **Metastasis.**
6. **Subependymoma** — non-enhancing well-defined benign tumour usually attached to the septum pellucidum. May be calcified with some heterogeneity on T_2W MRI.
7. **Meningioma.**
8. **Choroid plexus cysts/calcification.**
9. **Arteriovenous malformation.**
10. **Subependymal heterotopia** — nodules of ectopic grey matter.

FORAMEN OF MONRO

1. **Colloid cyst** — usually hyperdense on pre-contrast CT and high signal on T_1W MRI due to proteinaceous contents. T_2W signal variable. May cause obstruction of the lateral ventricles.
2. **Subependymal giant cell astrocytoma** — see 12.41.

THIRD VENTRICLE

1. **Craniopharyngioma** — see 12.48.
2. **Germinoma** — see 12.50.
3. **Metastasis.**
4. **Subependymoma.**
5. **Sarcoidosis** — see 12.47.

FOURTH VENTRICLE

1. **Metastasis.**
2. **Subependymoma.**
3. **Haemangioblastoma.**
4. **Inflammatory cyst (e.g. cysticercosis).**
5. **Choroid plexus papilloma.**

Further Reading

Guermazi A., De Kerviler E., Zagdanski A.-M. *et al.* (2000) Diagnostic imaging of choroid plexus disease. *Clin. Radiol.*, 55: 503–16.

Majos C., Coll S., Aguilera C. *et al.* (2000) Intraventricular mass lesions of the brain. *Eur. Radiol.*, 10: 951–61.

12.54 CEREBELLOPONTINE ANGLE MASS

1. **Vestibular schwannoma** — (acoustic neuroma), commonest CPA mass. On CT presents as a solid (small) or complex (large) enhancing mass with an intracanalicular component that expands the porus acousticus and internal auditory canal. MRI is the modality of choice and elegantly shows internal cystic degeneration ± haemorrhage within large lesions. Marked brainstem compression may occur and produce obstructive hydrocephalus. Intralabyrinthine tumours are rare and are best seen on contrast-enhanced MRI.
2. **Meningioma** — CPA meningiomas can be differentiated from vestibular schwannomas by virtue of their broad-based attachment to the petrous bone and more homogeneous signal. They are typically less bright on T_2W MRI and enhance uniformly. A small tongue of tissue may extend into the internal auditory canal, but there is usually no expansion. Peripheral 'dural tail' and hyperostosis suggests meningioma.
3. **Epidermoid** — low density on CT with lobulated margin. Usually same signal as CSF on MRI but relatively high signal on proton density, and diffusion-weighted imaging allows differentiation from arachnoid cyst. May be extensive and exert appreciable mass effect. Also occurs in the parasellar region. Rarely, epidermoids can be intradiploic.
4. **Trigeminal schwannoma** — similar in appearance to vestibular schwannoma, but arising from the fifth cranial nerve.
5. **Aneurysm** — large aneurysms arising from the vertebrobasilar system. See 12.9.
6. **Metastasis.**
7. **Skull base/temporal bone tumours** — e.g. glomus tumours, metastasis, cholesterol granuloma.
8. **Skull base infection** — Gradenigo's syndrome (osteomyelitis of the petrous apex) and malignant otitis externa.

Further Reading

Bonneville F., Sarrazin J.-L., Marsot-Dupuch K. *et al.* (2001) Unusual lesions of the cerebellopontine angle: a segmental approach. *RadioGraphics*, 21: 419–38.

12.55 INTERNAL AUDITORY CANAL ABNORMALITY

NEOPLASTIC

1. **Vestibular nerve schwannoma** — see 12.54.
2. **Meningioma** — see 12.54.
3. **Facial nerve schwannoma** — usually in the internal auditory canal or geniculate ganglion. Neuromas arising from the tympanic segment of the nerve may present with conductive deafness.
4. **Metastasis.**
5. **Haemangioma** — very high T_2W signal with avid enhancement.
6. **Lipoma** — high signal on pre-contrast T_1W MRI.

NON-NEOPLASTIC

1. **Bell's palsy** — pathological enhancement of the facial nerve can be seen on MRI.
2. **Postoperative** — postoperative dural enhancement can complicate the interpretation of imaging after acoustic neuroma surgery.
3. **Sarcoidosis*** — see 12.47.
4. **Langerhans cell histiocytosis*** — see 12.47 and 12.57.
5. **Other causes of meningeal enhancement** — see 12.26.

12.56 MIDDLE EAR MASS

INFLAMMATORY

1. **Acquired cholesteatoma** — a slowly expanding mass of epithelial debris originating within the middle ear. Local invasion (best assessed with CT) accounts for complications that include:
   (a) Cerebral abscess/meningitis (destruction of the tegmen).
   (b) Deafness (middle ear mass with ossicular destruction).
   (c) Facial paralysis (compromise of the intratympanic segment of the facial nerve or geniculate ganglion).
   (d) Severe vertigo and deafness (labyrinthine CSF leak caused by erosion of the lateral semicircular canal.
2. **Acute otitis media** — ascending infection from the nasopharynx produces acute middle ear infection. Untreated acute mastoiditis may result. CT shows opacified middle ear ± involvement of the entire mastoid and petrous air cell systems. May be complicated by cerebral abscess and facial palsy.
3. **Malignant otitis externa** — acute osteomyelitis of the temporal bone that occurs primarily in the elderly, diabetic and immunocompromised population. Local invasion occurs into the adjacent soft tissues and intracranial compartment. Extensive bone erosion is accompanied by soft-tissue swelling.
4. **Cholesterol granuloma** — non-specific chronic inflammation of the middle ear and mastoid. The middle ear is typically intact but the ossicles may be eroded. High signal on T_1W and T_2W MRI. Focal areas of internal low signal on T_2W MRI signify haemosiderin.
5. **Serous otitis media** — sterile fluid fills the middle ear and may opacify the entire mastoid air cell system. Identical in appearance to early acute otitis media, but the clinical presentation is quite different.
6. **Middle ear effusion** — obstruction of the eustachian tube results in middle ear effusion and conductive deafness (e.g. nasopharyngeal carcinoma).
7. **Tympanosclerosis** — deposits of fibrotic, often calcified, tissue in the middle ear, epitympanum and tympanic membrane. Presents as punctate or linear densities within the tympanic membrane or on the promontory. May appear as ill-defined calcified mass surrounding and ankylosing the ossicular chain.

NEOPLASTIC

1. **Glomus tympanicum** — reddish purple mass visible on otoscopy. CT shows soft-tissue mass centred on the cochlear promontory. Tumour or surrounding inflammation/serous fluid may opacify the entire middle ear. Tumours are often small as they present early with pulsatile tinnitus.
2. **Glomus jugulare** — extension from the jugular fossa. See 12.60.
3. **Facial nerve schwannoma.**
4. **Temporal bone mass** — see 12.57.

VASCULAR

1. **Aberrant internal carotid artery** — see 12.59.
2. **Dehiscent jugular bulb** — see 12.59.

Further Reading

Valvassori G.E., Mafee M.F. & Carter B.L. (1995). *Imaging of the Head and Neck*, Ch. 8. New York: Georg Thieme Verlag, pp. 83–103.

12.57 TEMPORAL BONE MASS

NEOPLASTIC

1. **Glomus** — jugulare and tympanicum. See 12.56 and 12.60.
2. **Meningioma.**
3. **Metastasis** — breast, lung, prostate, kidney.
4. **Myeloma/plasmacytoma*.**
5. **Lymphoma*** — usually orbit and paranasal sinuses.
6. **Nasopharyngeal carcinoma** — direct infiltration of the skull base.

7. **Carcinoma of the external auditory canal** — irregular soft-tissue mass within the external auditory canal plus ill-defined erosion of the periosteum and adjacent bone. Local invasion may be extensive.
8. **Carcinoma of the parotid gland** — local extension into the floor of the external auditory canal and inferior mastoid. May extend along the facial nerve.
9. **Rhabdomyosarcoma** — most common soft-tissue sarcoma in children. The head and neck is the most common site. Tumours usually involve the paranasal sinuses, orbit and pharynx. Bone destruction may be extensive.
10. **Chondrosarcoma** — rare slow-growing, locally aggressive at the petrous apex. Centred on the petroclival suture.
11. **Chordoma** — slow-growing locally invasive midline tumour centred on the clivus. Destructive expansile mass with internal calcification.

NON-NEOPLASTIC

1. **Cholesteatoma** — see 12.56.
2. **Cholesterol granuloma** — see 12.56.
3. **Apical petrositis** — purulent infection of the petrous apex results in destruction of the petrous apex (CT) with an inflammatory mass (MRI).
4. **Aneurysm** — fusiform aneurysm of the petrous carotid artery. CT demonstrates well-defined expansion of the carotid canal. Complex signal change on MRI must not be mistaken for a solid mass.
5. **Langerhans cell histiocytosis*** — normal bone is replaced by a mass of soft tissue that usually involves the mastoid bone. If there is extensive involvement of the temporal bone then differentiation from a malignant tumour such as rhabdomyosarcoma is difficult.

Further Reading

Fernandez-Latorre F., Menor-Serrano F., Alonso-Charterina S. *et al.* (2000) Langerhan's cell histiocytosis of the temporal bone in pediatric patients: imaging and follow-up. *Am. J. Roentgenol.*, 174: 217–22.

Valvassori G.E., Mafee M.F. & Carter B.L. (1995) *Imaging of the Head and Neck*, Ch. 10. New York: Georg Thieme Verlag, pp. 110–31.

12.58 TEMPORAL BONE SCLEROSIS

1. **Otosclerosis** — process involving the labyrinthine capsule, characterized by periods of demineralization and reparative sclerosis. Fenestral otosclerosis describes changes at the oval window. In the active phase the oval window is enlarged. The sclerotic phase sees bony obliteration of the window and footplate of the stapes. Cochlear otosclerosis is more easily recognized and results in ill-defined bone resorption (lucent halo surrounding the cochlea) and subsequent bone deposition. Bone demineralization and sclerosis may occur simultaneously, causing a mosaic pattern.
2. **Paget's disease*** — changes occur first within the petrous apex. An active stage of progressive demineralization is followed by irregular reconstruction that results in the formation of hypertrophied, irregularly mineralized bone. The otic capsule, labyrinth and internal auditory canal can all be involved.
3. **Fibrous dysplasia*** — the squamous temporal bone becomes thickened, the temporal air cells are obliterated and both the external and internal ear canals are stenosed. Changes are usually unilateral.
4. **Osteopetrosis*** — results in a homogeneous, non-pneumatized sclerotic temporal bone. The internal auditory canal is progressively narrowed and this may cause facial paralysis.
5. **Meningioma.**

Further Reading

Valvassori G.E., Carter B.L. & Mafee M.F. (1995) *Imaging of the Head and Neck*, Ch. 12. New York: Georg Thieme Verlag, pp. 143–57.

12.59 PULSATILE TINNITUS

ANATOMICAL VARIANTS

1. **Large/dehiscent jugular bulb** — flow through a normal jugular bulb may be perceived as pulsatile tinnitus, especially if the thin plate of bone between the wall of the jugular vein and middle ear is absent. If the bulb is dehiscent the jugular bulb may protrude into the middle ear and should not be mistaken for a glomus tumour.
2. **Intratympanic course of the internal carotid artery** — the inferior compartment of the middle ear is filled by the carotid artery as it runs slightly posterior and lateral to its normal course. Tracing the carotid canal on bone CT enables diagnosis.
3. **Persistent stapedial artery** — if the embryonic stapedial artery fails to regress it can be identified as it runs through the lumen of the stapes.

VASCULAR

1. **Dural arteriovenous fistula** — pulsatile tinnitus is a common presentation of fistulae into the transverse/sigmoid sinuses. Standard CT and MRI sequences are usually normal. Dynamic MR angiography or conventional catheter angiography is required for definitive diagnosis.
2. **Aneurysm of the petrous carotid** — usually there is fusiform expansion of the petrous segment of the internal carotid artery. This is best illustrated on bone CT through the carotid canal.
3. **Venous thrombosis** — incomplete thrombosis of the lateral sinus may result in turbulent flow that becomes audible. High-density material on CT represents acute thrombus. Loss of the normal venous flow void is the hallmark of MRI diagnosis. (See 12.3.)
4. **Arterial stenosis** — a high-grade arterial stenosis may also result in turbulent flow.

NEOPLASTIC

1. **Paraganglioma** — glomus jugulare/tympanicum. (See 12.56 and 12.60.)

Further Reading

Weissman U.L. & Hirsch B.E. (2000) Imaging of tinnitus. *Radiology*, 216: 342–9.

12.60 JUGULAR FORAMEN MASS

NEOPLASTIC

1. **Glomus jugulare** — ill-defined erosion ± expansion of the jugular foramen, jugular spine and surrounding bone by an enhancing mass. Tumour may extensively invade the temporal bone, infratemporal fossa and extend into the posterior fossa. Large intratumoral vessels present as flow voids within the mass on MRI ('salt and pepper' appearance). Hypervascular on angiography ± arteriovenous shunting.
2. **Schwannoma** — the jugular foramen is expanded, but the cortical outline is preserved. The tumour is well-defined, lobulated and enhances with contrast medium.
3. **Direct invasion** — nasopharyngeal carcinoma.
4. **Metastasis.**
5. **Meningioma.**
6. **Chondrosarcoma.**
7. **Langerhans cell histiocytosis*.**
8. **Lymphoma*.**

NON-NEOPLASTIC

1. **Normal large jugular bulb.**
2. **Venous thrombosis.**
3. **Skull base osteomyelitis** — e.g. malignant otitis externa.

Further Reading

Caldemeyer K.S., Mathews V.P., Azzarelli B. *et al.* (1997) The jugular foramen: a review of anatomy, masses, and imaging characteristics. *RadioGraphics,* 17: 1123–39.

Mafee M.F., Raofi B., Kumar A. *et al.* (2000) Glomus faciale, glomus jugulare, glomus tympanicum, glomus vagale, carotid body tumours, and simulating lesions: role of MR imaging. *Radiol. Clin. North Am.,* 38(5): 1059–76.

12.61 FORAMEN MAGNUM MASS

INTRINSIC CERVICOMEDULLARY LESION

1. **Glioma.**
2. **Ependymoma.**
3. **Demyelination.**
4. **Syrinx.**

ANTERIOR INTRADURAL

1. **Aneurysm.**
2. **Meningioma.**
3. **Schwannoma.**

POSTERIOR INTRADURAL

1. **Chiari malformations** — in Chiari 1, the obex and cervicomedullary junction are 'low'. Pointed tonsils show excessive descent through the foramen magnum (FM) and as a result there is crowding/compression of the neural structures at the FM, and a cord syrinx may develop. Absolute measures of tonsillar descent are less reliable than assessment of the overall morphology of the craniocervical junction.
2. **Secondary tonsillar descent** — large intracranial mass or severe brain swelling.
3. **Ependymoma** — see 12.42.
4. **Medulloblastoma** — see 12.42.

EXTRADURAL

1. **Inflammatory arthropathies** — e.g. rheumatoid arthritis. Soft-tissue pannus centred on the odontoid process + atlantoaxial instability/fixed subluxation.
2. **Skull base tumour** — chordoma, metastasis, myeloma, glomus jugulare.
3. **Osteomyelitis** — pyogenic, tuberculosis.

Further Reading

Osborn A.G. (1994) *Diagnostic Neuroradiology*, Ch. 12. St Louis: Mosby, pp. 507–9.

12.62 DIFFUSE SKULL BASE ABNORMALITY

NEOPLASTIC

1. **Metastases** — breast, bronchus and prostate.

   Patients may present with one of four clinical syndromes:
   Orbital syndrome — pain, diplopia, proptosis and external ophthalmoplegia.
   Parasellar and middle fossa syndrome — headache, ocular paresis without proptosis and facial numbness caused by invasion of the maxillary and mandibular divisions of the fifth cranial nerve. Radiological changes occur late.
   Jugular foramen syndrome — hoarseness and dysphagia. Radiological features often absent.
   Occipital condyle syndrome — stiffness and pain in the neck, worse on flexion.

2. **Multiple myeloma*.**
3. **Nasopharyngeal carcinoma.**
4. **Lymphoma*.**
5. **Meningioma.**
6. **Rhabdomyosarcoma.**

NON-NEOPLASTIC

1. **Fibrous dysplasia*.**
2. **Paget's disease*.**
3. **Osteomyelitis.**
4. **Langerhans cell histiocytosis*.**
5. **Renal osteodystrophy*.**
6. **Haemoglobinopathy** — e.g. sickle cell disease*.

Further Reading

Curtin H.D. & Chavali R. (1998) Imaging of the skull base. *Radiol. Clin. North Am.*, 36(5): 801–17.

12.63 SKULL VAULT LUCENCY WITH NO SURROUNDING SCLEROSIS

NORMAL

1. **Parietal foramina** — usually bilateral and symmetrical on either side of the sagittal suture, just anterior to the lambdoid suture. May be unilateral.
2. **Venous lakes and vascular channels** — emissary veins may have sclerotic margin.
3. **Pacchionian granulations** — near midline or dural venous sinus. The external table may be bowed.
4. **Frontal, temporal, occipital lucencies** — normal ageing calvarium.
5. **Prominent digital markings** — prominence of calvarial digital markings varies widely, particularly between the fourth and tenth years. They do not necessarily indicate raised intracranial pressure.
6. **Fontanelles.**

NEOPLASTIC (ADULTS)

1. **Multiple myeloma*** — diffuse involvement of the vault and skull base by multiple small 'punched out' lesions. May involve the mandible (metastases rarely do). Lesions are usually cold on radioisotope bone scan.
2. **Metastases** — breast, prostate, lung, kidney, leukaemia.
3. **Paget's sarcoma.**

NEOPLASTIC (CHILDREN)

1. **Metastases** — neuroblastoma (± periosteal new bone formation, 'hair-on-end' appearance and wide sutures) and leukaemia.
2. **Langerhans cell histiocytosis*** — eosinophilic granuloma typically produces a solitary round/ovoid 'punched out' lesion with serrated and bevelled edges. Sharply marginated with a sclerotic margin appearing as the lesion heals. A 'button sequestrum' of central bone within the lytic lesion may be seen. Lesions also within the mandible, temporal bone, orbits, spine, ribs, long bones and lungs.
   Hand–Schüller–Christian disease produces multiple ovoid/serpiginous lucencies that cover a large area of the calvarium ('geographical skull').

TRAUMATIC

1. **Leptomeningeal cyst** — skull fracture with dural tear allows herniation of arachnoid mater. The transmitted CSF pulsations prevent repair of the fracture and cause progressive widening and scalloping (growing fracture).
2. **Burr hole.**

METABOLIC

1. **Hyperparathyroidism*** — solitary 'brown' tumour or multiple small lytic lesions creating 'pepper pot skull'. Mandible common site for 'brown' tumour and there may be loss of the lamina dura around the teeth. Basilar invagination may occur.
2. **Osteoporosis** — age-related multifocal lucencies.

INFECTIVE

1. **Pyogenic** — usually related to sinus infection, mastoiditis, surgery or penetrating head injury.
2. **Tuberculosis** — may have central bony sequestrum.
3. **Hydatid.**
4. **Syphilis** — 'moth-eaten' appearance.

VASCULAR

1. **Haemangioma** — 'sunburst' pattern of radiating spicules without discreet margin. Sclerotic margin rare.
2. **Sinus pericranii** — abnormally large communication between the intracranial and extracranial venous circulations. May be congenital, traumatic or spontaneous. Presents as: (a) numerous small localized defects; (b) a discrete regular or irregular area of bone destruction; or (c) complete absence of bone.

OTHERS

1. **Osteoporosis circumscripta** — occurs in lytic phase of Paget's disease. Typically involves the lower frontal and occipital bones. Rare in the vertex. May cross sutures.
2. **Neurofibroma** — calvarial defect adjacent to left lambdoid suture.
3. **Intradiploic arachnoid cyst** — expanded diploic space with intact outer table.

Further Reading

Arana E. & Marti-Bonmati L. (1999) CT and MR imaging of focal calvarial lesions. *Am. J. Roentgenol.*, 172: 1683–8.

Keats T.E. (1996) *Atlas of Normal Roentgen Variants That May Simulate Disease, 6th edn.* St Louis: Mosby.

12.64 SKULL VAULT LUCENCY WITH SCLEROSIS

FIBROUS DYSPLASIA*

DEVELOPMENTAL

1. **Epidermoid** — scalloped appearance with thin sclerotic margins. Cortex expanded and thinned. There is no periosteal reaction, soft-tissue mass or central trabeculae.
2. **Encephalocoele/meningocoele** — midline defect with smooth sclerotic margin and overlying soft-tissue mass. Usually occurs in the occipital bone, but may occur in the frontal, parietal or basal bones.

NEOPLASTIC

1. **Haemangioma** — 'sunburst' pattern of radiating spicules without discrete margin. Sclerotic margin rare.
2. **Langerhans cell histiocytosis*** — sclerotic margin indicates healing. (See 12.57.)

INFECTIVE

1. **Chronic osteomyelitis** — sclerosis predominates.
2. **Frontal sinus mucocoele** — secondary to sinusitis.

12.65 GENERALIZED INCREASE IN SKULL VAULT DENSITY

1. **Paget's disease*** — multiple islands of dense bone. Later the differentiation between the inner and outer tables is lost and the skull vault is thickened (2–5× normal). Basilar invagination may occur. The sinuses may be involved, giving an appearance similar to leontiasis ossea. Loss of lamina dura may occur.
2. **Sclerotic metastases** — breast, prostate.
3. **Fibrous dysplasia*** — if the lesions are widespread throughout the skeleton, then the skull always has a lesion. However, if only the facial bones and base of skull are involved (leontiasis ossea), the rest of the skeleton is rarely affected. Younger age group than Paget's disease.
4. **Myelofibrosis** — there is endosteal thickening which causes narrowing of the diploe. The spleen is greatly enlarged.
5. **Renal osteodystrophy*** — osteosclerosis occurs in 25%. The skull and spine are commonly involved and can look similar to Paget's disease. ± Vascular calcification.
6. **Fluorosis** — mottling of the tooth enamel is a pronounced feature. The calvarium is a rare site for changes to be seen, the axial skeleton being the most frequent. Calcification of muscle attachments.
7. **Acromegaly** — enlarged frontal sinuses, prognathism, enlarged sella, thick vault.
8. **Phenytoin.**
9. **Chronic haemolytic anaemias.**
10. **Sclerosing bone dysplasias**
    (a) Osteopetrosis* — 'bone in bone' appearance in the spine. The mandible is not affected. 'Flask-shaped' femora.
    (b) Pyknodysostosis — particularly involves the skull base. Wormian bones. Wide sutures.
    (c) Pyle's disease — associated with metaphyseal splaying of the long bones.

Further Reading

Kaplan S.B., Kemp S.S. & Oh K.S. (1991) Radiographic manifestations of congenital anomalies of the skull. *Radiol. Clin. North Am.*, 29(2): 195–218.

12.66 LOCALIZED INCREASE IN SKULL VAULT DENSITY

WITHIN BONE

1. **Tumour**
   (a) Sclerotic metastasis — prostate, breast, neuroblastoma.
   (b) Osteoma.
   (c) Treated lytic metastasis.
   (d) Treated 'brown' tumour.
2. **Paget's disease*.**
3. **Fibrous dysplasia*.**
4. **Depressed bone fracture.**
5. **Hyperostosis frontalis interna.**

ADJACENT TO BONE

1. **Meningioma.**
2. **Calcified cephalhaematoma.**
3. **Hair braids.**
4. **Calcified sebaceous cyst.**

Further Reading

Avrahami E. & Even I. (2000) Osteoma of the inner table of the skull — CT diagnosis. *Clin. Radiol.*, 55: 435–8.

12.67 THICK SKULL

GENERALIZED

1. **Normal variant.**
2. **Phenytoin.**
3. **Microcephaly.**
4. **Shunted hydrocephalus.**
5. **Acromegaly** — frontal bossing, enlarged mandible, enlarged sella.
6. **Extramedullary haemopoiesis** — e.g. sickle-cell anaemia*.

FOCAL

1. **Normal variant.**
2. **Paget's disease*.**
3. **Hyperostosis frontalis interna** — typically bilateral and symmetrical thickening of the frontal bones of middle-aged/elderly women. May be localized and unilateral.
4. **Fibrous dysplasia*.**
5. **Meningioma.**
6. **Osteoma.**
7. **Metastasis** — e.g. prostate.

12.68 THIN SKULL

GENERALIZED

1. **Hyperparathyroidism*.**
2. **Osteogenesis imperfecta*.**
3. **Rickets*.**
4. **Chronic raised intracranial pressure.**
5. **Lacunar skull** — (luckenschadel), bone dysplasia of the membranous skull. Deep indentations or pits in the frontal and parietal regions that may traverse the full thickness of the skull. The defects are separated by thin rims of bone that have sharp edges, creating a 'soap bubble' appearance. Usually disappear by 6 months. Not associated with raised intracranial pressure.
6. **Cushing's disease.**

FOCAL

1. **Normal variants** — parietal, temporal and occipital squamae.
2. **Osteoporosis circumscripta.**
3. **Arachnoid cyst.**
4. **Slow-growing cortical tumour** — e.g. dysembryoplastic neuroepithelial tumour, ganglioglioma.
5. **Large intracranial cyst** — arachnoid and porencephalic cysts.

12.69 MULTIPLE WORMIAN BONES

Intrasutural ossicles common in infancy (lambdoid, posterior sagittal and temporosquamosal). Considered abnormal if large (6×4 mm or larger) and multiple (> 10). NB. Dahnert's mnemonic 'PORK CHOPS'.

1. **Idiopathic.**
2. **Pyknodysostosis.**
3. **Osteogenesis imperfecta*.**
4. **Rickets*.**
5. **Kinky hair (Menkes) syndrome.**
6. **Cleidocranial dysostosis.**
7. **Hypophosphatasia/hypothyroidism.**
8. **Otopalatodigital syndrome.**
9. **Primary acro-osteolysis (Hadju–Cheney), pachydermoperiostosis, progeria.**
10. **Down syndrome.**

Further Reading

Cremin B., Goodman H., Spranger J. *et al.* (1982) Wormian bones in osteogenesis imperfecta and other disorders. *Skeletal Radiol.*, 8: 35–8.
Dahnert W. (1993) *Radiology Review Manual,* 2nd edn. Baltimore: Williams and Wilkins.
Pryles C.V. & Khan A.J. (1979) Wormian bones. *Am. J. Dis. Child.*, 133: 380–2.

12.70 CRANIOSYNOSTOSIS

Premature closure of one or more sutures. May occur as an isolated primary abnormality, as part of a more complex syndrome, or secondary to systemic disease. Fusion of a suture results in arrested growth of the calvarium. Raised intracranial pressure may occur with closure of multiple sutures. CT with 3D reformatting offers the best evaluation of the skull sutures and also demonstrates the intracranial contents (e.g. malformations, hydrocephalus, arrested brain growth).

PRIMARY CRANIOSYNOSTOSIS

1. **Sagittal synostosis** — elongated narrow 'boat-shaped' skull (scaphocephaly/dolichocephaly).
2. **Unilateral coronal synostosis** — oblique appearance of the craniofacial structures with harlequin orbit (frontal plagiocephaly).
3. **Bilateral coronal synostosis** — 'short head', often seen with synostosis of other sutures (brachycephaly).
4. **Metopic synostosis** — triangular-shaped head (trigonocephaly).
5. **Unilateral lambdoid synostosis** — occipital plagiocephaly.
6. **Bilateral lambdoid synostosis** — occipital plagiocephaly with flattened occiput. Beware postural flattening of the occiput due to infants being placed to sleep on their backs to prevent sudden infant death syndrome. There is no sutural fusion in these cases.
7. **Cloverleaf skull (Kleeblattscheidel)** — synostosis of multiple paired sutures produces a 'trilobular skull'.

SYNDROMIC CRANIOSYNOSTOSIS

The most frequently described syndromes are the acrocephalo-syndactylies. This group of conditions includes Apert's, Carpenter's and Pfeiffer's syndromes. Each syndrome exhibits synostosis of multiple sutures with severe calvarial and facial malformations. Crouzon's syndrome differs in that there is no syndactyly.

SECONDARY

1. **Metabolic** — rickets, hyperthyroidism, hypophosphatasia.
2. **Inborn errors of metabolism** — Hurler's and Morquio's syndromes.
3. **Haematological disease** — thalassaemia, sickle-cell.

4. **Brain malformation** — holoprosencephaly, microcephaly.
5. **Iatrogenic** — shunted hydrocephalus.

Further Reading

Aviv R.I., Rodger E. & Hall C.M. (2002) Craniosynostosis. *Clin. Radiol.*, 57: 93–102.
Bensom M.L., Oliverio P.J., Yue N.C. *et al.* (1996) Primary craniosynostosis: imaging features. *Am. J. Roentgenol.*, 166: 697–703.
Boyle C.M. & Rosenblum J.D. (1997) Three-dimensional CT for pre- and post-surgical imaging of patients with craniosynostosis: correlation of operative procedure and radiologic imaging. *Am. J. Roentgenol.*, 169: 1173–7.
David D.J., Poswillo D. & Simpson D. (1982) *The Craniosynostoses.* Berlin: Springer-Verlag.
Fernbach S.K. (1998) Craniosynostosis 1998: concepts and controversies. *Pediatr. Radiol.*, 28: 722–8.

12.71 BASILAR INVAGINATION AND PLATYBASIA

BASILAR INVAGINATION

Basilar invagination describes an abnormal anatomical relationship between the cervical spine and the skull base. Essentially, there is superior extension of the spine into the skull base/foramen magnum and this may result in severe compression of the brainstem and hydrocephalus. McGregor's line extends from the posterior limit of the hard palate to the base of the occiput. The tip of the odontoid process should normally lie less than 5 mm above this line.

1. **Primary developmental/segmentation abnormality** — e.g. Klippel–Feil syndrome.
2. **Rickets/osteomalacia***.
3. **Paget's disease***.
4. **Fibrous dysplasia***.
5. **Osteogenesis imperfecta***.

PLATYBASIA

Platybasia describes a 'flattened skull base' and this may accompany basilar invagination. The basal angle describes the angulation between the floor of the anterior cranial fossa and the clivus. In platybasia the basal angle is less than 140°.

1. **Rickets/osteomalacia*.**
2. **Paget's disease*.**
3. **Fibrous dysplasia*.**
4. **Osteogenesis imperfecta*.**
5. **Hyperparathyroidism*.**

12.72 'HAIR-ON-END' SKULL VAULT

HAEMOLYTIC ANAEMIAS

1. **Sickle-cell anaemia*** — begins in the frontal region and can affect the entire calvarium above the internal occipital protuberance, since there is no marrow in this area. The diploic space is wide because of marrow hyperplasia.
2. **Thalassaemia*** — marrow hyperplasia in thalassaemia major is more marked than in any other anaemia. May be severe enough to cause hyperplasia of the facial bones, resulting in obliteration of the paranasal sinuses. (This does not occur in sickle-cell anaemia.)
3. **Others** — hereditary spherocytosis, elliptocytosis, pyruvate kinase deficiency and glucose-6-phosphate dehydrogenase deficiency.

NEOPLASTIC

1. **Haemangioma.**
2. **Meningioma** — only rarely when it breaks through the outer table.
3. **Metastases.**

OTHERS

1. **Cyanotic heart disease** — due to erythroid hyperplasia.
2. **Iron-deficiency anaemia** — severe childhood cases.

13 Obstetrics and gynaecology

Josephine McHugo

Obstetric ultrasound can broadly be divided into four sections:

1. Normality/abnormality of the first trimester.
2. Assessment of gestational age and fetal number.
3. Structural abnormalities.
4. Growth and fetal wellbeing throughout pregnancy.

For simplicity these will be dealt with separately, but an accurate knowledge of gestational age is essential before abnormal growth can be implied, and gestational age is often vital in assessing structural abnormalities.

Currently there is no convincing evidence that ultrasound is harmful to the developing fetus but thermal effect, particularly at the bone–soft tissue interface, is a theoretical risk. Ultrasound should therefore only be used for clinical indications and the investigation performed by appropriately trained personnel using appropriate equipment.

Further Reading

Salvensen K.A., Bakketeug L.S., Eis-nes S.H. *et al.* (1992) Routine ultrasonography *in utero* and school performance at 8–9 years. *Lancet,* 339: 85–91.

13.1 MEASUREMENTS FOR DATING (IN WEEKS POST LMP)

		range
Sac volume	5 wks	± 1.5 wks
Crown–rump length	$6\frac{1}{2}$ wks	± 0.7 wks
Biparietal diameter	12 wks	± 1 wk < 20 wks ± 1.5 wks at 20–26 wks ± 2–3 wks at 26–30 wks 3–4 wks after 30 wks
Femur length	12 wks	± 22 days > 34 wks
Cerebellar width	15–16 wks	
Foot length	14 wks	

From the above it can be seen that gestational age measurements are less variable in early pregnancy. Gestational age can be assessed up to approximately 22 weeks. After this, growth becomes the major factor in fetal size.

13.2 ULTRASOUND FEATURES OF A NORMAL INTRAUTERINE PREGNANCY

USING ABDOMINAL SCANNING

The earliest ultrasound sign of pregnancy is fundal endometrial thickening.

At 5 weeks

1. Gestational sac should be visible at the fundus.
2. The gestational sac is surrounded by an echo-dense ring.
3. Asymmetry of this ring is apparent.

At 6 weeks

Embryonic structures apparent (the yolk sac and developing amniotic sac).

At $6\frac{1}{2}$ weeks

Cardiac movement identifiable in the fetus.
Crown–rump length (CRL) approximately 5 mm.

These dates will not always apply in obese patients where ultrasound images are not ideal. In these cases ultrasound evidence of a normal pregnancy will not be seen so readily. The above appearances are easily seen using transvaginal scanning and the ultrasound findings of pregnancy are apparent approximately 1 week earlier.

Normal sac growth

A normal gestational sac grows at a rate of 0.7–1.75 mm/day (mean = 1.33) from 5 to 11 weeks.

USING TRANSVAGINAL ULTRASOUND

Gestational sac — seen as early as 32 days and present in all normal pregnancies with HCG level of 1000 $mIUml^{-1}$.

Yolk sac — seen in 100% of normal pregnancies with HCG level of 7200 $mIUml^{-1}$. Yolk sac first seen in every pregnancy between 36 and 40 days and when the gestational sac is between 6 and 9 mm.

Embryo with a heart beat — in all pregnancies greater than 40 days and when the gestational sac diameter is greater than 9 mm. The diagnosis of a failed pregnancy should, however, comply with the Royal College of Obstetrics and Gynaecology and the Royal College of Radiologists Guidelines before intervention is undertaken.

Failed pregnancy guidelines for diagnosis (royal college of obstetrics and gynaecology and the royal college of radiologists)

1. No fetal parts.
2. Gestational sac diameter > 20 mm.
3. CRL 6 mm, with no fetal heart activity.

Further Reading

Guidance on ultrasound procedures in early pregnancy (1995) Royal College of Obstetrics and Gynaecology and Royal College of Radiologists, London Ref. No. BFCR (95)8.

13.3 INDICATIONS FOR ULTRASOUND SCANNING IN THE FIRST TRIMESTER

COMMON

1. Threatened miscarriage.
2. Pelvic pain.
3. Suspected ectopic pregnancy.
4. Uncertain dates (LMP), discrepancy in the size of the uterus.
5. Evaluation of retained products post-spontaneous abortion.

LESS COMMON

1. Assessment of success of ovulation induction.
2. Assessment of multiple pregnancies.
3. Guidance for chorionic villus sampling.
4. Retained intrauterine contraceptive device.
5. Adjunct for therapeutic abortion.
6. Evaluation for pelvic masses in early pregnancy.

It should be noted that ultrasound should not simply be used to diagnose an uncomplicated pregnancy.

13.4 THREATENED MISCARRIAGE (ABORTION)

DEFINITION (CLINICAL)

Blood loss per vagina with a closed cervical os.

INCIDENCE

25% of pregnancies (clinically apparent).
50% of these go on to abort.
The incidence of chromosomal abnormality is high (up to 70%) in spontaneous miscarriage.
The prediction of a viable fetus identified by ultrasound being born live following blood loss relates to the fetal size CRL at the time of the ultrasound (which relates to the incidence of chromosomal abnormalities).
Fetal loss rate related to CRL:

Viable fetus 5–10 mm	loss rate 3–10%
Viable fetus 2–4 mm	loss rate 30%.

DEMONSTRATION OF A LIVING FETUS

90–97% favourable outcome.

ULTRASOUND FINDINGS IN THREATENED MISCARRIAGE (ABORTION)

1. Intact pregnancy approximately 50%. Fetal viability depends on imaging a fetal heart beat or fetal movements.
2. Anembryonic pregnancy 20–25%.
3. Missed abortion 25–30%.
4. Incomplete abortion 2–5%.
5. Ectopic pregnancy 1–3%.
6. Hydatidiform mole < 1%.

Further Reading

Trop I. & Levine D. (2001) Hemorrhage during pregnancy: sonography and MR imaging. *Am. J. Roentgenol.*, 176: 607–15.

13.5 ANEMBRYONIC PREGNANCY (BLIGHTED OVUM)

DEFINITION

A fertilized ovum in which development has been arrested. The majority (70%) have chromosomal abnormalities.

ULTRASOUND SIGNS OF AN 'EMPTY' SAC

1. No fetal parts seen with a sac diameter > 30 mm.
2. No yolk sac seen with a sac > 20 mm.
3. Irregular sac contour.
4. Abnormal implantation site.

13.6 ECTOPIC PREGNANCY

RISK FACTORS

1. Previous ectopic.
2. IUCD *in situ.*
3. History of pelvic inflammatory disease.
4. Previous tubal surgery.
5. Assisted conception therapies including *in vitro* fertilization.

ULTRASOUND FINDINGS

1. Ultrasound evidence of an intrauterine pregnancy excludes the diagnosis if there are no risk factors. (1:30 000 approximate rate of concomitant intrauterine and extrauterine pregnancy (heterotopic pregnancy). This increases to 1:7000 following ovulation induction.)
2. Endometrial thickening (decidual cast/pseudogestational sac).
3. Adnexal mass (complex).
4. Fluid in the pouch of Douglas.
5. Demonstration of a living fetus outside the uterus (demonstrated in approximately 10% of cases of ectopic pregnancy).
6. Absence of any ultrasound abnormality does not exclude the diagnosis (approximately 20% of proven cases have no ultrasound abnormalities).
7. HCG level > 1800 $mIUml^{-1}$ with no evidence of an intrauterine pregnancy strongly suggests an ectopic.
   Sensitivity 44%.
   Specificity 100%.

If no intrauterine gestation is identified on transabdominal scanning then transvaginal scanning is mandatory.

ULTRASOUND SIGNS AND ESTIMATES OF RISK OF AN ECTOPIC PREGNANCY

Ultrasound sign	*% Risk*
No intrauterine pregnancy	30%
Echogenic fluid in the pouch of Douglas	45%
Adenxal mass	78%
Adenxal ring structure	80%
Adenxal fetal parts	100%
Adenxal fetal parts with heart beat	100%

Further Reading

Kaakaji Y., Ngheim H.V., Nodell C. *et al.* (2000) Sonography of obstetric and gynecologic emergencies. Part II, obstetric emergencies. *Am. J. Roentgenol.*, 174: 641–9.

Kaakaji Y., Ngheim H.V., Nodell C. *et al.* (2000) Sonography of obstetric and gynecologic emergencies. Part II, gynecologic emergencies. *Am. J. Roentgenol.*, 174: 651–6.

13.7 ABSENT INTRAUTERINE PREGNANCY WITH POSITIVE PREGNANCY TEST

1. Ectopic.
2. Early intrauterine pregnancy < 5 weeks.
3. Recent complete/incomplete abortion.

13.8 ULTRASOUND SCREENING IN PREGNANCY

Routine dating scan (best performed at 11–13 weeks) should assess:

1. Viability.
2. Fetal number.
3. Chorionicity in multiple pregnancy.
4. Set gestation by measuring CRL.
5. Assess associated maternal uterine and adnexal pathology.
6. Nuchal translucency screening for chromosomal abnormalities is offered in some regions in the UK.

ROUTINE ANOMALY SCREENING

Minimum standards recommended by The Royal College of Obstetrics and Gynaecology:

1. Measure biparietal diameter, head circumference and femur length.
2. Head shape + internal structures, cavum septum pellucidum, cerebellum, ventricular size at the atrium < 10 mm.
3. Spine: longitudinal and transverse.
4. Abdominal shape and contents at the level of the stomach.
5. Abdominal shape and contents at the level of the kidneys and umbilicus.
6. Renal pelvis (< 5 mm AP measurement).
7. Longitudinal axis — thoracic abdominal appearances (diaphragm/bladder).
8. Thorax at the level of the four-chamber view.
9. Arms — Three bones and hand (not finger counting).
10. Legs — three bones and foot (not toe counting).
    Optimal standard: if resources allow the following could be added:
11. Cardiac outflows.
12. Face and lips.

Further Reading

Routine ultrasound screening in pregnancy. Protocol, standards and training. Royal College of Obstetrics and Gynaecology, www.rcog.org.uk/medical/ultrasound.html.

13.9 LIQUOR VOLUME

The liquor volume increases in normal pregnancy until approximately 34 weeks and then decreases towards term (approximately 400 ml at 20 weeks).

Assessment of liquor volume is usually subjective; < 2 cm pools in any direction indicates a reduction; > 8 cm indicates an increase. In these circumstances it is appropriate to measure the Amniotic Fluid Index (AFI). This is calculated by the sum of the maximum vertical depth of liquor that is free of fetal parts or loops of cord in the four lateral quadrants of the uterine cavity.

DIFFERENTIAL DIAGNOSIS OF ABNORMAL LIQUOR VOLUME

1. **Severe oligohydramnios**
   (a) Renal agenesis/bilaterally non-functioning kidneys.
   (b) Premature rupture of membranes.
   (c) Severe growth restriction.
2. **Moderate oligohydramnios**
   (a) Renal anomalies (bilateral).
   (b) Premature rupture of membranes.
   (c) Growth restriction.
3. **Polyhydramnios**
   (a) Diabetes (maternal).
   (b) Fetal anomaly (30% cases) — fetus may be hydropic.
   See 13.10.
   Cardiovascular decompensation.
   Obstructive malformations of the gastrointestinal tract, e.g. tracheo-oesophageal fistula, duodenal stenosis/atresia.
   Space-occupying lesion of the thorax resulting in disordered swallowing by compression of the oesophagus, e.g. diaphragmatic hernia, cystic adenomatoid lung.
   Anencephaly/other severe cranial anomalies resulting in disordered swallowing.
   (c) Rarer causes, e.g. bone dysplasias, neuromuscular abnormalities.

Further Reading

Sohaey R. (1998) Amniotic fluid and the umbilical cord: the fetal milieu and lifeline. *Semin. Ultrasound CT MRI*, 19(4): 355–69.

13.10 FETAL HYDROPS

Defined as skin oedema, plus at least one of the following: ascites, pleural or pericardial effusions.

In the fetus ascites and pericardial effusions occur earlier than pleural fluid in cardiac failure.

IMMUNE HYDROPS

1. **Rhesus incompatibility.**
2. **Other blood group incompatibility.**

NON-IMMUNE HYDROPS

(Late manifestations of many severe diseases.)

1. **Cardiovascular**
   (a) Arrhythmias.
   (b) Anatomical defects.
   (c) Cardiomyopathies.
2. **Chromosomal**
   (a) Trisomies.
   (b) Turner's syndrome.
   (c) Triploidy.
3. **Infections**
   (a) CMV (cytomegalovirus).
   (b) Toxoplasmosis.
   (c) Rubella.
   (d) Syphilis.
   (e) Other congenital infections.
4. **Twin pregnancies**
   (a) Twin-to-twin transfusion.
5. **Haematological**
   (a) Alpha-thalassaemia.
   (b) Arteriovenous shunts (large).
6. **Thoracic mass lesions,** e.g.
   (a) Diaphragmatic hernia.
   (b) Cystic adenomatoid malformation of the lung.
   (c) Pulmonary lymphangiectasia.
7. **Gastrointestinal**
   (a) Atresias.
   (b) Volvulus.
   (c) Perforation.

8. **Umbilicus/placenta**
   (a) Chorioangioma.
   (b) Fetomaternal transfusion.
9. **Urinary**
   (a) Congenital nephrosis.
10. **Miscellaneous**
   (a) Skeletal dysplasias.
   (b) Fetal tumours (usually related to high-output cardiac failure).

13.11 RAISED SERUM ALPHA-FETOPROTEIN (AFP)

This protein is produced by the fetus and crosses the placenta to enter the maternal blood. The level rises during normal pregnancy. Discrimination between normal and abnormal is best between 16 and 18 weeks when termination for lethal abnormalities can be offered.

1. **Wrong dates** — (a normal pregnancy which is more advanced).
2. **Twins.**
3. **Missed abortion.**
4. **CNS abnormalities**
   (a) Anencephaly.
   (b) Spina bifida (open).
   (c) Encephalocoele.
5. **Renal anomalies**
   (a) Renal agenesis.
   (b) Multicystic dysplasia.
   (c) Hydronephrosis.
6. **Anterior wall defects**
   (a) Omphalocoele.
   (b) Gastroschisis.

13.12 ULTRASOUND SIGNS SUGGESTING A CHROMOSOMAL ABNORMALITY AT 11–13 WEEKS

1. Nuchal translucency related to gestational and maternal age.
2. Cystic hygroma.
3. Hydrops.
4. Any condition listed in 13.13.

13.13 ULTRASOUND SIGNS SUGGESTING A CHROMOSOMAL ABNORMALITY AT THE 20-WEEK ANOMALY SCAN

1. **Cystic hygroma.**
2. **Hydrops.**
3. **Hydrocephalus.**
4. **Omphalocoele.**
5. **Gross renal anomalies.**
6. **Major structural cardiac defects** — particularly cushion defects.
7. **Multiple structural abnormalities involving separate systems.**
8. **Symmetrical growth restriction.**
9. **Severe growth retardation.**
10. **Duodenal stenosis/atresia.**
11. **Single umbilical artery** — associated with any structural anomaly.
12. **Abnormal placenta** — (cystic and thickened).
13. **Nuchal membrane** — $\geq$ 6 mm in the second trimester.

13.14 'SOFT' MARKERS OF CHROMOSOMAL DISORDERS

1. **Choroid plexus cysts.**
2. **Mild ventriculomegaly.**
3. **Echogenic foci in the cardiac ventricles.**
4. **Pyelectasis.**
5. **Echogenic bowel** — defined as greater than adjacent bone echogenicity.

Further Reading

Whittle M.J. (1997) Ultrasonographic "soft markers" of fetal chromosomal defects. *Br. Med. J.*, 314: 918.

13.15 CYSTIC STRUCTURES SEEN IN THE FETAL ABDOMEN

1. **Renal**
   (a) Multicystic dysplasia.
   (b) Hydronephrosis.
   (c) Bladder in outflow obstruction.
2. **Gut obstruction**
   (a) Duodenal (double bubble)
   (b) Jejunal (multiple fluid-filled loops)
   } with polyhydramnios.
3. **Ovarian cyst**
   (a) Simple.
   (b) Complex, associated with torsion.
4. **Mesenteric cysts.**
5. **Reduplication cysts.**
6. **Hepatic cysts.**
7. **Pancreatic cysts.**
8. **Lymphangioma.**

13.16 MAJOR STRUCTURAL ABNORMALITIES DIAGNOSABLE ANTENATALLY

Approximately 1:100 live births will have a congenital abnormality (often minor). Congenital abnormalities account for 30% of neonatal deaths and 5% deaths in the first year of life.

RENAL

1. **Hydronephrosis.**
2. **Multicystic dysplastic kidney.**
3. **Other causes of macrocysts** — in particular those associated with named syndromes: see 8.20.
4. **Autosomal recessive polycystic disease*** — bilaterally enlarged, highly reflective kidneys. (The tubular ectasia is usually too small to define, resulting in increased echogenicity.) Usually associated with oligohydramnios but this may not develop until the third trimester.
5. **Autosomal dominant polycystic disease*** — a few cases have been reported in which ultrasound has demonstrated cysts or large kidneys with accentuation of the corticomedullary junction.

CENTRAL NERVOUS SYSTEM

1. **Anencephaly** — 50–60% of all neural tube defects. Approximately 50% have an associated spinal anomaly.
2. **Spina bifida** — failure of fusion of the posterior vertebral arch. It may be open or closed (membrane covers the lesion).
   Myelocele — only CSF is present in the sac.
   Meningomyelocoele — neural tissue in the sac.
   Site: 90% lumbosacral; 6% thoracic; 3% cervical.
   Associated Arnold–Chiari malformation in 90% (100% with open lesions).
   US signs of the Arnold–Chiari malformation are:
   (a) Hydrocephalus.
   (b) Abnormally pointed frontoparietal region (lemon sign).
   (c) Abnormally shaped cerebellum (banana sign) due to downward displacement of the cerebellum into the foramen magna or upper cervical canal.

ANTERIOR ABDOMINAL WALL DEFECTS

1. **Gastroschisis** — a defect separate to the cord insertion through which both small and large bowel herniates. No covering membrane. Umbilical vessels not involved. Defect is usually on the right side and liver may, rarely, be involved. Low incidence of associated chromosome abnormalities. Incidence 1:10 000–1:15 000 live births. The long-term prognosis is good.
2. **Omphalocoele** — abdominal wall defect due to failure of small bowel to re-enter the abdomen. Membrane (amnion) covers the eventrated viscera (small bowel ± liver). Umbilical vessels pass through the defect. High incidence (30%) of chromosomal abnormalities. Other malformations in 30–60%. Incidence 1:2280–1:10 000. Poorer prognosis relating to the associated malformations and abnormal karyotype.

CONGENITAL DIAPHRAGMATIC HERNIA

Incidence: 1:2100–1:5000 live births.

High association (16–56%) with other anomalies:

Chromosomal abnormality	30%
Cardiac	13%
Neural tube defects	28%
Omphalocoele	20%
Renal	15%

Mortality is 80%; secondary to pulmonary hypoplasia and associated malformations and chromosomal disorders.

Mortality reduces to 50% in isolated lesions and normal chromosomes. (Karyotyping procedure is therefore indicated.)

US signs: Displaced heart with bowel within the thorax; polyhydramnios may occur in later pregnancy, usually after 25 weeks.

CARDIAC ANOMALIES

Major structural cardiac defects are potentially diagnosable antenatally.

The examination is best performed at 20 weeks with a repeat at 24 weeks. For screening, a four-chamber view is mandatory. Visualization of the outflow tracts will increase the sensitivity of the screening test.

A normal examination requires visualization of:

1. Four chambers with an intact ventricular septum.
2. Normal AV valves (off-set).
3. Normal semilunar valves.
4. Normal connections of the great vessels.

(A patent ductus arteriosus and foramen ovale are normal structures in the fetus.)

Fetal tachycardia (> 200 beats/min) has a high association with structural abnormalities.

Fetal bradycardia may be due to complete heart block, but is rarely associated with a structurally abnormal heart.

Complete heart block is associated with maternal SLE and positive Rho and anti-cardiolipin antibodies (maternal).

SKELETAL DYSPLASIAS

The diagnosis depends on identifying:

1. Abnormal bone growth for gestational age.
2. Abnormal bone architecture.

In the majority of cases of antenatally diagnosed skeletal dysplasia the femoral shortening is marked.

Lethal

1. **Achondrogenesis.**
2. **Thanatophoric dwarfism.**
3. **Asphyxiating thoracic dysplasia** — severe form.
4. **Short rib polydactyly syndromes.**
5. **Campomelic dysplasia.**
6. **Homozygous achondroplasia*.**

Sometimes lethal

1. **Chondroectodermal dysplasia.**
2. **Chondrodysplasia punctata** — rhizomelic type.
3. **Diastrophic dwarfism.**
4. **Metatropic dwarfism.**
5. **Osteogenesis imperfecta*.**
6. **Hypophosphatasia*** — infantile type.
7. **Osteopetrosis*** — AR congenital type.

Not usually lethal

1. **Achondroplasia*** — this shows a late fall in growth after 22–24 weeks.
2. **Spondyloepiphyseal dysplasia congenita.**
3. **Mesomelic dysplasia.**

Lethal with a narrow thorax

1. **Thanatophoric dysplasia.**
2. **Achondroplasia.**
3. **Hypochondroplasia.**
4. **Asphyxiating thoracic dysplasia.**
5. **Chondroectodermal dysplasia.**
6. **Short rib polydactyly syndromes.**
7. **Campomelic dysplasia.**

Further Reading

Emanuel P.G., Garcia G.I. & Angtuaco T.L. (1995) Prenatal detection of anterior abdominal wall defects with US. *RadioGraphics*, 15: 517–30.

Howe D.T., Shirry H., Kilby M.D. *et al.* (1996) Structural chromosome abnormalities and fetal outcomes in antenatally diagnosed congenital diaphragmatic hernia. *Prenat. Diagn.*, 16: 1003–9.

13.17 FETAL GROWTH

Fetal measurements of growth:

1. **Abdominal circumference (AC).**
2. **Head circumference (HC).**

GROWTH RESTRICTION

Definition

This remains problematic but is usually clinically defined as birth weight < 5th centile for gestation. This definition by weight is, however, imprecise as a baby may be severely growth-restricted if the appropriate weight was on the 90th centile but poor growth has resulted in the baby being born with a birth weight that is 10th centile. Therefore, postnatal growth restriction is more accurately diagnosed by skin fold thickness and other signs of poor nourishment.

Incidence

Approximately 5% of births.

Risk factors

Maternal:
- Hypertension.
- Renal disease.
- Heart disease.
- Autoimmune disease.

Placental insufficiency.
Multiple pregnancy.
Previous growth-retarded baby.
One-third of cases have no known risk factors. Perinatal mortality/morbidity is significantly increased by 4–8 × that of normally grown babies. Higher incidence of abnormal physical and neurological development.

TYPES OF GROWTH RESTRICTION

Type 1

Time of onset

Second trimester.

Form

Symmetrical, with the whole of the body being affected.

Causes

1. **Genetic** (low growth potential).
2. **Chromosomal abnormalities.**
3. **Malformations.**
4. **Intrauterine infections.**
5. **Severe placental insufficiency.**
6. **Drugs** — e.g. alcohol, smoking, etc.

Type 2

Time of Onset

Third trimester.

Form

Asymmetric, with the trunk being more affected than the head.

Causes

1. **Hypertension.**
2. **Maternal renal or vascular disease.**
3. **Placental insufficiency.**
4. **Idiopathic.**

Cases of early onset of growth restriction or cases where a structural anomaly is apparent in association with growth restriction should be karyotyped (amniocentesis/placental biopsy/fetal blood sample).

Asymmetrical growth results in an elevated HC:AC ratio.

Maternal uterine artery Doppler waveform can be abnormal in maternal renovascular disease and cases of abnormal placentation. In these cases there is an abnormal persistent notching in the uterine arteries (normally present in early pregnancy but absent by 24 weeks, representing normal invasion of the spiral arteries).

ACUTE FETAL COMPROMISE

This results in reduction in the amniotic fluid volume secondary to poor renal blood flow and reduced urine output.

Doppler measurements in the umbilical and middle cerebral arteries are used to assess redistribution of blood within the fetus. Doppler velocity wave form in the umbilical arteries shows changes that can indicate fetal compromise. The fetal circulation (aorta, neck vessel, etc.) similarly shows changes. (Increasing resistance to down stream flow will reduce the flow in diastole.) This is usually monitored in the umbilical arteries. An increasing resistive index demonstrates abnormality, and absent flow in diastole carries a very poor prognosis of fetal compromise and death.

13.18 NORMAL PLACENTAL DEVELOPMENT

	Gestation age (weeks)
Entire surface of the placenta is covered with villi.	Implantation to 6–7
Villous placenta (chorion frondosum) develops.	7–11
Atrophy of the remaining villi (chorion laeve).	7–11
Three layers of the placenta identifiable: 1. Basal plate 2. Placental substance 3. Chorionic plate	12

13.19 PLACENTA AND MEMBRANES IN TWIN PREGNANCIES

	Dizygotic (%)	Monozygotic (%)
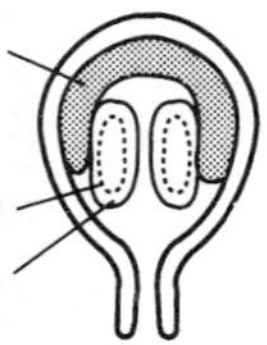 Dichorionic Diamniotic Single placenta	50	15
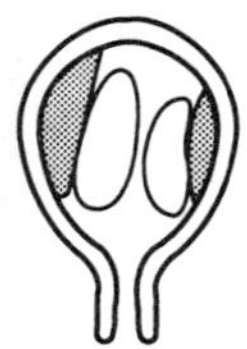 Dichorionic Diamniotic Separate placentae	50	15
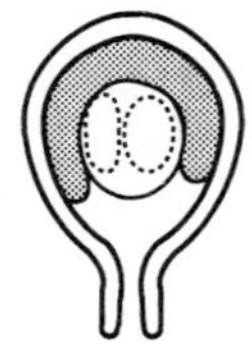 Monochorionic Diamniotic	0	70
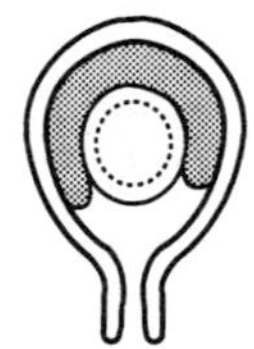 Monochorionic Monoamniotic	0	Rare <1%

13.20 ABNORMALITIES OF THE PLACENTA

PLACENTA PRAEVIA

Definition

A portion of the placenta covers the cervical os.

Incidence (on ultrasound)

20% at 20 weeks' gestation (termed low-lying if it does not completely and symmetrically cover the os).

0.5% at term (due to differential growth of the uterus and the development of the lower segment).

Incidence increases with:

1. Maternal age.
2. Multiparity.
3. Previous uterine surgery, e.g. caesarean section.

Classification

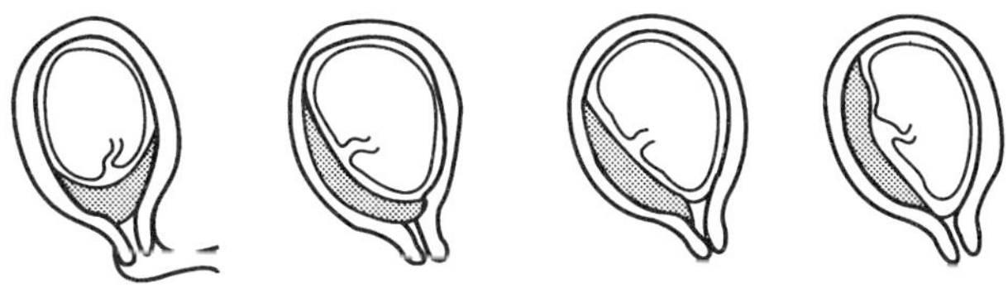

Symmetrical Complete praevia	Asymmetrical Complete praevia	Marginal Praevia	Low lying placenta

Associations

1. Maternal haemorrhage.
2. Abnormal presentation.
3. Intrauterine growth retardation.
4. Preterm delivery.
5. Increased perinatal mortality.

NB. Points 3–5 are related to premature detachment of the placenta.

13.21 PLACENTAL HAEMORRHAGE

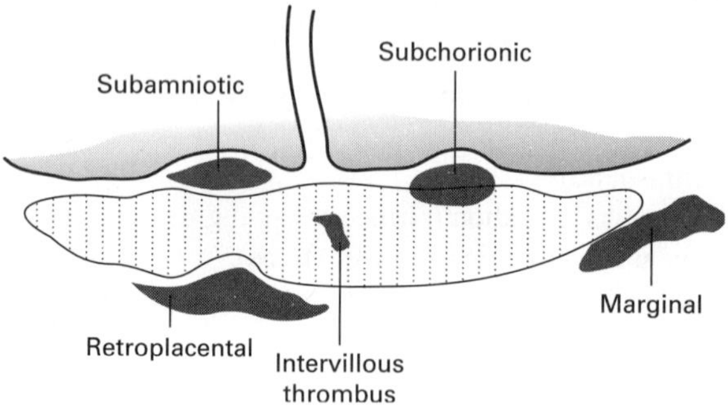

1. **Retroplacental** } both may result in abruption.
2. **Marginal**
3. **Preplacental** — may be either subamniotic or subchorionic but it is often impossible to distinguish this with US.
4. **Intervillous thrombosis** — on US, intraplacental sonolucencies. Incidence increases as the placenta matures. Differential diagnosis: maternal venous lakes.

PLACENTAL ABRUPTION

Definition

Premature separation of the normally sited placenta.

Incidence

Clinically apparent in 1% of pregnancies.

Classification

1. Marginal.
2. Retroplacental.

Maternal risk fators

1. Hypertension.
2. Vascular disease.
3. Smoking.
4. Drug abuse (cocaine etc.).
5. Fibroids.
6. Trauma.

Ultrasound signs

Variable, related to the size, site and time since the event. Acutely, a hyper-reflective focus relative to the placenta which becomes echo-free by 8–14 days. Placental thickness at the site of haemorrhage increases by > 4–4.5 cm.

Outcome

< 20 weeks gestation. 80% normal outcome.

Major placental separation in later pregnancy is a clinical diagnosis.

13.22 CAUSES OF A THICKENED PLACENTA (> 4 CM)

1. **Diabetes.**
2. **Rhesus isoimmunization.**
3. **Fetal hydrops.**
4. **Triploidy.**
5. **Intrauterine infections.**

13.23 CAUSES OF A THIN PLACENTA

1. **Intrauterine growth restriction** (IUGR).

13.24 GESTATIONAL TROPHOBLASTIC DISEASE

Definition

Proliferative disease of the trophoblast.

Classification

1. Hydatidiform mole.
2. Invasive mole.
3. Choriocarcinoma.

Incidence

Geographical variation.
1:1200–2000 pregnancies in USA.
1:100 hospital patients in Indonesia.

Risk factors

Increasing maternal age.
Previous hydatidiform mole.

Genetics

Two distinct genetic types.

1. Complete (classic) mole 46XX of paternal origin.
2. 46 XY of paternal origin (rare).

Ultrasound appearances

Large echogenic mass occupying the uterine cavity with numerous small fluid-filled spaces < 15 mm.

(These features are classically seen in the second trimester.)

No fetal parts except in a partial mole.

First trimester may simulate a missed abortion or an embryonic pregnancy.

Raised human chorionic gonadotrophin (HCG) – in 100% of cases.

Association

Theca-lutein cysts (multiseptate). In 20–50% of patients.

Differential diagnosis

1. Missed abortion with hydropic degeneration of the placenta.
2. Retained products.

INCOMPLETE MOLE

Ultrasound features

1. Fetal parts seen.
2. Thickened placenta with multiple fluid spaces.
3. Multiple fetal anomalies.
4. Severe intrauterine growth retardation.

INVASIVE MOLE

Develops in approximately 12–15% of cases.

METASTATIC CHORIOCARCINOMA

5–8% of cases.

CHORIOCARCINOMA

50% associated with a molar pregnancy.
25% following abortion.
22% following a normal pregnancy.
3% following an ectopic.

13.25 THE NORMAL UTERUS

SIZE

(length × depth × width).

Nulliparous postpubertal — 7 × 4 × 5 cm.

Multiparity — increases the uterine size approximately 1 cm in all directions.

Postmenopausal — the size of the uterus progressively reduces following the menopause.

The neonatal uterus is larger than the prepubertal uterus due to maternal hormones. The endometrial cavity is visualized in 97% of babies and endometrial fluid in 23%.

In childhood the cervix is larger than the uterine body.

The endometrium thickens during the normal menstrual cycle.

A very thin endometrial echo is apparent in the pre- and post-menopausal patient. This endometrial echo should be regular and surrounded by a low reflective myometrial layer in the post-menopausal state.

13.26 ENDOMETRIAL THICKNESS

NORMAL

Proliferative phase — 3–5 mm; seen as a thin continuous line early and then as an interrupted line.

Secretory phase — 5–6 mm.

Postmenopausal — <4 mm.

INCREASED

1. **Early intrauterine pregnancy.**
2. **Ectopic pregnancy.**
3. **Oestrogen excess** — e.g. polycystic ovary syndrome.
4. **Endometrial carcinoma/hyperplasia**
5. **Endometrial polyp**

(4 and 5:) 4 mm is abnormal in postmenopausal women. Usually irregular.

6. **Ultrasound screening for endometrial carcinoma** — a cut-off value of 3 mm gives a negative predictive value of 99% for carcinoma, positive likelihood ratio of 1.61 and negative likelihood ratio of 0.00, i.e. this is an excellent screening test to exclude endometrial carcinoma.

Further Reading

Dijkhuizen F.P., Brolmann H.A., Potters A.E. *et al.* (1996) The accuracy of transvaginal ultrasonography in the diagnosis of endometrial abnormalities. *Obstet. Gynecol.*, 87: 345–9.

13.27 ENLARGED UTERUS

1. **Pregnancy.**
2. **Leiomyoma.**
3. **Carcinoma (endometrial).**
4. **Sarcoma** — rare.
5. **Congenital uterine abnormality** — uterus didelphys.

13.28 THE NORMAL OVARY

VOLUME

Length × width × depth × 0.5223 = volume of an ellipse.
Volume increases from the antenatal period to puberty.

Child	1 ml
Normal postpubertal state	5.3–7.6 ml (excluding a dominant follicle)
Normal post-menopausal state	4.3 ml (range 1.5–10.3 ml)

Progressively reduces in size following the menopause.

In the normal menstrual cycle one follicle becomes dominant with a follicular growth of 2 mm/day.

OVULATION

Occurs at a follicular size of 20–24 mm (maximum diameter) in normal cycles. Smaller in clomiphene cycles; smaller still in Pergonal cycles.

ULTRASOUND SIGNS OF OVULATION

1. Collapse of the follicle.
2. Free fluid in the pouch of Douglas.
3. Echo-free zone around the endometrium — myometrial oedema.

DEFINITION OF SIMPLE CYSTIC STRUCTURES IN THE OVARY

Developing follicle	0.4–1.4 cm
Mature follicle	1.5–2.9 cm
Follicular cyst	> 3 cm

13.29 OVARIAN MASSES

Ultrasonography is 80–90% accurate in demonstrating the size, consistency and location of pelvic masses. Gross morphology correlates well with ultrasound but poorly with histology. Therefore histological correlation is essential for persisting complex ovarian masses.

Intraovarian Doppler velocities (PI < 1) in a morphologically abnormal ovary markedly increase the odd ratio of malignancy. This differentiation holds true for post-menopausal women but is less accurate in pre- or peri-menopausal women. In this group the corpus luteum is a highly vascular structure with PI < 1 being normal post-ovulation.

SIMPLE CYSTIC STRUCTURES

Definition: thin regular cyst wall with no nodules and anechoic fluid. If the ultrasound features do not fit the above criteria then the cyst should be considered complex.

1. **Follicular cyst** — may be functional, i.e. hormone secreting.
2. **Cystadenoma.**
3. **Polycystic ovaries**
   (a) large volume, >7 ml (30% of case have normal-sized ovaries).
   (b) multiple (> 10) cysts, 5–8 mm in diameter, peripherally placed.
   (c) echogenic stroma relative to the myometrium. (a) and (b) are seen in 35–40% of cases. 30% have normal volume ovaries, 25% have hyperechoic ovaries and 5% have enlarged ovaries with no cysts. ↑ Risk of carcinoma of the endometrium.

COMPLEX (Mainly cystic)

1. **Cystadenocarcinoma.**
2. **Dermoid.**
3. **Abscess.**
4. **Endometriosis.**
5. **Ectopic pregnancy.**

COMPLEX (Mainly solid)

1. **Cystadenocarcinoma.**
2. **Dermoid.**

3. **Granulosa cell tumour.**
4. **Ectopic pregnancy.**

SOLID

1. **Metastases.**
2. **Adenocarcinoma.**
3. **Solid teratoma** — malignant.
4. **Fibroma.**
5. **Lymphoma*.**
6. **Arrhenoblastoma.**

Further Reading

Callen P.W. (2000) *Ultrasonography in Obstetrics and Gynaecology,* 4th edn. Philadelphia: Saunders.

Dewbury K., Meire H., Cosgrove D. *et al.* (eds) (2000) *Clinical Ultrasound,* Vol. 13. Obstetrics and Gynaecology, 2nd edn. Edinburgh: Churchill Livingstone.

Jeong Y.-Y., Outwater E.K. & Kang H.K. (2000) Imaging evaluation of ovarian masses. *RadioGraphics,* 20: 1445–70.

Kawamoto S., Urban B.A. & Fisman E.K. (1999) CT of epithelial ovarian tumours. *RadioGraphics,* 19: S85–102.

Ko S.-F., Wan Y.-L., Ng S.-H. *et al.* (1999) Adult ovarian granulosa cell tumours: spectrum of sonographic and CT findings with pathologic correlation. *Am. J. Roentgenol.,* 172: 1227–33.

Nyberg D.A., Hill L.M., Böhm-Vélez M. *et al.* (1992) *Transvaginal Ultrasound.* St Louis: Mosby Year Book.

Outwater E.K., Siegelman E.S. & Hunt J.L. (2001) Ovarian teratomas: tumour types and imaging characteristics. *RadioGraphics,* 21: 475–90.

Rumack C.M., Wilson S.R. & Charboneau J.W. (1997) *Diagnostic Ultrasound,* 2nd edn. St Louis: Mosby.

Twining P., McHugo J.M., Pilling D.S. (1999) *Textbook of Fetal Abnormalities.* Edinburgh: Churchill Livingstone.

Woodward J., Sohaey R. & Mezzetti T.P. Jr (2001) Endometriosis: radiologic–pathologic correlation. *RadioGraphics,* 21: 193–216.

14 Evaluating statistics – explanations of terminology in general use

1. **Reliability**: reproducibility of results. (These may be from the same observer or from different observers.) Assessment of this can be built into a study of diagnostic accuracy of a technique, or evaluated beforehand.
2. **Accuracy**: 'proportion of results (positive and negative) which agree with the final diagnosis'.

   $$\text{i.e. } \frac{\text{true positives + true negatives}}{\text{total number of patients in the study.}}$$

   NB. This does not take false positive and false negatives into account, and is therefore less meaningful than sensitivity and specificity.
3. **Sensitivity**: 'proportion of diseased patients who are reported as positive'.

   $$\text{i.e. } \frac{\text{true positives}}{\text{total number of final diagnosis positive.}}$$

4. **Specificity**: 'proportion of disease-free patients who are reported as negative'.

   $$\text{i.e. } \frac{\text{true negatives}}{\text{total number of final diagnosis negative.}}$$

5. **Positive predictive value**: 'proportion of patients reported positive who have the disease'.

   $$\text{i.e. } \frac{\text{true positives}}{\text{true positives + false positives.}}$$

6. **Negative predictive value**: 'proportion of patients reported negative who do not have the disease'.

   $$\text{i.e. } \frac{\text{true negatives}}{\text{true negatives + false negatives.}}$$

   Differences in the prevalence of the disease in different studies can affect sensitivity and specificity. For example, if a study is conducted in a tertiary referral hospital the patients will be highly selected and this can alter the way that subtle abnormalities are interpreted as there is a high likelihood of disease being present.

Predictive values are now in common use to indicate the usefulness of an imaging test. However, these depend on sensitivity, specificity *and* prevalence and therefore only apply to settings with a similar prevalence. Formulae are available for calculation of predictive values for different prevalences — see Further Reading.

7. **Receiver operating characteristic (ROC) curves**: In many situations it is not possible to be definitely positive or definitely negative when reporting. With this method approximately five or six levels of certainty may be used in reporting (e.g. 1 = definitely positive, 2 = probably positive, etc.). Using each of these levels in turn as the point of cut-off between a 'definitely positive' and a 'definitely negative' result, the sensitivity and specificity for each level are then plotted in the form of a graph of sensitivity against 1 – specificity. The area under the curve will be 1.0 for a perfect technique (or observer) and 0.5 for an absolutely useless technique (or observer!) (see Figure).

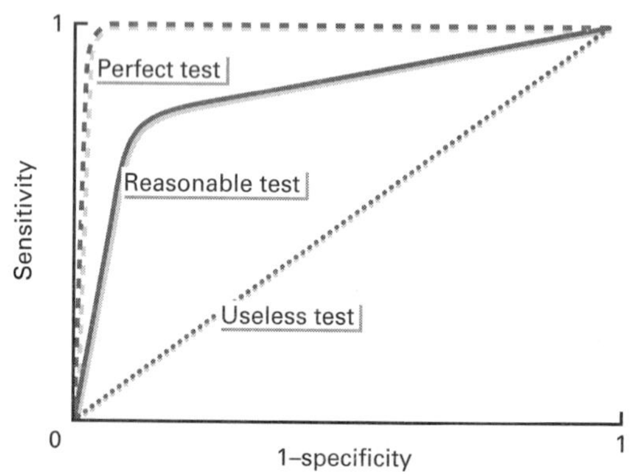

Further Reading

Freedman L.S. (1987) Evaluating and comparing imaging techniques: a review and classification of study designs. *Br. J. Radiol.*, 60: 1071–81.

Part 2

ACHONDROPLASIA

A primary defect of enchondral bone formation. AD (but 80% are spontaneous mutations).

SKULL

1. Large skull. Small base. Small sella. Steep clivus. Small funnel-shaped foramen magnum.
2. Hydrocephalus — of variable severity.

THORAX

1. Thick, stubby sternum.
2. Short ribs with deep concavities to the anterior ends.

AXIAL SKELETON

1. Decreasing interpedicular distance caudally in the lumbar spine.
2. Short pedicles with a narrow sagittal diameter of the lumbar spinal canal.
3. Posterior scalloping.
4. Anterior vertebral body beak at T12/L1/L2.

PELVIS

1. Square iliac wings.
2. 'Champagne-glass' pelvic cavity.
3. Short, narrow sacrosciatic notch.
4. Horizontal sacrum articulating low on the ilia.

APPENDICULAR SKELETON

1. Rhizomelic micromelia with bowing of long bones.
2. Widened metaphyses.
3. Ball-and-socket epiphyseal/metaphyseal junction.
4. Broad and short proximal and short proximal and middle phalanges.
5. Trident-shaped hands.

ACQUIRED IMMUNE DEFICIENCY SYNDROME (AIDS) IN ADULTS

A. CHEST

> 50% present with pulmonary symptoms.

Bronchoscopy, lavage ± transbronchial biopsy should be considered in all patients as CXR is not pathognomonic.

The presence of mediastinal/hilar nodes or pleural effusions is serious and often indicates a serious complication such as infection (TB, fungal) or tumour (lymphoma, Kaposi's). Mediastinal/hilar nodes are not a common feature of AIDS or pneumocystis.

1. **Opportunist infections**
   (a) *Pneumocystis carinii* — most common life-threatening infection. Affects 60% of all AIDS patients at least once, and 25% of initial episodes are fatal (it requires intubation, 90% fatality).
   CXR
   Normal at presentation in one-third.
   Typically: bilateral perihilar and/or basal reticulonodular infiltrates; rapid progression to alveolar consolidation in 3–5 days.
   Less commonly:
      (i) asymmetrical, upper lobe
      (ii) 10–30% have cystic parenchymal changes which (in 30%) are complicated by pneumothorax
      (iii) mediastinal/hilar nodes (in 18% on CT)
      (iv) miliary nodules or solitary nodule (mimics rounded consolidation; may cavitate)
      (v) pleural effusion, but more common in mycobacterial and bacterial infections and neoplasia.
   CT
   Extensive ground-glass attenuation ± thickened interlobular septa and focal consolidation.
   (b) CMV found in 80% of autopsies but rarely the only pathogen.
   CXR
   Typically indistinguishable from *Pneumocystis* or fibrosis.
   (c) *Mycobacterium* affects 10%, and can occur long before other features of AIDS.
   (d) Bacterial, e.g. *Haemophilus influenzae* and *Streptococcus*.

2. **Neoplasms**
   (a) Kaposi's sarcoma — lung involvement occurs in 20% of Kaposi's, and is almost always preceded by cutaneous and/or visceral involvement. It can mimic the appearance of an opportunist infection. Transbronchial and open lung biopsy is often not diagnostic.
   (b) Pulmonary lymphoma — rare. Non-Hodgkin's > Hodgkin's.

B. ABDOMEN

1. **Dysphagia** — common. Usually due to candidiasis, but occasionally caused by viral oesophagitis or Kaposi's sarcoma.
2. **Diarrhoea** — common. Usually CMV colitis if mild, or *Cryptosporidium* (protozoa) if severe. The latter produces thick mucosal folds and mild dilatation with a predilection for the duodenum and jejunum. *Giardia*, *Clostridium difficile* and *Mycobacterium* may also occur.
3. **Retroperitoneal/mesenteric lymphadenopathy**
   (a) Progressive generalized lymphadenopathy syndrome — i.e. two or more extrainguinal nodes persisting for more than 3 months with no obvious cause. Biopsy reveals benign hyperplasia, and CT shows clusters of small nodes < 1 cm in diameter in the mesentery and retroperitoneum.
   (b) Kaposi's sarcoma (KS) — commonest AIDS-related tumour. Cutaneous KS usually precedes involvement of the gut and viscera. Duodenum is the commonest site but may be multicentric and involve gut and liver.
   (c) Lymphoma — usually aggressive form of non-Hodgkin's lymphoma. Peripheral nodes are present in 50% and extranodal involvement is common, particularly bowel, viscera and marrow.
   (d) *Mycobacterium*.
4. **AIDS cholangiopathy** — right upper quadrant pain, nausea, vomiting and fever. Due to infection by CMV or *Cryptosporidium*. Gallbladder wall thickening, pericholecystic fluid, intrahepatic and extrahepatic bile duct strictures, diverticula, intraluminal filling defects and strictures of the juxta-ampullary pancreatic duct.
5. **HIV nephropathy** — proteinuria and rapidly progressive renal failure. Usually, globally enlarged kidneys.
6. **Pyelonephritis and renal abscesses.**

C. CNS

See 12.14

Further Reading

Boiselle P.M., Crans S.A. Jr & Kaplan M.A. (1999) The changing face of *Pneumocystis carinii* pneumonia in AIDS patients. *Am. J. Roentgenol.*, 172: 1301–9.

Kuhlman J.E. (1999) Imaging pulmonary disease in AIDS: state of the art. *Eur. Radiol.*, 9: 395–408.

Logan P.M. & Finnegan M.M. (1998) Pictorial review: pulmonary complications in AIDS: CT appearances. *Clin. Radiol.*, 53: 567–73.

Major N.M. & Tehranzadeh J. (1997) Musculoskeletal manifestations of AIDS. *Radiol. Clin. North Am.*, 35: 1167–90.

Provenzale J.M. & Jinkins J.R. (1997) Brain and spine imaging findings in AIDS patients. *Radiol. Clin. North Am.*, 35: 1127–66.

Redvanly R.D. & Silverstein J.E. (1997) Intra-abdominal manifestations of AIDS. *Radiol. Clin. North Am.*, 35: 1083–126.

Reeders J.W. & Goodman P.C. (2001) *Radiology of AIDS.* Heidelberg: Springer.

Richards P.J., Armstrong P., Parkin J.M. *et al.* (1998) Chest imaging in AIDS. *Clin. Radiol.*, 53: 554–66.

ACQUIRED IMMUNE DEFICIENCY SYNDROME (AIDS) IN CHILDREN

The majority of cases are due to transmission from an infected mother (i.v. drug user, partner of an i.v. drug user, or past history of contact with a bisexual partner) or from transfusions (in the neonatal period or because of diseases such as thalassaemia and haemophilia). 50% of those infected congenitally will present in the first year of life.

AIDS in children differs from AIDS in adults in the following ways:

1. Shorter incubation period.
2. Children are more likely to have serious bacterial infections or CMV.
3. They develop pulmonary lymphoid hyperplasia (PLH)/lymphocytic interstitial pneumonia (LIP), which is rare in adults.
4. They almost never develop Kaposi's sarcoma.
5. They are less likely to be infected with *Toxoplasma*, *Mycobacterium tuberculosis*, *Cryptococcus* and *Histoplasma*.
6. Two patterns of presentation and progression can be recognized:
   (a) In the first year of life with serious infections and encephalopathy. Poor prognosis.
   (b) Preschool and school age with bacterial infections and lymphoid tissue hyperplasia. Survival is longer, to adolescence.

Prognostic factors are severity of disease in the mother, the age of onset and the severity at onset.

GENERALIZED FEATURES

Failure to thrive; weight loss; fever; generalized lymphadenopathy; hepatosplenomegaly; recurrent infections; chronic diarrhoea; parotitis.

CHEST

1. *Pneumocystis carinii* pneumonia (PCP) — may be localized initially but typically there is rapid progression to generalized lung shadowing which is a mixed alveolar and interstitial infiltrate. 50% of infections occur at age 3–6 months. Two-thirds of infections are the first and only infective episode.
2. Cytomegalovirus (CMV) pneumonia.
3. LIP/PLH — in 50% of patients. Insidious onset of clinical symptoms. CXR shows a diffuse, symmetrical reticulonodular or nodular pattern (2–3 mm in diameter) which is most easily seen at the bases and periphery of the lungs ± hilar or mediastinal

lymphadenopathy. The nodules consist of collections of lymphocytes and plasma cells without any organisms. Children with LIP are more likely to have generalized lymphadenopathy, salivary gland enlargement and finger clubbing than those whose CXR changes due to opportunistic infection, and the prognosis for LIP is better. Longstanding LIP may be complicated by lower lobe bronchiectasis or cystic lung disease (resembling that seen in histiocytosis).

4. Mediastinal or hilar adenopathy may be secondary to PLH, *M. tuberculosis*, *M. avium intracellulare*, CMV, lymphoma or fungal infection.
5. Cardiomyopathy, dysrhythmias and unexpected cardiac arrest.

ABDOMEN

1. Hepatosplenomegaly — due to chronic active hepatitis, hepatitis A or B, CMV, Epstein–Barr virus (EBV) and *M. tuberculosis*, generalized sepsis, tumour (fibrosarcoma of the liver) or congestive cardiac failure.
2. Oesophagitis — *Candida*, CMV or herpes simplex.
3. Chronic diarrhoea — in 40–60% of children. Infectious agents are only infrequently found but include *Candida*, CMV and *Cryptosporidium*. Radiological findings are non-specific and include a malabsorption type pattern with thickening of bowel wall and mucosal folds and dilatation. Fine ulceration may be seen.
4. Pneumatosis coli.
5. Mesenteric, para-aortic and retroperitoneal lymphadenopathy — due to *M. avium intracellulare*, lymphocytic proliferation (lymph node syndrome), Kaposi's sarcoma or lymphoma.
6. HIV nephropathy — children may present with proteinuria, fluid and electrolyte imbalances and/or acute or chronic renal failure. Ultrasound shows enlarged echogenic kidneys and CT shows enlarged pyramids. Simple cysts may be present.
7. Urinary tract infection — in up to 50% of AIDS patients. May be due to common organisms or unusual agents e.g. CMV, *Cryptococcus*, *Candida*, *Aspergillus*, *Mycobacteria* and *Pneumocystis*.

HEAD

1. HIV encephalopathy is divided into two types:
   (a) Progressive encephalopathy comparable to adult AIDS dementia complex. There is step-wise deterioration of mental status and higher functions. It is associated with severe immune deficiency.

(b Static encephalopathy, associated with better higher functions but failure to reach appropriate milestones.

Imaging may show:

(a) Cerebral atrophy — worse with progressive encephalopathy.
(b) Non-enhancing white matter of ↓ attenuation (CT) or ↑ T_2W signal (MRI) in the frontal lobes, periventricular regions and centrum semiovale.

2. Intracranial calcifications — in up to 33% of HIV-infected children. Usually bilateral and symmetrical and most commonly seen in the globus pallidus and putamen; less commonly in the subcortical frontal white matter and cerebellum. Usually not seen before 10 months of age; early calcifications are more likely because of congenital infections.
3. Malignancy — most commonly high-grade B cell lymphoma associated with EBV infection.
4. Cerebrovascular accidents.
5. Infections:
   (a) Progressive multifocal leukoencephalopathy — difficult to distinguish from HIV encephalopathy, but tends to be more focal, asymmetrical and commoner in the posterior parietal lobe.
   (b) Toxoplasmosis — enhancing mass lesions with surrounding oedema in the basal ganglia and corticomedullary junction of the periventricular white matter.
   (c) Meningitis — due to fungi, *Mycobacteria* spp. and *Nocardia*, in addition to the more usual causes of meningitis.
   (d) CMV.
6. Chronic otitis media and sinusitis.

Further Reading

Haller J.O. (1997) AIDS-related malignancies in pediatrics. *Radiol. Clin. North Am.*, 35(6): 1517–38.

Haller J.O. & Cohen H.L. (1994) Pediatric HIV infection: an imaging update. *Pediatr. Radiol.*, 24: 224–30.

Miller C.R. (1997) Pediatric aspects of AIDS. *Radiol. Clin. North Am.*, 35: 1191–222.

Stoane J.M., Haller J.O. & Orentlicher R.J. (1996) The gastrointestinal manifestations of pediatric AIDS. *Radiol. Clin. North Am.*, 34(4): 779–90.

Safriel Y.I., Haller J.O., Lefton D.R. *et al.* (2000) Imaging of the brain in the HIV-positive child. *Pediatr. Radiol.*, 30: 725–32.

Zinn H.L. & Haller J.O. (1999) Renal manifestations of AIDS in children. *Pediatr. Radiol.*, 29: 558–61.

ACROMEGALY

The effect of excessive growth hormone on the mature skeleton.

SKULL

1. Thickened skull vault.
2. Enlarged paranasal sinuses and mastoids.
3. Enlarged pituitary fossa because of the eosinophilic adenoma.
4. Prognathism (increased angle of mandible).

THORAX AND SPINE

1. Increased sagittal diameter of the chest with a kyphosis.
2. Vertebral bodies show an increase in the AP and transverse dimensions with posterior scalloping.

APPENDICULAR SKELETON

1. Increased width of bones but unaltered cortical thickness.
2. Tufting of the terminal phalanges, giving an 'arrow-head' appearance.
3. Prominent muscle attachments.
4. Widened joint spaces — especially the metacarpophalangeal joints: due to cartilage hypertrophy.
5. Premature osteoarthritis.
6. Increased heel pad thickness (> 21.5 mm in female; > 23 mm in male).
7. Generalized osteoporosis.

ALKAPTONURIA

The absence of homogentisic acid oxidase leads to the accumulation of homogentisic acid and its excretion in sweat and urine. The majority of cases are AR.

AXIAL SKELETON

1. Osteoporosis.
2. Intervertebral disc calcification — predominantly in the lumbar spine.
3. Disc-space narrowing with vacuum phenomenon.
4. Marginal osteophytes and end-plate sclerosis.
5. Symphysis pubis — joint-space narrowing, chondrocalcinosis, eburnation and, rarely, bone ankylosis.

APPENDICULAR SKELETON

1. Large joints show joint-space narrowing, bony sclerosis, articular collapse and fragmentation, and intra-articular loose bodies.
2. Calcification of bursae and tendons.

EXTRASKELETAL

Ochronotic deposition in other organs may have the following results:

1. Cardiovascular system — atherosclerosis, myocardial infarction, calcification of aortic and mitral valves.
2. Genito-urinary system — renal calculi, nephrocalcinosis, prostatic enlargement with calculi.
3. Upper respiratory tract — hoarseness and dyspnoea.
4. Gastrointestinal tract — dysphagia.

ANEURYSMAL BONE CYST

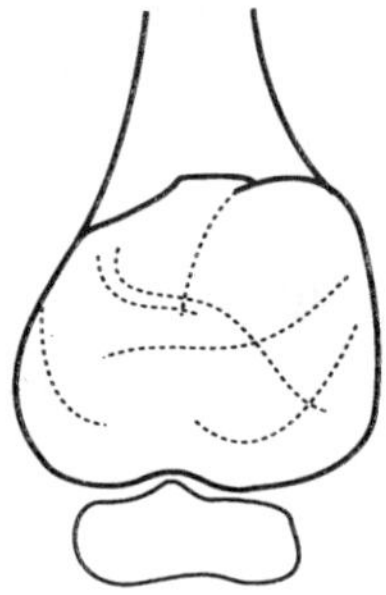

1. Age — 10–30 years (75% occur before epiphyseal closure).
2. Sites — ends of long bones, especially in the lower limbs. Also flat bones and vertebral appendages.
3. Appearances:
   (a) Arises in unfused metaphysis or in metaphysis and epiphysis after fusion.
   (b) Well-defined lucency with thin but intact cortex.
   (c) Marked expansion (ballooning).
   (d) Thin internal strands of bone.
   (e) ± New bone in the angle between original cortex and the expanded part.
   (f) Fluid/fluid level(s) on CT and MRI.
   (g) In the spine they involve the posterior elements.

ANKYLOSING SPONDYLITIS

A mesenchymal disease mainly manifest as an inflammatory arthritis affecting synovial and cartilaginous joints and as an enthesopathy.

AXIAL SKELETON

1. Involved initially in 70-80%. Initial changes in the sacroiliac joints followed by the thoracolumbar and lumbosacral regions. The entire spine may be involved eventually.

2. The radiological changes in the sacroiliac joints (see 3.13) are present at the time of the earliest spinal changes.
3. Discovertebral junction:
   (a) Osteitis — resulting in the squaring of vertebral bodies.
   (b) Syndesmophytes — eventually leading to the 'bamboo spine' (see 2.14).
   (c) Disc calcification.
   (d) Erosions and destruction — which can be central, peripheral or extensive (pseudarthrosis).
   (e) Osteoporosis — with longstanding disease.
   (f) Kyphosis.
4. Apophyseal joints haziness, erosions, subchondral
5. Costotransverse joints
6. Costovertebral joints } sclerosis and eventually ankylosis.
7. Posterior ligament calcification and ossification.

APPENDICULAR SKELETON

1. Involved initially in 10–20% but eventually in 50% of cases. Mild and transient. Asymmetrical involvement of few joints, most frequently hips and shoulders.
2. Similar changes to rheumatoid arthritis, but synovitis is more discrete and less severe. Subchondral bone sclerosis and chondral ossification lead to bony ankylosis. (In adult rheumatoid arthritis, bony ankylosis only occurs in the carpus and tarsus.)
3. No periarticular osteoporosis.

EXTRASKELETAL

1. Iritis in 20% — more frequent with a peripheral arthropathy.
2. Pulmonary upper lobe fibrosis and cavitation (1%).
3. Heart disease — aortic incompetence, conduction defects and pericarditis.
4. Amyloidosis.
5. Inflammatory bowel disease.

ASBESTOS INHALATION

Lung and/or pleural disease caused by the inhalation of asbestos fibres. Disease is more common with crocidolite (blue asbestos) than chrysotile (white asbestos). Pleural disease alone 50%; pleura and lung parenchyma 40%; lung parenchyma alone 10%.

PLEURA

1. Plaques or pleural thickening. Most frequent in the lower half of the thorax and tend to follow rib contours. Parietal pleura is affected. Do not occur with less than 20 years' exposure.
2. Calcified plaques (in 10–15%) — probably related to the type of fibre. Usually diaphragmatic.
3. Effusions (in 20%) — frequently recurrent, usually bilateral and often associated with chest pain. Usually associated with pulmonary involvement.

LUNG PARENCHYMA

1. Small nodular and/or reticular opacities which progress through three stages:
   (a) Fine reticulation in the lower zones → ground-glass appearance.
   (b) More prominent interstitial reticulation in the lower zones.
   (c) Reticular shadowing in the mid and upper zones with obscured heart and diaphragmatic outlines.
2. Large opacities (1 cm or greater), associated with widespread interstitial fibrosis.

COMPLICATIONS

1. Carcinoma of the bronchus — 6–10× increased incidence in smokers with asbestosis and accounts for 35% of deaths.
2. Mesothelioma — 80% of all mesotheliomas are associated with asbestosis. Accounts for 10% of deaths.
3. Peritoneal mesothelioma.
4. Gastrointestinal carcinomas.
5. Laryngeal carcinoma.

Further Reading

Peacock C., Copley S.J. & Hansell D.M. (2000) Asbestos-related benign pleural disease. *Clin. Radiol.*, 55: 422–32.

CALCIUM PYROPHOSPHATE DIHYDRATE DEPOSITION DISEASE

1. Three manifestations which occur singly or in combination:
   (a) Crystal-induced acute synovitis (pseudogout).
   (b) Cartilage calcification (chondrocalcinosis).
   (c) Structural joint abnormalities (pyrophosphate arthropathy).
2. Associated conditions are hyperparathyroidism and haemochromatosis (definite) and gout, Wilson's disease and alkaptonuria (less definite).
3. Chondrocalcinosis involves:
   (a) Fibrocartilage — especially menisci of the knee, triangular cartilage of the wrist, symphysis pubis and annulus fibrosus of the intervertebral disc.
   (b) Hyaline cartilage — especially the wrist, knee, elbow and hip.
4. Synovial membrane, joint capsule, tendon and ligament calcification.
5. Pyrophosphate arthropathy is most common in the knee, wrist, metacarpophalangeal joint and acromioclavicular joint. It has similar appearances to osteoarthritis but with several differences:
   (a) Unusual articular distribution — the wrist, elbow and shoulder are uncommon sites for osteoarthritis.
   (b) Unusual intra-articular distribution — the patellofemoral compartment of the knee and the radiocarpal compartment of the wrist.
   (c) Numerous, prominent subchondral cysts.
   (d) Marked subchondral collapse and fragmentation with multiple loose bodies simulating a neuropathic joint.
   (e) Variable osteophyte formation.

CHONDROBLASTOMA

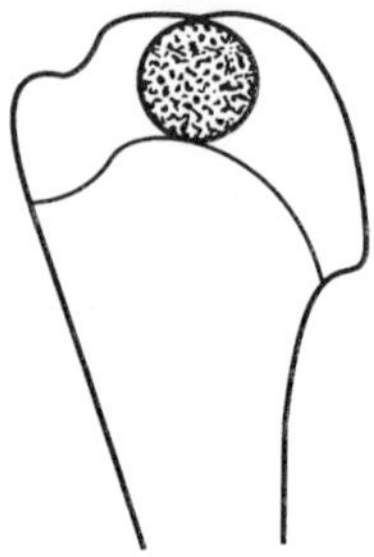

1. Age — 5–20 years.
2. Sites — proximal humerus, distal femur and proximal tibia (50% occur in the lower limb).
3. Appearances:
   (a) Arises in the epiphysis prior to fusion and may expand to involve the metaphysis.
   (b) Well-defined lucency with a thin sclerotic rim.
   (c) Internal calcification in 60%.
   (d) Florid surrounding marrow oedema on MRI.

CHONDROMYXOID FIBROMA

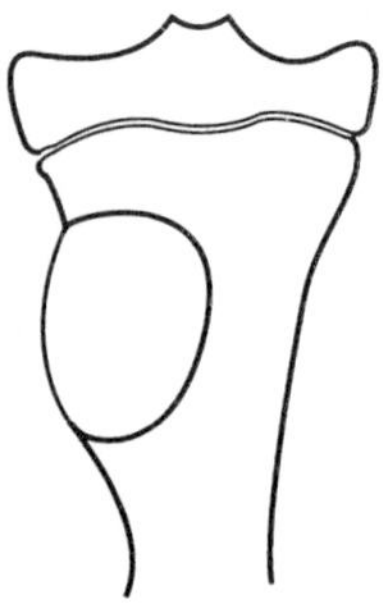

1. Age — 10–30 years.
2. Sites — proximal tibia (50%); also femur and ribs.
3. Appearances:
   (a) Metaphyseal ± extension into epiphysis, but never only in the epiphysis.
   (b) Round or oval, well-defined lucency with a sclerotic rim.
   (c) Eccentric expansion.
   (d) Internal calcification is uncommon.

CHONDROSARCOMA

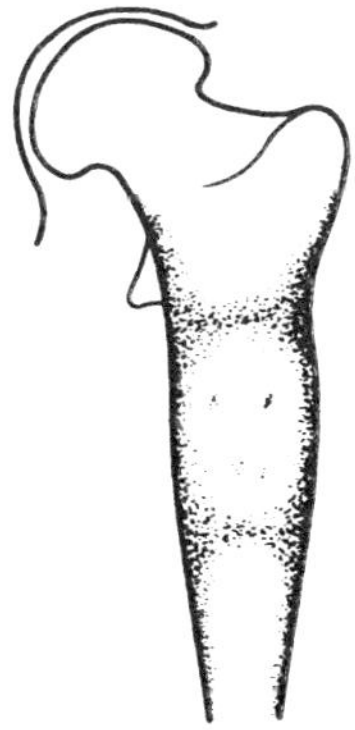

Central

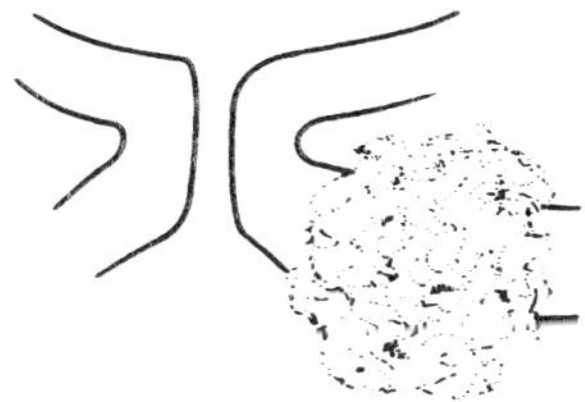

Peripheral

CENTRAL

1. Age — 30–60 years.
2. Sites — femur and humerus.
3. Appearances:
   (a) Metaphyseal or diaphyseal.
   (b) Lucent, expansile lesion with a sclerotic margin.
   (c) Endosteal cortical thickening or thinning.
   (d) ± Cortical destruction and a soft tissue mass.
   (e) 'Pop-corn', 'ring and arc' or 'dot and comma' internal calcification.

PERIPHERAL

1. Age — 30–60 years.
2. Sites — pelvic and shoulder girdle, upper femur and humerus.
3. Appearances:
   (a) Soft-tissue mass, often arising from the cartilage tip of an osteochondroma. A cartilage cap >2 cm in thickness, as measured by ultrasound, CT or MRI, is considered suspicious of malignant change.
   (b) Multiple calcific densities.
   (c) Ill-defined margins.
   (d) In the later stages, destruction of underlying bone.

Further Reading

Murphey M.D., Flemming D.J., Boyea S.R. *et al.* (1998) Enchondroma versus chondrosarcoma in the appendicular skeleton: differentiating features. *RadioGraphics*, 18: 1213–37.

CLEIDOCRANIAL DYSPLASIA

AD. One-third are new mutations.

SKULL

1. Brachycephaly. Wormian bones. Frontal and parietal bossing.
2. Wide sutures and fontanelles with delayed closure.
3. Broad mandible. Small facial bones. Delayed eruption and supernumerary teeth.
4. Basilar invagination.

THORAX

1. Aplasia or hypoplasia of the clavicles, usually the lateral portion but occasionally the middle portion.
2. Small, high scapulae.
3. Neonatal respiratory distress because of thoracic cage deformity.

PELVIS

1. Absent or delayed ossification of the pubic bones, producing apparent widening of the symphysis pubis.

APPENDICULAR SKELETON

1. Short or absent fibulae.
2. Coxa vara or coxa valga.
3. Congenital pseudarthrosis of the femur.
4. Hand:
   (a) Long second and fifth metacarpals; short second and fifth middle phalanges.
   (b) Cone-shaped epiphyses.
   (c) Tapered distal phalanges.
   (d) Supernumerary ossification centres.

COAL MINER'S PNEUMOCONIOSIS

The effect of the inhalation of coal dust in coal workers.

SIMPLE

1. Small round opacities, 1–5 mm in size. Widespread throughout the lungs but sparing the extreme bases and apices.
2. Less well defined than silicosis.
3. Generally less dense than silicosis, but calcification occurs in at least a few of the nodules in 10% of older coal workers.
4. 'Egg-shell' calcification of lymph nodes in 1%.

COMPLICATED, I.E. PROGRESSIVE MASSIVE FIBROSIS

See Silicosis.

COMPLICATIONS

See Silicosis.

CROHN'S DISEASE

Colon and small bowel are affected equally. Gastric involvement is uncommon and is usually affected in continuity with disease in the duodenum. Oesophageal involvement is rare.

SMALL BOWEL

1. Terminal ileum is the commonest site.
2. Asymmetrical involvement and skip lesions are characteristic. The disease predominates on the mesenteric border.
3. Aphthoid ulcers — the earliest sign in the terminal ileum and colon.
4. Fissure ulcers — typically they are distributed in a longitudinal and transverse fashion. They may progress to abscess formation, sinuses and fistulae.
5. Blunting, thickening or distortion of the valvulae conniventes — the earliest sign in the small bowel proximal to the terminal ileum. Caused by hyperplasia of lymphoid tissue, producing an obstructive lymphoedema of the bowel wall.
6. 'Cobblestone' pattern — two possible causes:
   (a) A combination of longitudinal and transverse fissure ulcers bounding intact mucosa.
   (b) The bulging of oedematous mucosal folds that are not closely attached to the underlying muscularis.
7. Separation of bowel loops — due to thickened bowel wall.
8. Strictures — may be short or long, single or multiple. Significant clinical obstruction is less commonly observed.
9. Pseudosacculation.

COLON

1. Asymmetrical involvement and skip lesions. The rectum is involved in 30–50%.
2. Aphthoid ulcers.
3. Deeper fissure ulcers which may produce a 'cobblestone' pattern.
4. Strictures.
5. Pseudosacculation.
6. Inflammatory pseudopolyps.
7. The ileocaecal valve may be thickened, narrowed and ulcerated.

COMPLICATIONS

1. Fistulae.
2. Perforation — usually localized and results in abscess formation.
3. Toxic megacolon.
4. Carcinoma:
   (a) Colon — less common than in ulcerative colitis, but this may be because more patients with Crohn's disease undergo colectomy at an early stage.
   (b) Small bowel — 300× increased incidence.
5. Lymphoma.
6. Associated conditions:
   (a) Erythema nodosum.
   (b) Arthritis:
      (i) Spondyloarthritis mimicking ankylosing spondylitis. It follows a course independent of the bowel disease and precedes it in 25% of cases.
      (ii) Enteropathic synovitis, the activity of which parallels the bowel disease. The weight-bearing joints of the lower limbs, wrist and fingers are affected.
   (c) Cirrhosis.
   (d) Chronic active hepatitis.
   (e) Gallstones.
   (f) Oxalate urinary tract calculi.
   (g) Pericholangitis.
   (h) Cholangiocarcinoma.
   (i) Sclerosing cholangitis.

Further Reading

Ali S.I. & Carty H.M. (2000) Paediatric Crohn's disease: a radiological overview. *Eur. Radiol.*, 10: 1085–94.

Wills J.S., Lobis I.F. & Denstman F.J. (1997) Crohn disease. State of the art. *Radiology*, 202: 597–610.

CUSHING'S SYNDROME

Cushing's syndrome results from increased endogenous or exogenous cortisol.

Spontaneous Cushing's syndrome is rare and due to:

Pituitary disease (Cushing's disease). 80%

90% of these are due to adenoma and 20% have radiological evidence of an intrasellar tumour.

Adrenal disease	— adenoma.	20%
	— carcinoma.	
Ectopic ACTH, e.g. from a carcinoma of the bronchus.		

Iatrogenic Cushing's syndrome is common and due to high doses of corticosteroids. The effects of excessive amounts of corticosteroids are:

1. Growth retardation in children.
2. Osteoporosis.
3. Pathological fractures which show excessive callus formation during healing; vertebral end-plate fractures, in particular, show prominent bone condensation.
4. Avascular necrosis of bone.
5. Increased incidence of infection — including osteomyelitis and septic arthritis (the knee is affected most frequently).
6. Hypertension.
7. Water retention resulting in oedema.

CYSTIC FIBROSIS

AR condition (gene located in the middle of the long arm of chromosome 7) in which the basic problem is one of excessively viscid mucus. 1 in 2000 live births.

CARDIOPULMONARY

1. Overinflation — the earliest sign in children and due to mucus plugging of small bronchioles. Focal air trapping is better recognized on HRCT done in expiration.
2. Bronchial wall thickening (submucosal infiltration by acute and chronic inflammatory cells) and mucus-filled bronchi.
3. Atelectasis — subsegmental, segmental or lobar (especially the right upper lobe).
4. Nodular and reticulonodular appearance due to obstruction of small airways. Centrilobular nodules on HRCT. The early changes are most marked in the right upper lobe.
5. Bronchiectasis.
6. Recurrent pneumonia.
7. Cystic air spaces — either ectatic bronchi or focal emphysema.
8. 'Honeycomb lung' (q.v.) ± pneumothorax (rare before puberty).
9. Low incidence of pleural effusion or empyema at all ages.
10. Cor pulmonale — more common in the older age group and often precedes death.

GASTROINTESTINAL

1. Meconium ileus (10%), meconium peritonitis and meconium ileus equivalent (5–10%).
2. Thickened mucosal folds, nodular filling defects and small bowel dilatation.

HEPATOBILIARY

1. Hepatomegaly with parenchymal changes on ultrasound, CT and MRI.
2. Fatty liver, cirrhosis and portal hypertension.
3. Gallstones, contracted gallbladder, dilatation of intrahepatic bile ducts, intrahepatic bile duct strictures and retention of radionuclide on dynamic biliary scintigraphy.

PANCREAS

1. Calcification and calculi.
2. Fibrosis and/or fatty replacement. A number of patterns may be observed on MRI:
   (a) An enlarged pancreas with complete fatty replacement, low signal septations ± lobulated outline.
   (b) A small atrophic pancreas with partial fatty replacement.
   (c) Diffuse pancreatic atrophy without fatty replacement.
   (d) Complete pancreatic fibrosis (low signal on T_1W and T_2W).

SKELETAL

1. Retarded maturation.
2. Clubbing and hypertrophic osteoarthropathy.

SINUSES

1. Chronic sinusitis — opaque maxillary antra in nearly all children over 2 years of age.
2. Nasal polyps (10–15%).
3. Mucocoele.

Further Reading

King L.J., Scurr E.D., Murugan N. *et al.* (2000) Hepatobiliary and pancreatic manifestations of cystic fibrosis: MR imaging appearances. *RadioGraphics*, 20: 767–77.
Ruzal-Shapiro C. (1998) Cystic fibrosis. An overview. *Radiol. Clin. North Am.*, 36(1): 143–61.
Wood B.P. (1997) Cystic fibrosis: 1997. *Radiology*, 204: 1–10.

DOWN'S SYNDROME (trisomy 21)

CRANIOFACIAL

1. Brachycephaly and microcephaly.
2. Hypoplasia of facial bones and sinuses.
3. Wide sutures and delayed closure. Multiple wormian bones.
4. Hypotelorism.
5. Dental abnormalities.

CENTRAL NERVOUS SYSTEM

1. Bilateral basal ganglia calcification.

AXIAL SKELETON

1. Increased height and decreased AP diameter of lumbar vertebrae.
2. Atlantoaxial subluxation.
3. Atlanto-occipital subluxation.
4. Hypoplasia of the posterior arch of C1.
5. Incomplete fusion of vertebral arches of the lumbar spine.

PELVIS

1. Flared iliac wings with small acetabular angles resulting in an abnormal iliac index (iliac angle + acetabular angle).

CHEST

1. Congenital heart disease (40%) — mainly endocardial cushion defects and aberrant right subclavian artery.
2. Eleven pairs of ribs.
3. Two ossification centres for the manubrium (90%).

HANDS

1. Short tubular bones, clinodactyly (50%) and hypoplasia of the middle phalanx of the little finger (60%).

GASTROINTESTINAL

1. Umbilical hernia.

2. Duodenal atresia or stenosis.
3. Tracheo-oesophageal fistula.
4. Anorectal anomalies.

Further Reading

Stein S.M., Kirchner S.G., Horev G. *et al.* (1991) Atlanto-occipital subluxation in Down syndrome. *Pediatr. Radiol.*, 21: 121–4.

ENCHONDROMA

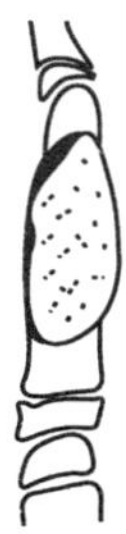

1. Age — 10–50 years.
2. Sites — hands and wrists predominate (50%). Any other bones formed in cartilage.
3. Appearances:
   (a) Diaphyseal or diametaphyseal.
   (b) Well-defined lucency with a thin sclerotic rim.
   (c) Often expansile; cortex preserved.
   (d) Internal ground-glass appearance ± calcification
   (e) Especially in long bones, may be multilocular.
   (f) Pathological fracture — a frequent presenting complaint of enchondromas of the hands or feet.

SYNDROMES

Ollier's disease — multiple enchondromas.
Maffucci's syndrome — enchondromas + soft-tissue haemangiomas.

EOSINOPHILIC GRANULOMA

See Langerhans cell histiocytosis.

EWING'S SARCOMA

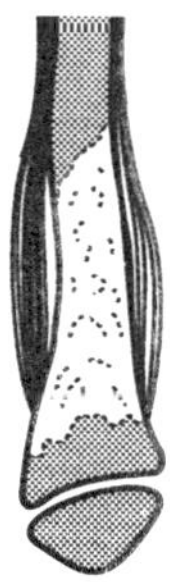

1. Age — 5–15 years.
2. Sites — femur, pelvis and shoulder girdle.
3. Appearances:
   (a) Diaphyseal or, less commonly, metaphyseal.
   (b) Ill-defined medullary destruction.
   (c) ± Small areas of new bone formation.
   (d) Periosteal reaction — lamellated (onion skin), Codman's angle or 'sunray' spiculation.
   (e) Soft-tissue extension (best appreciated on MRI).
   (f) Metastases to other bones and lungs.

EXTRINSIC ALLERGIC ALVEOLITIS

An allergic reaction in the alveoli of sensitized individuals following repeated exposure to one of a number of specific antigens (see 4.21).

ACUTE EXPOSURE

1. Symptoms 4–8 hours after exposure (dyspnoea, dry cough, fever, malaise and myalgia).
2. The chest X-ray may be normal.
3. When radiological changes are present they usually parallel the severity of clinical symptoms. Changes consist of:
   (a) Ground-glass, nodular or miliary shadows, between one and several millimetres in diameter, diffusely throughout both lungs but with some sparing of the apices and bases. Usually poorly defined.
   (b) Alveolar shadows, particularly in the lower zones, following heavy exposure to antigen.
   (c) Septal lines.
   (d) Hilar lymphadenopathy is rare but may be more frequent in mushroom-worker's lung.
4. Removal from antigen exposure results in resolution of the radiological changes over between one and several weeks.

CHRONIC EXPOSURE

1. Persistent exposure to low doses of antigen.
2. The diffuse nodular pattern is replaced by the changes characteristic of diffuse interstitial fibrosis.
   (a) Reticular pattern
   (b) Loss of lung volume
   (c) 'Honeycomb' pattern
   } but with marked upper zone predominance.

FIBROUS DYSPLASIA

Unknown pathogenesis. Medullary bone is replaced by fibrous tissue.

1. Diagnosis usually made between 3 and 15 years.
2. May be monostotic or polyostotic. In polyostotic cases the lesions tend to be unilateral; if bilateral then asymmetrical.
3. Most frequent sites are femur, pelvis, skull, mandible, ribs (most common cause of a focal expansile rib lesion) and humerus. Other bones are less frequently affected.
4. Radiological changes include:
   (a) A cyst-like lesion in the diaphysis or metaphysis with endosteal scalloping ± bone expansion. No periosteal new bone. The epiphysis is only involved after fusion. Thick sclerotic border: 'rind' sign. Internally the lesion shows a ground-glass appearance ± irregular calcifications together with irregular sclerotic areas.
   (b) Bone deformity, e.g. shepherd's crook deformity of the proximal femur.
   (c) Growth disparity.
   (d) Accelerated bone maturation.
   (e) Skull shows mixed lucencies and sclerosis, mainly on the convexity of the calvarium and the floor of the anterior fossa.
   (f) Leontiasis ossea is a sclerosing form affecting the face ± the skull base and producing leonine facies. In such cases extracranial lesions are rare. Involvement may be asymmetrical.
5. Associated endocrine abnormalities include:
   (a) Sexual precocity (+ skin pigmentation) — in 30% of females with the polyostotic form. This constitutes the McCune–Albright syndrome.
   (b) Acromegaly, Cushing's syndrome, gynaecomastia and parathyroid hyperplasia (all rare).

GIANT CELL TUMOUR

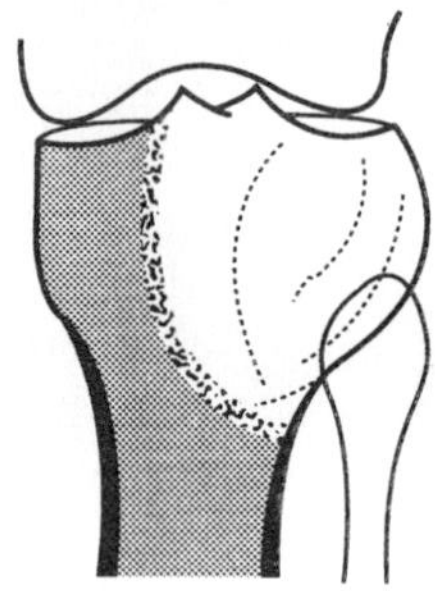

1. Age — 20–40 years (only 3% occur before epiphyseal closure).
2. Sites — long bones, distal femur especially; occasionally the sacrum or pelvis. Spine rarely.
3. Appearances:
   (a) Epiphyseal and metaphyseal, i.e. subarticular.
   (b) A lucency with an ill-defined endosteal margin.
   (c) Eccentric expansion ± cortical destruction and soft-tissue extension.
   (d) Cortical ridges or internal septa produce a multilocular appearance.
   (e) Fluid levels on CT or MRI.
   (f) 30% local recurrence rate and, rarely, pulmonary metastases.

Further Reading

Lee M.J., Sallomi D.F., Munk P.L. *et al.* (1998) Pictorial review: giant cell tumours of bone. *Clin. Radiol.*, 53: 481–9.

Manaster B.J. & Doyle A.J. (1993) Giant cell tumours of bone. *Radiol. Clin. North Am.*, 31(2): 299–323.

Murphey M.D., Nomikos G.C., Flemming D.J. *et al.* (2001) Imaging of giant cell tumour and giant cell reparative granuloma of bone: radiologic–pathologic correlation. *RadioGraphics*, 21: 1283–1309.

GOUT

Caused by monosodium urate monohydrate or uric acid crystal deposition. Idiopathic (in the majority of patients) or associated with many other disorders, e.g. myeloproliferative diseases, drugs and chronic renal disease. Idiopathic gout may be divided into three stages.

ASYMPTOMATIC HYPERURICAEMIA

1. No radiological signs but renal calculi or arthritis will develop in 20%.

ACUTE GOUTY ARTHRITIS

1. Monoarticular or oligoarticular; occasionally polyarticular.
2. Predilection for joints of the lower extremities, especially the first metatarsophalangeal joint (70%), intertarsal joints, ankles and knees. Other joints are affected in longstanding disease.
3. Soft-tissue swelling and joint effusion during the acute attack, with disappearance of the abnormalities as the attack subsides.

CHRONIC TOPHACEOUS GOUT

1. In 50% of patients with recurrent acute gout.
2. Eccentric, asymmetrical nodular deposits of calcium urate (tophi) in the synovium, subchondral bone, helix of the ear and in the soft tissues of the elbow, hand, foot, knee and forearm. Calcification of tophi is uncommon; ossification is rare.
3. Joint space is preserved until late in the disease.
4. Little or no osteoporosis until late, when there may be disuse osteoporosis.

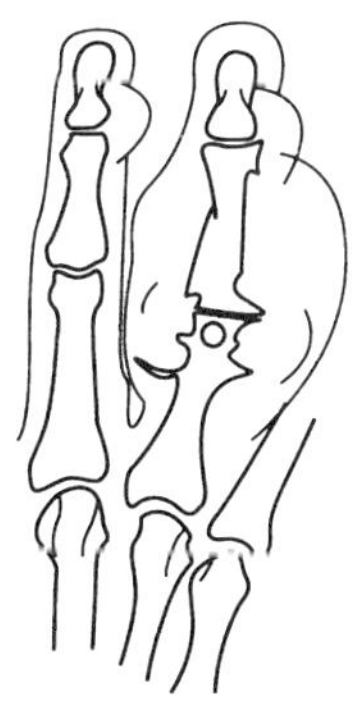

5. Bony erosions are produced by tophaceous deposits and may be intra-articular, periarticular or well away from the joint. The latter two may be associated with an obvious soft-tissue mass. Erosions are round or oval, with the long axis in line with the bone. They may have a sclerotic margin. Some erosions have an overhanging lip of bone, which is strongly suggestive of the condition.
6. Severe erosive changes result in an arthritis mutilans.

COMPLICATIONS

1. Urolithiasis — in 10% of gout patients (higher in hot climates).
2. Renal disease:
   (a) Acute urate nephropathy — precipitation of uric acid in the collecting ducts. Usually follows treatment with cytotoxic drugs.
   (b) Chronic urate nephropathy — rare.

HAEMANGIOMA OF BONE

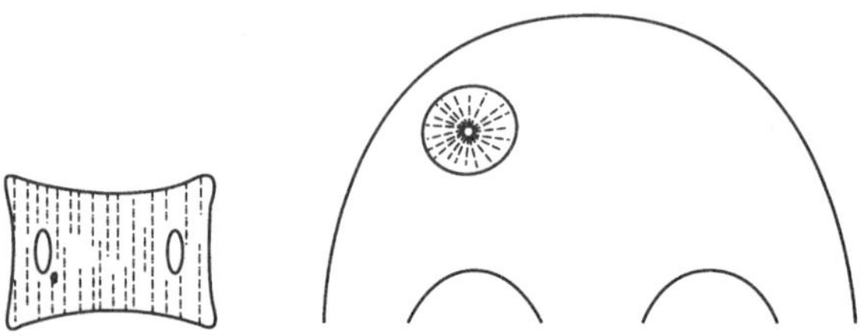

1. Age — 10–50 years.
2. Sites — vertebra (dorsal lumbar) or skull vault.
3. Appearances:
   (a) Vertebra — coarse vertical striations, usually affecting only the body but the appendages are, uncommonly, also involved.
   (b) Skull — radial spiculation ('sunburst') within a well-defined vault lucency. 'Hair-on-end' appearance in tangential views.
   (c) High signal on T_1W and T_2W MRI because of high fat content.

HAEMOCHROMATOSIS

A genetically determined primary abnormality of iron metabolism. Also occurs secondary to alcohol cirrhosis or multiple blood transfusions, e.g. in thalassaemia or chronic excessive oral iron ingestion.

Clinically — cirrhosis, skin pigmentation, diabetes (bronze diabetics), arthropathy and, later, ascites and cardiac failure.

BONES AND JOINTS

1. Osteoporosis.
2. Chondrocalcinosis — due to calcium pyrophosphate dihydrate deposition (q.v.).
3. Arthropathy — resembles the arthropathy of calcium pyrophosphate deposition disease (q.v.), but shows a predilection for the metacarpophalangeal joints (especially the second and third), the midcarpal joints and the carpometacarpal joints. It also exhibits distinctive beak-like osteophytes and is less rapidly progressive.

LIVER AND SPLEEN

1. Mottled increased density of liver and spleen due to the deposition of iron.

HAEMOPHILIA

Classical (Factor VIII deficiency) or Christmas disease (Factor IX deficiency). Both are X-linked recessive traits, i.e. manifest in males and carried by females.

JOINTS

1. Knee, elbow, ankle, hip and shoulder are most frequently affected.
2. Soft-tissue swelling due to haemarthrosis which may appear to be unusually dense owing to the presence of haemosiderin in the chronically thickened synovium.
3. Periarticular osteoporosis.
4. Erosion of articular surfaces, with subchondral cysts.
5. Preservation of joint space until late.
6. Accelerated maturation and growth of epiphyses resulting in disparity of size between epiphysis and diaphysis.
7. Contractures.

BONES

1. Osteonecrosis — especially in the femoral head and talus.
2. Haemophilic pseudotumour — in the ilium, femur and tibia most frequently.
   (a) Intraosseous — a well-defined medullary lucency with a sclerotic margin. It may breach the cortex. ± Periosteal reaction and soft-tissue component.
   (b) Subperiosteal — periosteal reaction with pressure resorption of the cortex and a soft-tissue mass.
3. Fractures — secondary to osteoporosis.

SOFT TISSUES

1. Pseudotumour — slow-growing.
2. Ectopic ossification.

Further Reading

Stoker D.J. & Murray R.O. (1974) Skeletal changes in haemophilia and other bleeding disorders. *Semin. Roentgenol.*, 9: 185–93.

HOMOCYSTINURIA

AR, inborn error of metabolism. A lack of cystathionine synthetase results in the accumulation of homocystine and methionine, with a deficiency of cystathionine and cystine.

1. Mental defect (60%).
2. Tall stature, slim build and arachnodactyly, with a morphological resemblance to Marfan's syndrome.
3. Pectus excavatum or carinatum, kyphoscoliosis, genu valgum and pes cavus.
4. Osteoporosis.
5. Medial degeneration of the aorta and elastic arteries.
6. Arterial and venous thromboses.
7. Lens subluxation — usually downward.

HURLER'S SYNDROME

A mucopolysaccharidosis transmitted as an AR trait. Clinical features become evident at the end of the first year: dwarfism, mental retardation, coarse facial features, corneal opacification, deformed teeth and hepatosplenomegaly. Respiratory infections and cardiac failure usually lead to death in the first decade.

CRANIOFACIAL

1. Scaphocephalic macrocephaly.
2. J-shaped sella (prominent sulcus chiasmatus).

CENTRAL NERVOUS SYSTEM

1. Hydrocephalus due to cystic arachnoiditis in the hypothalamic region.
2. Symmetrical low attenuation of white matter on CT (high signal on T_2W, MRI).

AXIAL SKELETON

1. Oval vertebral bodies with an antero-inferior beak.
2. Kyphosis and a thoracolumbar gibbus.
3. Posterior scalloping with widened interpedicular distance.
4. Short neck.

APPENDICULAR SKELETON

1. Thickened diaphyses.
2. Angulated, oblique growth plates, e.g. those of the distal radius and ulna are angled toward each other.
3. Coxa valga (common). Genu valgum (always).
4. Trident hands with a coarse trabecular pattern. Proximal tapering of metacarpals.

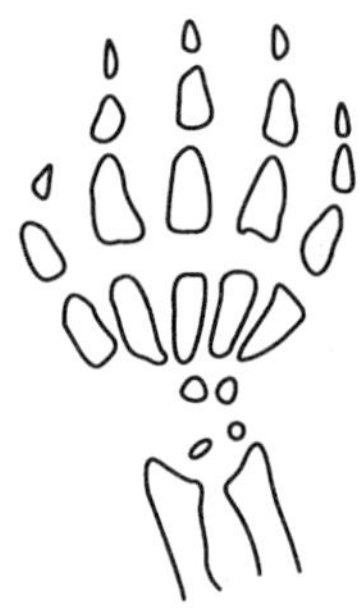

CARDIOVASCULAR SYSTEM

1. Cardiac failure due to intimal thickening of coronary arteries or valves.

NB. Hunter's syndrome is very similar clinically and radiologically, but the differences are:

(a) X-linked recessive transmission (i.e. no affected females).
(b) Later onset (2–6 years) and slower progression (death in the second or third decade).
(c) No corneal clouding.

HYPERPARATHYROIDISM, PRIMARY

CAUSES

1. Adenoma of one gland (90%). (2% of adenomas are multiple.)
2. Hyperplasia of all four glands (5%). (More likely if there is a family history.)
3. Carcinoma of one gland.
4. Ectopic parathormone — e.g. from a carcinoma of the bronchus.
5. Multiple endocrine adenopathy syndrome (type 1) — hyperplasia or adenoma associated with pituitary adenoma and pancreatic tumour.

BONES

1. Osteopenia — uncommon. When advanced there is loss of the fine trabeculae and sometimes a ground-glass appearance.
2. Subperiosteal bone resorption — particularly affecting the radial side of the middle phalanx of the middle finger, medial proximal tibia, lateral and occasionally medial end of clavicle, symphysis pubis, ischial tuberosity, medial femoral neck, dorsum sellae, superior surface of ribs and proximal humerus. Severe disease produces terminal phalangeal resorption and, in children, the 'rotting fence-post' appearance of the proximal femur.
3. Diffuse cortical change — cortical tunnelling eventually leading to a 'basketwork' appearance. 'Pepper-pot skull'.
4. Brown tumours — the solitary sign in 3% of cases. Most frequent in the mandible, ribs, pelvis and femora.
5. Bone softening — basilar invagination, wedged or codfish vertebrae, kyphoscoliosis, triradiate pelvis. Pathological fractures.

SOFT TISSUES

1. Calcification in soft tissues, pancreas, lung and arteries.

JOINTS

1. Marginal erosions — predominantly the distal interphalangeal joints, the ulnar side of the base of the little-finger metacarpal and the hamate. No joint-space narrowing.
2. Weakened subarticular bone, leading to collapse.
3. Chondrocalcinosis (calcium pyrophosphate dihydrate deposition disease) and true gout.
4. Periarticular calcification, including capsular and tendon calcification.

KIDNEY

1. Nephrocalcinosis.
2. Calculi (in 50%).

HYPERCALCAEMIA

1. Asymptomatic (in 15%) or overt (in 8%).

GASTROINTESTINAL TRACT

1. Peptic ulcer.
2. Pancreatitis.

Further Reading

Hayes C.W. & Conway W.F. (1991) Hyperparathyroidism. *Radiol. Clin. North Am.*, 29(1): 85–96.

HYPOPARATHYROIDISM

1. Short stature, dry skin, alopecia, tetany ± mental retardation.
2. Skeletal changes affecting the entire skeleton.
3. Minimal, generalized increased density of the skeleton, but especially affecting the metaphyses.
4. Calcification of paraspinal ligaments (secondary to elevation of plasma phosphate, which combines with calcium, resulting in heterotopic calcium phosphate deposits).
5. Basal ganglia calcification — uncommon.

HYPOPHOSPHATASIA

AR. Deficiency of serum and tissue alkaline phosphatase, with excessive urinary excretion of phosphoethanolamine. 50% die in early infancy.

NEONATAL FORM

1. Most severely affected. Stillborn or die within 6 months.
2. Clinically — hypotonia, irritability, vomiting respiratory insufficiency, failure to thrive, convulsions and small stature with bowed legs.
3. Radiologically:
   (a) Profoundly deficient mineralization with increased liability to fractures.
   (b) Irregular lack of metaphyseal mineralization affecting especially the wrists, knees and costochondral junctions.

INFANTILE FORM

1. Initially asymptomatic, but between 2 weeks and 6 months shows the same symptoms as the neonatal form. Most survive.
2. Radiologically:
   (a) Cupped and frayed metaphyses with widened growth plates.
   (b) Demineralized epiphyses.
   (c) Defective mineralization of skull, including sutures which appear widened.
   (d) Premature sutural fusion → craniostenosis with brachycephaly.

CHILDHOOD FORM

1. Presents 6 months to 2 years with bowed legs, genu valgum, delayed walking, bone pain, dental caries and premature loss of teeth.
2. Radiologically:
   (a) Mild rickets.
   (b) No craniostenosis.

ADULT FORM

1. Osteomalacia — both clinically and radiologically.

HYPOTHYROIDISM, CONGENITAL

APPENDICULAR SKELETON

1. Delayed appearance of ossification centres which may be:
   (a) Slightly granular.
   (b) Finely stippled.
   (c) Coarsely stippled.
   (d) Fragmented.
   The femoral capital epiphyses may be divided into inner and outer halves.
2. Delayed epiphyseal closure.
3. Short long bones with slender shafts, endosteal thickening and dense metaphyseal bands.
4. Coxa vara with shortened femoral neck and elevated greater trochanter.

SKULL

1. Brachycephaly.
2. Multiple wormian bones.
3. Delayed development of vascular markings and diploic differentiation.
4. Delayed sutural closure.
5. Poorly developed sinuses and mastoids.

AXIAL SKELETON

1. Kyphosis at the thoracolumbar junction, usually associated with a hypoplastic or 'bullet-shaped' body of LV1 or LV2.

The bone changes may have completely regressed in adults.

JUVENILE IDIOPATHIC ARTHRITIS

A heterogeneous group of conditions which begin in childhood (age < 16 years) and involve persistent inflammation of one or more joints (for at least 6 weeks).

OLIGOARTICULAR OR MONOARTICULAR ONSET (45%)

1. Most commonly presents at 1–5 years.
2. Four or less joints involved at the onset — knees, ankles and hips most commonly.
3. ± Iridocyclitis.

POLYARTICULAR ONSET (23%)

1. Rh F negative — 21% of total. Rh F positive — 2% of total; F>M; onset > 11 years.
2. Arthritis predominates with a similar distribution to the systemic onset, but also including the small joints of the fingers and toes. The cervical spine is involved frequently and early.
3. Prolonged disease leads to growth retardation and abnormal epiphyseal development.

SYSTEMIC ONSET

1. Most common at 1–5 years. M = F.
2. Severe extra-articular clinical manifestations include pyrexia, rash, lymphadenopathy and hepatosplenomegaly.
3. Joint involvement is late, but eventually a polyarthritis affects especially the knees, wrists, carpi, ankles and tarsi.

PSORIATIC ARTHRITIS (13%)

1. M > F.

ENTHESITIS-RELATED ARTHRITIS (10%)

1. Distal > proximal joints.
2. HLA B27 positive.
3. M > F. > 8 years.

RADIOLOGICAL CHANGES

1. Joint effusion — early finding.
2. Periarticular soft-tissue swelling — early finding.
3. Osteopenia — juxta-articular, diffuse or band-like in the metaphyses, the latter particularly in the distal femur, proximal tibia, distal radius and distal tibia.
4. Periostitis — common. Mainly periarticular in the phalanges, metacarpals and metatarsals, but when diaphyseal will eventually result in enlarged rectangular tubular bones.
5. Growth disturbances — epiphyseal overgrowth; premature fusion of growth plates; short broad phalanges, metacarpals and metatarsals; hypoplasia of the temporomandibular joint; leg length discrepancy.
6. Subluxation and dislocation — common in the wrist and hip. Atlantoaxial subluxation is most frequent in seropositive juvenile onset rheumatoid arthritis. Protrusio acetabuli of the hip.
7. Bony erosions — late manifestation; predominantly knees, hands and feet.
8. Joint-space narrowing — late manifestations due to cartilage loss.
9. Bony ankylosis — late finding; especially carpus, tarsus and cervical spine.
10. Epiphyseal compression fractures.

Further Reading

Cohen P.A., Job-Deslandre C.H., Lalande G. (2000) Overview of the radiology of juvenile idiopathic arthritis (JIA). *Eur. J. Radiol.*, 33: 94–101.

Davidson J. (2000) Juvenile idiopathic arthritis: a clinical overview. *Eur. J. Radiol.*, 33: 128–34.

Johnson K. & Gardner-Medwin J. (2002) Childhood arthritis: classification and radiology. *Clin. Radiol.*, 57: 47–58.

Wihlborg C., Babyn P., Ranson M. *et al.* (2001) Radiologic mimics of juvenile rheumatoid arthritis. *Pediatr. Radiol.*, 31: 315–26.

LANGERHANS CELL HISTIOCYTOSIS

A disease characterized by intense proliferation of reticulohistiocytic elements. Younger patients have more disseminated disease. There are three clinical subgroups.

EOSINOPHILIC GRANULOMA

1. Accounts for 60–80% of histiocytosis.
2. Commonest in 4–7-year olds, who present with bone pain, local swelling and irritability.
3. 50–75% have solitary lesions. When multiple, usually only two or three. Long bones, pelvis, skull and flat bones are the most common sites involved. 20% of solitary lesions become multiple.
4. Radiological changes in the skeleton include:
   (a) Well-defined lucency in the medulla ± thin sclerotic rim. ± Endosteal scalloping. True expansion is uncommon except in ribs and vertebral bodies. ± Overlying periosteal reaction.
   (b) Multilocular lucency, without expansion, in the pelvis.
   (c) Punched-out lucencies in the skull vault with little or no surrounding sclerosis. May coalesce to give a 'geographical skull'.
   (d) Destructive lesions in the skull base, mastoids, sella or mandible ('floating teeth').
   (e) Vertebra plana, with intact intervertebral discs.
5. Lung involvement in < 10% and associated with a worse prognosis.
   (a) Hilar lymphadenopathy.
   (b) Miliary shadowing.
   (c) 'Honeycomb lung'.

HAND–SCHÜLLER–CHRISTIAN DISEASE

1. Commonest in 1–3-year olds.
2. Osseous lesions together with mild to moderate visceral involvement which includes lymphadenopathy, hepatosplenomegaly, skin lesions, diabetes insipidus, exophthalmos and pulmonary disease.
3. Bone lesions are similar to eosinophilic granuloma, but more numerous and widely distributed.

LETTERER–SIWE DISEASE

1. Major visceral involvement with less prominent bone involvement during the first year of life.
2. Bone lesions are poorly defined.

LYMPHOMA

INTRATHORACIC LYMPHADENOPATHY

1. 66% of patients with Hodgkin's disease have intrathoracic disease and 99% of these have intrathoracic lymphadenopathy.
2. 40% of patients with non-Hodgkin's lymphoma have intrathoracic disease and 90% of these have intrathoracic lymphadenopathy.
3. Nodes involved are (in order of frequency) anterior mediastinal, paratracheal, tracheobronchial, bronchopulmonary and subcarinal. Involvement tends to be bilateral and asymmetrical, although unilateral disease is not uncommon.
4. Nodes show a rapid response to radiotherapy, and 'egg-shell' calcification of lymph nodes may be observed following radiotherapy.

PULMONARY DISEASE

1. More common in Hodgkin's disease than non-Hodgkin's lymphoma.
2. Very unusual without lymphadenopathy, but may be the first evidence of recurrence after radiotherapy.
3. Most frequently one or more large opacities with an irregular outline. ± Air bronchogram.
4. Collapse due to endobronchial lymphoma or, less frequently, extrinsic compression. (Collapse is less common than in bronchial carcinoma.)

5. Lymphatic obstruction → oedema or lymphangitis carcinomatosa.
6. Miliary or larger opacities widely disseminated throughout the lungs.
7. Cavitation — eccentrically within a mass and with a thick wall. (More common than in bronchial carcinoma.)
8. Calcification following radiotherapy.
9. Soft-tissue mass adjacent to a rib deposit.
10. Pleural and pericardial effusions.

GASTROINTESTINAL TRACT

Involvement may be the primary presentation (5% of all lymphomas) or be a part of generalized disease (50% at autopsy). In descending order of frequency, the stomach, small intestine, rectum and colon may be involved.

STOMACH

1. Primary lymphoma accounts for 2.5% of all gastric neoplasms, and 2.5% of lymphomas present with a stomach lesion. Non-Hodgkin's lymphoma accounts for 80%.
2. The radiological manifestations comprise:
   (a) Diffuse mucosal thickening and irregularity ± decreased distensibility and peristaltic activity. ± Multiple ulcers.
   (b) Smooth nodular mass ± central ulceration. Surrounding mucosa may be normal or show thickened folds.
   (c) Single or multiple ulcers with irregular margins.
   (d) Thickening of the wall with narrowing of the lumen. If the distal stomach is involved there may be extension into the duodenum.
   (e) Duodenal ulcer associated with a gastric mass.

SMALL INTESTINE

1. Usually secondary to contiguous spread from mesenteric lymph nodes. Primary disease only in non-Hodgkin's lymphoma.
2. Usually more than one of the following signs is evident:
   (a) Irregular mucosal infiltration → thick folds ± nodularity.
   (b) Irregular polypoid mass ± barium tracts within it or central ulceration.
   (c) Annular constriction — usually a long segment.
   (d) Aneurysmal dilatation, with no internal mucosal pattern.
   (e) Polyps — multiple and small or solitary and large. The latter may induce an intussusception.
   (f) Multiple ulcers.
   (g) Non-specific malabsorption pattern.

(h) Fistula.
(i) Perforation.

COLON AND RECTUM

1. Rarely involved. Caecum and rectum more frequently involved than the rest of the colon.
2. Radiologically the disease may show:
   (a) Polypoidal mass — which may induce an intussusception.
   (b) Diffuse infiltration of the wall.
   (c) Constricting annular lesion.

RETROPERITONEAL LYMPHADENOPATHY

1. CT has largely replaced lymphangiography, having a similar accuracy for retroperitoneal nodes and the ability to show mesenteric nodes, nodes above the cisterna chyli and extranodal pathology.
2. Although CT cannot identify lymphoma in normal size nodes, the false negative rate is low.
3. Normal lymph nodes are 3–10 mm in diameter. Abdominal lymph nodes are definitely abnormal if > 10 mm diameter. A localized cluster of lymph nodes 6–10 mm in diameter should be considered highly suspect.
4. Lymphadenopathy should be considered in the presence of:
   (a) A small number of discretely enlarged lymph nodes.
   (b) A conglomerate group of contiguous lymph nodes of similar size to the aorta or SVC.
   (c) A large mass in which individual lymph nodes cannot be recognized.

SKELETON

1. Radiological involvement in 10–20% of patients with Hodgkin's disease (50% at autopsy).
2. Involvement arises either from direct spread from contiguous lymph nodes or infiltration of bone marrow (spine, pelvis, major long bones, thoracic cage and skull are sites of predilection).
3. Patterns of bone involvement are:
   (a) Predominantly osteolytic.
   (b) Mixed lytic and sclerotic.
   (c) Predominantly sclerotic — *de novo* or following radiotherapy to a lytic lesion.
   (d) 'Moth-eaten' — characteristic of round cell malignancies.

4. In addition, the spine may show:
   (a) Anterior erosion of a vertebral body caused by involvement of an adjacent paravertebral lymph node.
   (b) Solitary dense vertebral body (ivory vertebra).
5. Hypertrophic osteoarthropathy.

CENTRAL NERVOUS SYSTEM

1. Primary lymphoma (usually non-Hodgkin's B cell) shows increased incidence in HIV/AIDS and immunodeficiency states (Wiskott–Aldrich syndrome, IgA deficiency, X-linked lymphoproliferative syndrome and following organ transplantation). The cerebrum (deep hemispheric periventricular white matter), corpus callosum, brainstem and cerebellum are affected (in order of frequency). Two patterns may be recognized:
   (a) In immunocompetent patients there is a large, round or oval space-occupying lesion showing increased attenuation (CT), intermediate- to low-signal (T_1W MRI), isointense or hyperintense signal relative to grey matter (T_2W MRI) and surrounding oedema. Marked homogeneous enhancement (although avascular at angiography).
   (b) In patients with HIV, a supratentorial mass frequently involves the corpus callosum, basal ganglia and other deep cerebral nuclei. Enhancement is variable and often bizarre. Multifocal lesions in 50%. Ependymal seeding in one-third, but meningeal disease is infrequent.
2. Systemic lymphoma typically presents as leptomeningeal disease.

Further Reading

Craig O. & Gregson R. (1981) Primary lymphoma of the gastrointestinal tract. *Clin. Radiol.*, 32: 63–71.

Erdag N., Bhorade R.M., Alberico R.A. *et al.* (2001) Primary lymphoma of the central nervous system. Typical and atypical CT and MR imaging appearances. *Am. J. Roentgenol.*, 176: 1319–26.

Felson B. (ed.) (1980) The lymphomas and leukaemias. Part I. *Semin. Roentgenol.*, 15(3).

Felson B. (ed.) (1980) The lymphomas and leukaemias. Part 2. *Semin. Roentgenol.*, 15(4).

Libshitz H.I. (ed.) (1990) Imaging the lymphomas. *Radiol. Clin. North Am.*, 28(4).

Parker BR (1997) Leukaemia and lymphoma in childhood. *Radiol. Clin. North Am.*, 35: 1495–516.

Rehm P.K. (2001) Radionuclide evaluation of patients with lymphoma. *Radiol. Clin. North Am.*, 39(5): 957–78.

MARFAN'S SYNDROME

A connective tissue disorder transmitted as an AD trait, but with variable expression. 25% spontaneous mutations. Multisystem defects due to defective fibrillin, a component of microfibrils which is found in mesenchymal tissues.

SKELETAL SYSTEM

1. Pectus excavatum or carinatum.
2. Disproportionate tall stature (upper segment:lower segment < 0.86 or span:height 1.05).
3. Arachnodactyly (metacarpal index 8.4–10.4).
4. Scoliosis (> 20°) or spondylolisthesis.
5. Joint laxity.
6. Dislocations of sternoclavicular joint and hip and perilunate dislocation.
7. Pes planus with valgus ankle.
8. Protrusio acetabula.
9. Rib notching.
10. Narrow facies with a narrow, high arched palate.

OCULAR SYSTEM

Ectopia lentis — usually upwards.

CARDIOVASCULAR SYSTEM

1. Aortic sinus dilatation and aortic regurgitation.
2. Cystic medial necrosis of the aorta; aortic dissection.
3. Ascending aortic dilatation ± dissection. Less commonly aneurysms of the descending thoracic or abdominal aorta or pulmonary artery.
4. Mitral valve abnormalities — large annulus, regurgitation and prolapse.

DURA

1. Lumbosacral dural ectasia.

LUNGS

1. Pulmonary emphysema and bullae.

DIFFERENTIAL DIAGNOSIS

1. Familial Marfan-like habitus (< 2 s.d. above normal).
2. Familial ectopia lentis.
3. Familial aortic aneurysm/dissection.
4. MASS phenotype (myopia, mitral valve prolapse, aortic root dilatation, striae, skeletal involvement).
5. Congenital contractural arachnodactyly (Beal syndrome).

Further Reading

De Paepe A., Devereux R.B., Dietz H.C. *et al.* (1996) Revised diagnostic criteria for the Marfan syndrome. *Am. J. Med. Genet.*, 62: 417–26.

MORQUIO'S SYNDROME

A mucopolysaccharidosis transmitted as an AR trait. Clinical presentation during the second year, with decreased growth, progressive skeletal deformity, corneal opacities, lymphadenopathy, cardiac lesions and deafness.

AXIAL SKELETON

1. Universal vertebra plana. Wide discs.
2. Hypoplastic dens.
3. Hypoplastic dorsolumbar vertebra which may be displaced posteriorly.
4. Central anterior vertebral body beaks.
5. Short neck.
6. Dorsal scoliosis and dorsolumbar kyphosis.

APPENDICULAR SKELETON

1. Defective irregular ossification of the femoral capital epiphyses leading to flattening.
2. Genu valgum.
3. Short, wide tubular bones with irregular metaphyses. Proximal tapering of the metacarpals.
4. Irregular carpal and tarsal bones.

CARDIOVASCULAR SYSTEM

1. Late-onset aortic regurgitation.

MULTIPLE ENDOCRINE NEOPLASIA (MEN) SYNDROMES

AD.

MEN I (WERNER'S SYNDROME)

1. Hyperparathyroidism (90%).
2. Pancreatic islet cell tumours (60%).

   Gastrinomas (60%) — usually slow-growing: → Zollinger–Ellison syndrome.
   Insulinomas — symptoms of hypoglycaemia.
   VIPomas — secreting vasoactive intestinal peptide → explosive, watery diarrhoea with hypokalaemia and achlorhydria.
   Glucagonomas — produce a syndrome of diabetes mellitus, necrolytic migratory erythema, anaemia, weight loss and thromboembolic complications.

3. Pituitary tumours (5%) — hormone-secreting and non-secreting.
4. Thyroid adenoma.
5. Adrenal adenoma.
6. Carcinoid tumour.

MEN IIA (SIPPLE'S SYNDROME)

1. Medullary carcinoma of the thyroid (100%).
2. Phaeochromocytoma (50%).
3. Hyperparathyroidism (10%).

MEN IIB

1. Marfanoid appearance (100%).
2. Multiple mucosal neuromas (100%).
3. Medullary carcinoma of the thyroid (100%).
4. Phaeochromocytoma (50%).

MULTIPLE MYELOMA/PLASMACYTOMA

Plasma cell neoplasms of bone are solitary (plasmacytoma; 3% of all plasma cell tumours) or multiple (multiple myeloma; 94% of all plasma cell tumours). 3% of all plasma cell tumours are solely extraskeletal.

PLASMACYTOMA

1. A well-defined, grossly expansile bone lesion arising, most commonly, in the spine, pelvis or ribs.
2. It may also exhibit soft-tissue extension, internal septa or pathological fracture.

MULTIPLE MYELOMA

Radiological manifestations are skeletal and extraskeletal.

Skeletal

1. 80–90% have an abnormal skeleton at the time of diagnosis.
2. The skeleton may:
   (a) Be normal — uncommon.
   (b) Show generalized osteopenia only — rare.
   (c) Show osteopenia with discrete lucencies.
      (i) The lucencies are usually:
         - widely disseminated at the time of diagnosis (spine, pelvis, skull, ribs and shafts of long bones)
         - uniform in size (cf. metastases, which are usually of varying size)
         - well-defined, with a narrow zone of transition.
      (ii) Vertebral body collapse, occasionally with disc destruction. ± Paravertebral shadow. Involvement of pedicles is late.
      (iii) Rib lesions tend to be expansile and associated with extrapleural soft-tissue masses.
      (iv) Pathological fractures occur and healing is accompanied by much callus.
   (d) Show a permeating, mottled pattern of bone destruction similar to other round cell malignancies, e.g. Ewing's sarcoma, anaplastic metastatic carcinoma, leukaemia and reticulum cell sarcoma.
   (e) Show multiple sclerotic lesions which mimic osteoblastic metastases (2%).

Extraskeletal

1. Hypercalcaemia (30%).
2. Soft-tissue tumours in sinuses, the submucosa of the pharynx and trachea, cervical lymph nodes, skin and gastrointestinal tract.
3. Hepatosplenomegaly.

Further Reading

Meszaros W.T. (1974) The many facets of multiple myeloma. *Semin. Roentgenol.*, 9: 21–8.

MYASTHENIA GRAVIS

An autoimmune disorder characterized by muscle weakness and fatiguability. Confirmed clinically by a positive response to intravenous edrophonium chloride (Tensilon test) and the presence of acetylcholine receptor antibodies.

1. Thymus is normal or involuted in 20%, hyperplastic in 65% and 15% have a thymoma. Hyperplasia is more common in the young; thymoma more common after the fourth decade.
2. 60% of thymomas are benign and well-encapsulated; 40% are locally invasive and show subpleural deposits.

Further Reading

Moore N.R. (1989) Imaging in myasthenia gravis. *Clin. Radiol.*, 40: 115–6.

NEUROFIBROMATOSIS

NEUROFIBROMATOSIS 1 (NF-1; VON RECKLINGHAUSEN DISEASE)

90% of all cases. Prevalence 1 in 4000 persons. 50% are new mutations, 30% are AD. Gene is located on chromosome 17. May be diagnosed if two or more of the following criteria are present:

- Six or more *café-au-lait* spots > 5 mm in diameter in prepubertal patients and > 15 mm in postpubertal patients.
- Two or more neurofibromas.
- Axillary freckling.
- One plexiform neurofibroma.
- Two or more iris hamartomas (Lisch nodules).
- Optic glioma.
- Typical bone lesions such as sphenoid dysplasia or tibial pseudarthrosis.
- One or more first-degree relatives with NF-1.

NEUROFIBROMATOSIS 2 (NF-2)

10% of all cases. Rare in childhood. Prevalence 1 in 50 000 persons. AD with the gene located on chromosome 22. Manifestations include VIIIth nerve tumours or schwannomas, other intracranial or spinal tumours such as neurinomas and meningiomas. May be diagnosed if one of the following criteria are present:

- Bilateral VIIIth nerve tumours.
- Unilateral VIIIth nerve tumour in association with any two of the following: meningioma, neurofibroma, schwannoma, juvenile posterior subcapsular cataracts.
- Unilateral VIIIth nerve tumour with other spinal or brain tumour as above in a first-degree relative.

Skull

1. Dysplastic sphenoid — absent greater wing ± lesser wing (empty orbit), absent posterolateral wall of the orbit. May result in proptosis.
2. Lytic defects in the calvarium, especially in or near the lambdoid suture.
3. Enlargement of foramina.

4. Mandibular abnormalities.
5. Enlarged internal auditory meati — due to acoustic neuromas or dural ectasia without associated neuroma.

Brain (see also 12.38)

1. Focal or multifocal ↓ T_1W and/or ↑ T_2W signal without mass effect, most often in the basal ganglia, cerebellum and cerebral peduncles. No enhancement. ?Due to hamartomas. More common in younger patients and in those with an optic glioma. Tendency to regress after teenage years.
2. Tumours:
   (a) Optic tract, chiasm and nerve gliomas (common). 10–30% of optic gliomas are associated with NF-1. The association is higher with optic nerve gliomas, and bilateral optic nerve gliomas are found almost exclusively in NF-1. Optic nerve glioma is not found in NF-2.
   (b) Optic nerve sheath meningiomas (rare).
   (c) Cranial nerve (V–XII) schwannomas. Frequently multiple and bilateral in NF-2. Acoustic neuromas (schwannomas) are bilateral in at least 90% of NF-2.
   (d) Brainstem and supratentorial gliomas.
   (e) Intracranial meningiomas — often multiple in NF-2.
3. Macrocephaly.
4. Hydrocephalus, of insidious onset — usually due to aqueduct stenosis caused by gliosis but may be secondary to a tumour.
5. Cerebral and cerebellar calcification. Heavy calcification of the choroid plexuses is rare but classic.
6. Arachnoid cyst.
7. Arterial occlusive disease, including moyamoya.

Spine

1. Scoliosis (typically acute and thoracic) and kyphosis.
2. Dural ectasia with posterior scalloping.
3. Absent or hypoplastic pedicles.
4. Spondylolisthesis.
5. Lateral meningocoele (rare).
6. Multiple neurofibromas (enhancing) ± dumbbell. Enlargement of intervertebral foramina. Most common in the cervicothoracic region.
7. Paraspinal plexiform neurofibromas.

Thorax

1. Rib notching, 'twisted ribbon' ribs and splaying of ribs.
2. Interstitial pulmonary fibrosis progressing to a 'honeycomb' lung.

Appendicular skeleton

1. Overgrowth or, less commonly, undergrowth of long bones.
2. Overtubulation or undertubulation (due to cortical thickening).
3. Anterior and lateral bowing of the tibia with irregular periosteal thickening is common and is usually evident in the first year. It frequently progresses to no. 4.
4. Pseudarthrosis.
5. Intraosseous neurofibromas present as subperiosteal or cortical lucencies with a smooth expanded outer margin.
6. Cortical pressure resorption from an adjacent soft-tissue neurofibroma.
7. Cortical defects may also be due to dysplastic periosteum.
8. Association of non-ossifying fibromas and neurofibromatosis.

Other

1. Soft-tissue neurofibromas and plexiform neurofibromas. The latter may be associated with partial gigantism.
2. Renal artery stenosis or aneurysm.
3. Phaeochromocytoma (in 1%).
4. Osteomalacia.

Further Reading

Klatte E.C., Franken E.A. & Smith J.A. (1976) The radiographic spectrum in neurofibromatosis. *Semin. Roentgenol.,* 11: 17–33.

Menor F., Martí-Bonmatí L., Mulas F. *et al.* (1991) Imaging considerations of central nervous system manifestations in paediatric patients with neurofibromatosis type 1. *Pediatr. Radiol.,* 21: 389–94.

Murphey M.D., Smith W.S., Smith S.E. *et al.* (1999) Imaging of musculoskeletal neurogenic tumors: radiologic–pathologic correlation. *RadioGraphics,* 19:1253–80.

Rossi S.E., Erasmus J.J., McAdams H.P. *et al.* (1999) Thoracic manifestations of neurofibromatosis-1. *Am. J. Roentgenol.,* 173: 1631–8.

NEUROPATHIC ARTHROPATHY

Disease	*Sites of involvement*
Diabetes mellitus	Metatarsophalangeal, tarsometatarsal and intertarsal joints
Steroid treatment	Hips and knees
Syringomyelia	Shoulder, elbow, wrist and cervical spine
Tabes dorsalis	Knee, hip, ankle and lumbar spine
Congenital insensitivity to pain	Ankle and intertarsal joints
Myelomeningocoele	Ankle and intertarsal joints
Leprosy	Hands (interphangeal), feet (metatarsophalangeal) and lower limbs
Chronic alcoholism	Metatarsophalangeal and interphalangeal joints

Radiological changes include:

1. Variable progression, but often rapid. In the early stages can resemble osteoarthritis.
2. Joint effusion.
3. Osteochondral fractures and fragmentation of articular surfaces.
4. Intra-articular bony debris.
5. Excessive callus formation.
6. Subluxations and dislocations.
7. Bone density is normal but in diabetes and syringomyelia superadded infection is not uncommon, resulting in juxta-articular osteoporosis.
8. Bone resorption can produce a 'cup and pencil' appearance.

Further Reading

Jones E.A., Manamaster B.J., May D.A. *et al.* (2000) Neuropathic osteoarthropathy: diagnostic dilemmas and differential diagnosis. *RadioGraphics*, 20: 5279–93.

NON-ACCIDENTAL INJURY

SKELETAL

1. Fractures in 11–55% and significantly more common in the younger child. Typically multiple, in varying stages of healing and explained by an implausible history.
2. Shaft fractures are more common than metaphyseal fractures although the latter are characteristic.
3. Metaphyseal fractures are due to tractional and torsional stresses on limbs and histologically there is a transmetaphyseal disruption of the most immature metaphyseal primary spongiosa. The most subtle indication of injury is a transverse lucency within the subepiphyseal region of the metaphysis. It may be visible in only one projection and its appearance is influenced by the severity of the bony injury, the degree of displacement of the fragments and the chronicity of the process. Peripherally the fracture line may undermine and isolate a thicker fragment of bone and it is this thick peripheral margin of bone that produces the corner fractures and bucket handle configurations.
4. Rib fractures comprise 5–27% of all fractures in abused children. Posterior rib fractures have a higher specificity for abuse than anterolateral fractures. In the absence of prematurity, birth injury, metabolic disorders, bone dysplasias and major trauma, e.g. road traffic accidents, rib fractures may be considered specific for abuse. The majority are occult.
5. Skull fractures which are linear and in the parietal bone are most common; more complex fractures may be suggestive of non-accidental injury.
6. In infants and young children certain fractures have a high specificity for abuse owing to their unusual locations. These include scapular injuries, injuries involving the small bones of the hands and feet and spinal injuries.
7. Dislocations are rarely encountered in abused children. Malalignment of bones sharing an articulation usually indicates a growth plate injury rather than dislocation. When dislocations do occur they are likely to be secondary to massive injury and are accompanied by adjacent fracture.

INTRACRANIAL INJURIES

Shaking is the most important mechanism in the production of intracranial injury in child abuse. The spectrum of injuries includes:

(a) Subdural haematoma, especially posterior interhemispheric collections due to tearing of the small bridging veins which cross the subdural space.
(b) Intraventricular haemorrhage — when gross is usually associated with massive intracranial injury.
(c) Subarachnoid haemorrhage.
(d) Cerebral oedema — generalized or focal and is the most common CT alteration in all types of paediatric head injury.
(e) Contusional tears — pathognomonic of shaking in the first 6 months of life.
(f) Cerebral contusion — seen usually along the cerebral convexities, particularly in the frontal and parasagittal regions, conforming to the sites of greatest stress during acceleration–deceleration movements.
Commonly associated with subdural haematomas.
(g) Cerebral atrophy — depending on the site of the original injury may be focal or diffuse and evident as early as 1 month following the acute injury.
(h) Post-traumatic hydrocephalus.

VISCERAL TRAUMA

Commonly occurs after the child is able to move about. Mortality of 50% for visceral injuries associated with child abuse. The most likely mechanism of injury is a direct blow or the effect of rapid deceleration after being hurled. The most common injuries involve the hollow viscera, mesenteries, liver and pancreas.

Further Reading

Chapman S. (1990) Radiological aspects of non-accidental injury. *J. R. Soc. Med.*, 83: 67–71.
Hymel K.P., Rumack C.M., Hay T.C. *et al.* (1997) Comparison of intracranial computed tomographic (CT) findings in pediatric abusive and accidental head trauma. *Pediatr. Radiol.*, 27: 743–7.
Jaspan T., Narborough G., Punt J.A. *et al.* (1992) Cerebral contusional tears as a marker of child abuse — detection by cranial sonography. *Pediatr. Radiol.*, 22: 237–45.
Kleinman P. (1998) *Diagnostic Imaging of Child Abuse*, 2nd edn. St Louis: Mosby.
Merten, D.F., Radkowski M.A. & Leonidas J.C. (1983) The abused child: a radiological reappraisal. *Radiology*, 148: 377–81.
Rao P. & Carty H. (1999) Non-accidental injury: review of the radiology. *Clin. Radiol.*, 4: 11–24.
Strouse P.J., Close B.J., Marshall K.W. *et al.* (1999) CT of bowel and mesenteric trauma in children. *RadioGraphics*, 19: 1237–50.
Worlock P., Stower M. & Barbor P. (1986) Patterns of fractures in accidental and non-accidental injury in children: a comparative study. *Br. Med. J.*, 293: 100–3.

NON-OSSIFYING FIBROMA (FIBROUS CORTICAL DEFECT)

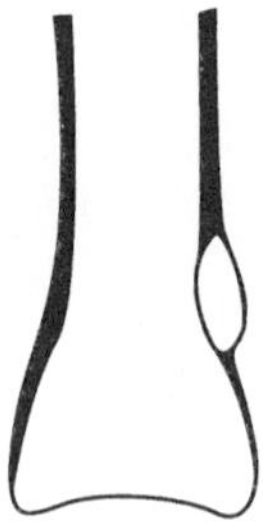

1. Age — 10–20 years.
2. Sites — femur and tibia.
3. Appearances:
   (a) Diametaphyseal, becoming diaphyseal as the bone grows.
   (b) Well-defined lucency with a sclerotic margin.
   (c) Eccentric ± slight expansion; in thin bones, e.g. fibula, it occupies the entire width of the bone.

OCHRONOSIS

See Alkaptonuria.

OSTEOBLASTOMA

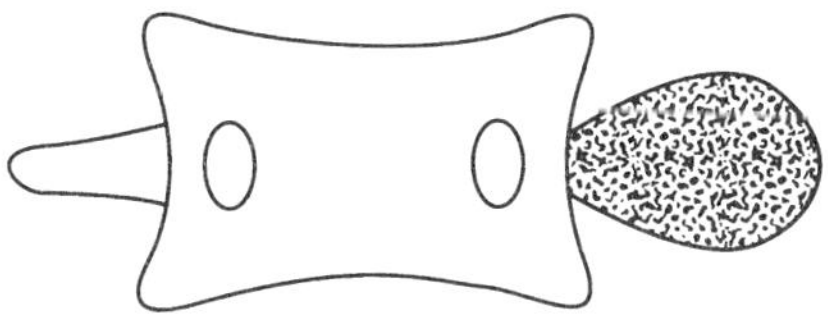

1. Age — 10–20 years.
2. Sites — vertebra (neural arch predominantly) and, less commonly, in the long bones.
3. Appearances:
   (a) Well-defined lucency with a sclerotic rim.
   (b) May be expansile, but the cortex is preserved.
   (c) ± Internal calcification.
   (d) May be purely sclerotic in the spine.
   (e) In long bones it is metaphyseal or diaphyseal.

OSTEOCHONDROMA (exostosis)

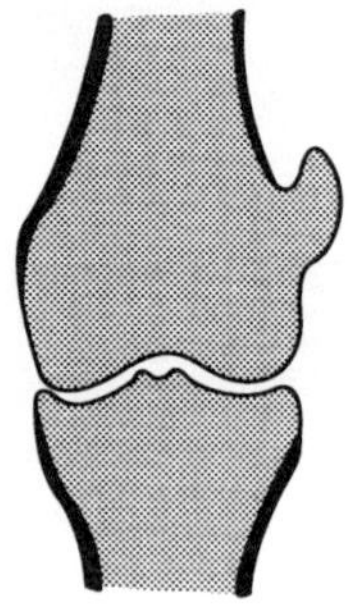

1. Age — 10–20 years. M < F.
2. Sites — distal femur, proximal tibia, proximal humerus, pelvis and scapula. When there are multiple osteochondromas the condition is termed diaphyseal aclasis (AD).
3. Appearances:
   (a) Metaphyseal.
   (b) Well-defined eccentric protrusion with the parent cortex and trabeculae continuous with that of the tumour.
   (c) Tumour is usually directed away from the end of the bone and migrates away from the end as growth proceeds.
   (d) The cartilage cap is not visible in childhood, but becomes calcified in the adult.
   (e) If large → failure of correct modelling.
4. Complications:
   (a) Cosmetic deformity.
   (b) Bony deformity.
   (c) Fracture.
   (d) Vascular compromise.
   (e) Peripheral nerve and spinal cord compression.
   (f) Bursa formation.
   (g) Malignant transformation. Rapid growth of a stable lesion suggests transformation to a chondrosarcoma (less than 1% of solitary, 5–25% of multiple osteochondromas).

Further Reading

Lee K.C.Y., Davies A.M. & Cassar-Pullicino V.N. (2002) Imaging the complications of osteochondromas. *Clin. Radiol.*, 57: 18–28.

Murphey M.D., Choi J.J., Kransdorf M.J. *et al.* (2000) Imaging of osteochondroma: variants and complications with radiologic–pathologic correlation. *RadioGraphics*, 20: 1407–34.

Woertler K., Lindner N., Gosheger G. *et al.* (2000) Osteochondroma: MR imaging of tumor-related complications. *Eur. Radiol.*, 10: 832–40.

OSTEOGENESIS IMPERFECTA

A clinically heterogeneous condition due to disorders of collagen. There are several distinct genetic entities and the current classification is as shown below.

TYPE 1

Osseous fragility (variable from minimal to severe), blue sclerae, presenile deafness due to otosclerosis (in 20%). Multiple fractures and intracranial bleeding may result in stillbirth or perinatal death. Gracile, osteoporotic bones, often with deformity secondary to fractures and mechanical stresses. Rapid fracture healing ± exuberant callus. Flattened or biconcave vertebral bodies. Wormian bones, although these may be obliterated in adulthood. AD.

Subgroup A: with normal teeth.

Subgroup B: with dentinogenesis imperfecta.

TYPE II

Lethal perinatal. Extremely severe osseous fragility.

Subgroup A: extremely osteopenic skull; broad beaded ribs; short, broad 'concertina' shaped long bones; platyspondyly. New mutation, AD.

Subgroup B: better ossification of skull; thin, wavy ribs with only a few fractures; short, broad 'concertina'-shaped long bones; vertebral body height similar to or greater than disc space. AR.

Subgroup C: poor ossification of skull; thin, irregularly-shaped ribs, short, poorly modelled long bones with multiple angulations; normal vertebral body height. AR or new AD mutation.

TYPE III

Rare. Moderate to severe osseous fragility; normal sclerae; severe deformity of long bones and spine result in severe dwarfing; cystic expansion of ends of long bones with increasing age. Wormian bones. Markedly elongated lumbar pedicles. White sclerae. AR, or new AD mutation.

TYPE IV

Rare. Osseous fragility with normal sclerae and severe deformity of long bones and spine. AD.

Further Reading

Sillence D.O. (1981) Osteogenesis imperfecta. An expanding panorama of variants. *Clin. Orthop.*, 159: 11–25.

Sillence D.O., Senn A. & Danks D.M. (1979) Genetic heterogeneity in osteogenesis imperfecta. *J. Med. Genet.*, 16: 101–16.

Smith R., Francis M.J.O. & Houghton G.R. (1983) *The Brittle Bone Syndrome: Osteogenesis Imperfecta.* Butterworth: London.

Thompson E.M., Young I.D., Hall C.M. & Pembrey M.E. (1987) Recurrence risk and prognosis in severe sporadic osteogenesis imperfecta. *J. Med. Genet.*, 24: 390–405.

OSTEOID OSTEOMA

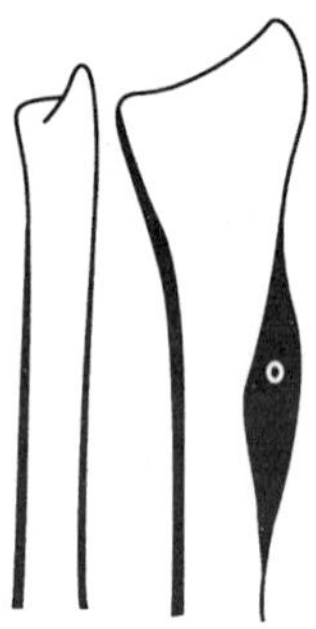

Cortical

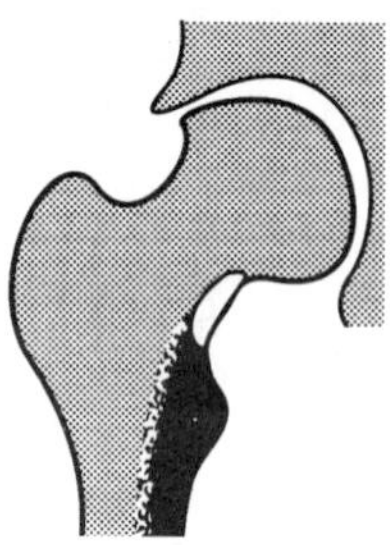

Cancellous

1. Age — 10–30 years.
2. Sites — most commonly femur and tibia.
3. Appearances:

   Cortical

   (a) Central lucent nidus (< 1 cm) ± dense calcified centre.
   (b) Dense surrounding bone.
   (c) Eccentric bone expansion ± periosteal reaction.

   Cancellous

   (a) Usually femoral neck.
   (b) Lucent lesion with bone sclerosis a distance away. The head and neck may be osteoporotic.

OSTEOMALACIA

Increased uncalcified osteoid in the mature skeleton.

1. Decreased bone density.
2. Looser's zones — bilaterally symmetrical transverse lucent bands of uncalcified osteoid which, later in the disease, have sclerotic margins. Common sites are the scapulae, femoral necks and shafts, pubic rami and ribs.
3. Coarsening of the trabecular pattern with ill-defined trabeculae.
4. Bone softening — protrusio acetabuli, bowing of long bones, biconcave vertebral bodies and basilar invagination.

Further Reading

Pitt M.J. (1991) Rickets and osteomalacia are still around. *Radiol. Clin. North Am.*, 29(1): 97–118.

OSTEOPETROSIS

A defect of bone resorption caused by decreased osteoclastic activity. A number of forms have been recognized.

BENIGN OR TARDA, AD

1. Often asymptomatic individuals in whom a chance diagnosis is made on radiographs taken for some other purpose. Some have a mild anaemia and there may be cranial nerve compressions. Predisposition to fractures. Tooth extraction may be complicated by osteomyelitis.
2. Increasing bone sclerosis during childhood, with some sparing of the peripheral skeleton.
3. 'Bone-within-bone' appearance — usually disappearing by the end of the second decade.
4. 'Rugger jersey' spine.

MALIGNANT OR CONGENITA, AR

1. Manifestations during infancy — failure to thrive and evidence of marrow failure due to bone overgrowth, i.e. anaemia, thrombocytopenia and hepatosplenomegaly. Pathological fractures. Cranial nerve palsies due to bony compression. Death in the first decade.
2. Generalized bone sclerosis with transverse metaphyseal bands.
3. 'Bone-within-bone' appearance.
4. 'Rugger jersey' spine.
5. Later, flask-shaped ends of the long bones.

INTERMEDIATE, AR

WITH RENAL TUBULAR ACIDOSIS, AR

1. Presents in early childhood with failure to thrive and hypotonia due to renal tubular acidosis. Anaemia, cranial nerve lesions and fractures are variable features.
2. Radiology is similar to the benign form but tends to normality in later childhood. Basal ganglia and periventricular calcification are consistent findings which differentiate this form from the others.

Further Reading

Beighton P. (1988) *Inherited Disorders of the Skeleton.* Edinburgh: Churchill Livingstone, pp. 163–9.

Beighton P. & Cremin B.J. (1980) *Sclerosing Bone Dysplasias.* Berlin: Springer–Verlag, pp. 19–31.

OSTEOSARCOMA

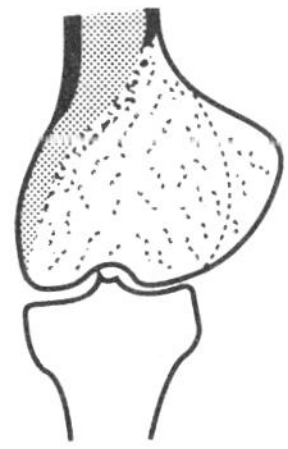

1. Age — 10–25 years with a second peak in the seventh decade (flat bones).
2. Sites — distal femur, proximal tibia, proximal humerus and pelvis.
3. Predisposing factors — Paget's disease, radiotherapy, osteochondroma, fibrous dysplasia, retinoblastoma, osteopetrosis and bone infarct.
4. Association — bilateral retinoblastoma.
5. Appearances:
   (a) Metaphyseal; epiphyseal (< 1%) and diaphyseal (10%) are unusual.
   (b) May be predominantly lytic, sclerotic or mixed.
   (c) Wide zone of transition with normal bone.
   (d) Cortical destruction with soft-tissue extension.
   (e) ± Internal calcification of bone.
   (f) Periosteal reaction — 'sunray' spiculation, lamellated and/or Codman's triangle.
6. Unusual variants
   (a) Telangiectatic — 5% of osteosarcomas. Aggressive. Characterized by large blood-filled cavities and thin septations within the tumour. Similar presentation to conventional osteosarcoma but pathological fracture is more common. Diaphyseal > metaphyseal. Majority in femur and tibia. Usually entirely osteolytic. Fluid/fluid levels on CT and MRI.
   (b) Small cell — 1% of osteosarcomas. Similar appearance and presentation to conventional osteosarcoma but prognosis is much worse.
   (c) Low grade or intraosseous well-differentiated — 1–2%. Older age at presentation and more chronic history. More benign-looking radiological appearance.
   (d) Parosteal — 5%. Attached to the surface of the bone by a stalk (early) or a broad base (late) with a tendency to encircle it. Older age group, 20–40 years. Femur is most common site.
   (e) Extraskeletal — buttocks and thighs. Ossification or calcification in a soft-tissue mass.
   (f) Multicentric — rapidly fatal.

Further Reading

Bloem J.L. & Kroon H.M. (1993) Osseous lesions. *Radiol. Clin. North Am.*, 31(2): 261–78.
Murphey M.D., Robbin M.R., McRae G.A. *et al.* (1997) The many faces of osteosarcoma. *RadioGraphics*, 17: 1205–31.

PAGET'S DISEASE

A condition characterized by excessive abnormal remodelling of bone. Increasing prevalence with age: rare in patients less than 40 years old, 3% of the population in middle age and 10% of the population in old age. The disease predominates in the axial skeleton — spine (75%), skull (65%), pelvis (40%) — and proximal femur (75%). (The percentages represent patients with Paget's disease in whom these sites are affected.) Monostotic disease does occur. There are three stages.

ACTIVE (OSTEOLYTIC)

1. Skull — osteoporosis circumscripta, especially in the frontal and occipital bones.
2. Long bones — a well-defined, advancing radiolucency with a V-shaped margin which begins subarticularly.

OSTEOLYTIC AND OSTEOSCLEROTIC

1. Skull — osteoporosis circumscripta with focal areas of bone sclerosis.
2. Pelvis — mixed osteolytic and osteosclerotic areas.
3. Long bones — epiphyseal and metaphyseal sclerosis with diaphyseal lucency.

INACTIVE (OSTEOSCLEROTIC)

1. Skull — thickened vault. 'Cotton wool' areas of sclerotic bone. The facial bones are not commonly affected (cf. fibrous dysplasia).
2. Spine — especially the lumbar spine. Enlargement of vertebrae and coarsened trabeculae. Cortical thickening produces the 'picture frame' vertebral body. Ivory vertebra.
3. Pelvis — widening and coarsened trabeculation of the pelvic ring, with splitting of the iliopectineal line may progress to widespread changes in the pelvis which are commonly asymmetrical.
4. Long bones — sclerosis due to coarsened, thickened trabeculae. Cortical thickening with encroachment on the medullary canal. The epiphyseal region is nearly always involved.

COMPLICATIONS

1. Bone softening — bowed bones, basilar invagination and protrusio acetabuli.
2. Fractures — transverse with a predilection for the convex aspect of the bone and which usually only partially traverse the bone.
3. Sarcomatous change — in 1% of patients (5–10% if there is widespread involvement). Femur, pelvis and humerus most commonly affected. Osteogenic sarcoma (50%), fibrosarcoma (25%) and chondrosarcoma (10%) are the most common histological diagnoses. They are predominantly lytic.
4. Degenerative joint disease — most frequent in the hip and knee.
5. Neurological complications — nerve entrapment and spinal cord compression.
6. High output cardiac failure.
7. Extramedullary haemopoiesis.
8. Osteomyelitis.

PARANEOPLASTIC SYNDROMES

ENDOCRINE DISORDERS

1. Cushing's syndrome — carcinoma of the bronchus, malignant epithelial thymoma, islet cell carcinoma, small cell carcinoma, medullary thyroid carcinoma, ovarian carcinoma.
2. Hypercalcaemia — osseous metastases; carcinoma of lung, oesophageal carcinoma, squamous carcinomas of the head and neck, lymphoma and leukaemia.
3. Hypocalcaemia and osteomalacia — non-ossifying fibroma, giant cell tumour, osteoblastoma (and fibrous dysplasia, neurofibromatosis and melorrheostosis bone).

4. Hypoglycaemia — sarcomas, mesothelioma, lymphoma, gastrointestinal carcinomas, adrenal cortical carcinoma.
5. Hyperglycaemia — glucagon-producing islet cell tumour, enteroglucagon-producing renal carcinoma.
6. Inappropriate antidiuretic hormone — carcinoma of bronchus, adenocarcinomas of the gastrointestinal tract.
7. Carcinoid syndrome — adenocarcinoma of pancreas, islet cell tumours, small cell carcinoma of the lung, medullary carcinoma of the thyroid, APUD (amine precursor uptake and decarboxylation) tumours.
8. Gynaecomastia — non-seminomatous tumours of the testis, liver and renal cell carcinomas, carcinoma of bronchus.
9. Hyperthyroidism — hydatidiform mole or choriocarcinoma, non-seminomatous tumours of testis.
10. Hypertension — phaeochromocytoma, neuroblastoma, aldosterone-secreting tumours, renal tumours (Wilms' tumour, renal cell carcinoma, haemangiopericytoma).

HAEMATOLOGICAL DISORDERS

1. Polycythaemia — renal tumours (Wilms' tumour, renal cell carcinoma), liver cell carcinoma, cerebellar haemangioblastoma, uterine fibroids, renal cystic disease.
2. Red cell aplasia — thymoma, carcinomas of the bronchus, stomach or thyroid.
3. Haemolytic anaemia — lymphoid malignancies, carcinomas of the ovary, stomach, colon, bronchus, cervix and breast.
4. Thrombocytosis and leukocytosis — bone marrow metastases.

DIGESTIVE DISORDERS

1. Zollinger–Ellison syndrome — non-beta cell adenomas or carcinomas of the pancreas or duodenum, mucinous adenocarcinoma of the ovary.
2. Multiple endocrine neoplasia (MEN) (q.v.).
3. Tumour-related diarrhoea — Zollinger–Ellison syndrome, carcinoid syndrome, non-beta cell tumour of the pancreas, vasoactive intestinal peptide-secreting tumours (VIPomas).

RENAL DYSFUNCTION

1. Nephrotic syndrome — lymphoma, carcinomas of the bronchus, stomach, colon and ovary.
2. Tubular dysfunction — multiple myeloma.

MUSCULOSKELETAL DISORDERS

1. Hypertrophic osteoarthropathy (see 1.38) — carcinoma of bronchus, metastases, lymphomas, pleural fibroma.
2. Dermatomyositis — carcinomas of the breast, bronchus, ovary or stomach, leukaemia, lymphoma and sarcomas.

SKIN DISORDERS

1. Acanthosis nigricans — adenocarcinoma of the stomach.
2. Pellagra-like lesions — carcinoid syndrome.
3. Porphyria cutanea tarda — liver cell carcinoma or adenoma.
4. Pemphigus vulgaris — adenocarcinoma of the pancreas.

NEUROLOGICAL DISORDERS

1. Progressive multifocal leukoencephalopathy — leukaemia, lymphoma, myeloma.
2. Cerebellar atrophy — carcinomas of the lung, breast, ovary and kidney; lymphomas.
3. Central pontine myelinolysis — leukaemia.
4. Myelopathy — visceral carcinomas.
5. Myasthenia gravis — thymoma, thymic hyperplasia.
6. Myasthenic syndrome — small cell carcinoma of the lung (Lambert–Eaton syndrome).
7. Opsimyoclonus (dancing eyes) neuroblastoma (usually cervicothoracic).

Further Reading

Taybi H. & Lachman R.S. (1996) *Radiology of Syndromes, Metabolic Disorders, and Skeletal Dysplasias*, 4th edn. St Louis: Mosby, pp. 693–5.

PERTHES' DISEASE (LEGG–CALVE–PERTHE DISEASE)

1. Idiopathic childhood avascular necrosis of the femoral head.
2. M > F. Age 4–8 years.
3. The epiphysis appears small and sclerotic and the joint space may be widened. Demineralization is seen, particularly in the metaphyseal area of the neck, which may appear rarefied. There is no articular cortex destruction.
4. Later a subchondral fracture may be seen as a radiolucent crescent. A subcortical fracture may be seen on the anterior articular surface (frog lateral view).
5. Femoral neck cysts may be seen.
6. Fragmentation develops and this may lead to coxa plana.
7. Femoral head remodelling leads to coxa magna.
8. Delayed bony maturation may occur.
9. As with other causes of avascular necrosis MRI is more sensitive, particularly in the early stage of the disease process when plain films are normal.

PIGMENTED VILLONODULAR SYNOVITIS

1. Benign proliferative disorder of synovium.
2. Knee (80%) > hip > ankle > shoulder.
3. Young adults (third and fourth decades).
4. Also known as giant cell tumour of tendon sheath when it affects tendons in the hands and feet. It is the second commonest soft-tissue mass of the hands and feet after ganglion.

5. Radiographs:
   (a) Normal or periarticular soft-tissue swelling.
   (b) Bone density preserved.
   (c) Joint space preserved until late in the disease.
   (d) Well-defined erosions on both sides of the joints.
   (e) Erosions are more prominent when joint capsule is tight (e.g. hip).
6. MRI:
   (a) Diffuse nodular thickening of the synovium with low signal intensity due to haemosiderin deposition.
   (b) Localized intra-articular variant typically affects Hoffa's fat.

Further Reading

Llauger J., Palmer J., Rosón N. *et al.* (1999) PVNS and giant cell tumor of the tendon sheath. *Am. J. Roentgenol.*, 172: 1087–91.

PLASMACYTOMA

See Multiple myeloma/plasmacytoma.

POLYCYSTIC DISEASE, AUTOSOMAL RECESSIVE

Polycystic kidneys, with periportal hepatic fibrosis and bile duct obstruction. In general, the relative severity of renal and liver disease is inversely proportional to each other in individual patients. Four subgroups: perinatal, neonatal, infantile and juvenile, based on age at presentation, kidney size and clinical course. Infants presenting in the perinatal period have renal failure and/or respiratory distress because of elevated diaphragms. The majority die in a few days. Disease in the neonatal group is milder. Children present in the first month and most die within the first year. The infantile group have both renal and hepatic disease. The juvenile form presents between 6 months and 5 years with portal hypertension, but little renal impairment.

RENAL DISEASE

1. In neonates and infants, bilateral, large, smooth kidneys. Abdominal distension on AXR with bowel gas displaced medially. Severe disease is associated with pulmonary hypoplasia.
2. Markedly hyperechoic kidneys on ultrasound with loss of corticomedullary differentiation. There may be a thin rim of compressed normal parenchyma. May be some macrocysts.
3. Dense striated nephrograms (because of dilated tubules) on IVU and CT. Calyces are not usually demonstrated but are normal.
4. Increased signal on T_2W MRI.
5. In older children kidneys may be normal or show changes similar to, but milder than, the neonatal form.

LIVER DISEASE

1. Heterogeneous or diffuse increased echogenicity on ultrasound ± periportal echogenicity. Usually no bile duct dilatation.
2. Signs of portal hypertension — varices, splenomegaly, etc.

Further Reading

Avni E., Guissard G., Hall M. *et al.* (2002) Hereditary polycystic kidney diseases in children: changing sonographic patterns through childhood. *Pediatr. Radiol.*, 32: 169–74.

Lonergan G.J., Rice R.R. & Suarez E.S. (2000) Autosomal recessive polycystic kidney disease: radiologic–pathologic correlation. *RadioGraphics*, 20: 837–55.

POLYCYSTIC DISEASE, AUTOSOMAL DOMINANT

Presents in third–fourth decade. Unpredictable effect on renal function, but accounts for 10–15% of all patients on renal dialysis. Also diagnosed by screening family members (antenatally and postnatally) or identified as an incidental finding.

KIDNEYS

1. Bilateral, but asymmetrical, enlarged lobulated kidneys. Unilateral in 8%.
2. Multiple smooth defects in the nephrogram with elongation and deformity of calyces giving a 'spider leg' appearance. Cysts may produce filling defects in the renal pelvis.
3. Multiple cysts on ultrasound, CT and MRI.
4. Calcifications in the walls of the cysts are common and stones develop in 20–35% of patients.
5. Increased incidence of renal cell carcinoma (may be bilateral) when on dialysis.
6. There are a number of criteria for positive ultrasound screening examinations. That proposed by Ravine *et al.* (1994) is:
   - two renal cysts (unilateral or bilateral) in patients with a family history and age < 30 years.
   - at least two renal cysts in each kidney in patients with a family history and age 30–59 years.
   - at least four renal cysts in each kidney in patients with a family history and age > 60 years.

OTHER ORGANS

1. Cystic changes in the liver (in 75% by 60 years of age) and, less commonly, in the pancreas (10%) and spleen.
2. Colonic diverticula.
3. Subarachnoid haemorrhage (2–11%) due to intracranial aneurysm (18–26%). Cerebrovascular accidents unrelated to aneurysms are more common.
4. Structural abnormalities of cardiac valves.

Further Reading

Ravine D., Gibson R.N. & Walker R.G. (1994) Evaluation of ultrasonographic diagnostic criteria for autosomal dominant polycystic kidney disease 1. *Lancet*, 343: 824–7.

PSEUDOHYPOPARATHYROIDISM

End organ unresponsiveness to parathormone. X-linked dominant transmission.

1. Short stature, round face, thickset features, mental retardation and hypocalcaemia.
2. Short fourth and fifth metacarpals and metatarsals.
3. Basal ganglia calcification (50%).
4. Soft-tissue calcification.

PSEUDOPSEUDOHYPOPARATHYROIDISM

Similar clinical and radiological features to pseudohypoparathyroidism but with a normal plasma calcium.

PSORIATIC ARTHROPATHY

Occurs in 5% of psoriatics and may antedate the skin changes. There are five clinical and radiological types.

1. Polyarthritis with predominant involvement of the distal interphalangeal joints.
2. Seronegative polyarthritis simulating rheumatoid arthritis.
3. Monoarthritis or asymmetrical oligoarthritis.
4. Spondyloarthritis which can mimic ankylosing spondylitis.
5. Arthritis mutilans (commonly associated with severe skin changes).

The radiological changes comprise:

1. Involvement of synovial and cartilaginous joints and entheses.
2. Joints most frequently affected are the interphalangeal joints of the hands and feet, the metacarpophalangeal and metatarsophalangeal joints, the sacroiliac joints and those in the spine. The large joints are relatively spared. Involvement is asymmetrical.
3. Preserved bone density.
4. Soft-tissue swelling — periarticular or fusiform of a digit.
5. The joint space is narrowed in the large joints and widened in the small joints because of severe destruction of subchondral bone.
6. Erosions which are initially periarticular and progress to involve the entire articular surface. 'Cup and pencil' deformity. Severe destructive changes result in an arthritis mutilans. Erosions also occur at entheses.
7. Bony proliferation: (a) adjacent to the erosions; and (b) at tendon and ligament insertions.
8. Periosteal new bone — particularly in the hands and feet.
9. Ankylosis — especially at the interphalangeal joints of the hands and feet.
10. Distal phalangeal tuft resorption — almost always with severe nail changes.
11. Sacroiliitis and spondylitis with paravertebral ossification.

PULMONARY EMBOLIC DISEASE

Clinical conditions which predispose to venous thromboembolism are:

1. Surgical procedures, especially major abdominal and gynaecological surgery and hip operations.
2. Trauma.
3. Prolonged bed-rest.
4. Neoplastic disease.
5. Pregnancy and the puerperium.
6. Oestrogens.

Pulmonary embolism is massive if more than 50% of the major pulmonary arteries are involved and minor if less than 50% are involved. Duration of embolism in the pulmonary arteries may be acute (< 48 hours), subacute (several days or weeks) or chronic (months or years).

ACUTE OR SUBACUTE MASSIVE EMBOLISM

1. The CXR is most commonly normal.
2. Asymmetrical oligaemia — often best diagnosed by comparison with a previous CXR. The main pulmonary artery may be enlarged.
3. CT pulmonary angiography shows an intraluminal well-defined filling defect.

ACUTE MINOR

1. Although segmental oligaemia ± dilatation of the segmental artery proximal to the obstruction may be observed, this is uncommon and the CXR is often normal.
2. Pulmonary infarction follows in about 33%. The signs are non-specific but include:
   (a) Subpleural consolidation — segmental or subsegmental. Single or multiple.
   (b) Segmental collapse and later linear (plate) atelactasis.
   (c) Pleural reaction with a small effusion.
   (d) Elevation of the hemidiaphragm on the affected side.
   (e) Cavitation of the infarct.
3. Infarction is more common on the right side and in the lower zones.

NB. The ventilation–perfusion radionuclide lung scan is an extremely useful investigation for the diagnosis of pulmonary embolism, especially as the CXR is so commonly normal. The characteristic abnormality is a segmental perfusion defect at the periphery of the lung with no corresponding ventilation defect, i.e. a mismatched defect. This is pathognomonic of pulmonary embolism. When the CXR shows collapse or infarction the lung scan shows a corresponding ventilation and perfusion defect, i.e. a matched effect. This is a non-specific finding seen with any pulmonary mass lesion.

CHRONIC

1. 'Plump' hila with peripheral arterial pruning, i.e. the signs of pulmonary arterial hypertension.
2. ± Multiple areas of linear atelectasis.

Further Reading

Gefter W.B. (ed.) (1997) Pulmonary thromboembolic disease. *Semin. Ultrasound CT MRI,* 18(3).

Kerr I.H., Simon G. & Sutton G.C. (1971) The value of the plain radiograph in acute massive pulmonary embolism. *Br. J. Radiol.,* 44: 751–7.

Padley S.P. (2002) Lung scintigraphy vs spiral CT in the assessment of pulmonary emboli. *Br. J. Radiol.,* 75: 5–8.

Worsley D.F. & Alavi A. (2001) Radionuclide imaging of acute pulmonary embolism. *Radiol. Clin. North Am.,* 39(5): 1035–52.

REITER'S SYNDROME

Sexually transmitted or following dysentery. Males predominate.

1. Urethritis ± cystitis ± prostatitis.
2. Circinate balanitis (30%).
3. Conjunctivitis (30%).
4. Keratoderma blennorrhagica.
5. Arthritis (radiological changes in 80% of cases):
   (a) Involvement of synovial and cartilaginous joints and entheses.
   (b) Asymmetrical involvement of the lower limbs — most commonly the knees, ankles, small joints of the feet and calcaneum. The spine and sacroiliac joints are involved less frequently.
   (c) Soft-tissue swelling.
   (d) Osteoporosis is a feature of the acute disease but not of recurrent or chronic disease.
   (e) Erosions which are initially periarticular and progress to involve the central portion of the articular surface.
   (f) Periosteal new bone.
   (g) New bone formation at ligament and tendon insertions.
   (h) Sacroiliitis and spondylitis with paravertebral ossification.

RENAL OSTEODYSTROPHY

Due to renal glomerular disease: most bilateral reflux nephropathy pyelonephritis and chronic glomerulonephritis. It consists of osteomalacia or rickets + secondary hyperparathyroidism + osteosclerosis.

CHILDREN

1. Changes most marked in the skull, pelvis, scapulae, vertebrae and metaphyses of tubular bones.
2. Vertebral sclerosis may be confined to the upper and lower thirds of the bodies ‘rugger jersey’ spine.
3. Soft-tissue calcification — less common than in adults.
4. Rickets — the epiphyseal plate is less wide and the metaphysis is less cupped than in vitamin D-dependent rickets.
5. Secondary hyperparathyroidism — subperiosteal erosions and a ‘rotting fence-post’ appearance of the femoral necks. ± Slipped upper femoral epiphysis.
6. Delayed skeletal maturation.

ADULTS

1. Hyperparathyroidism (q.v.).
2. Soft-tissue calcification is common, especially in arteries.
3. Osteosclerosis, including ‘rugger jersey’ spine.
4. Osteomalacia is mainly evident as Looser’s zones.

RHEUMATOID ARTHRITIS

A multisystem collagen disorder in which joint disease is variably associated with other systemic manifestations.

1. A symmetrical arthritis of synovial joints, especially the metacarpophalangeal and proximal interphalangeal joints of the hands and feet, wrists, knees, ankles, elbows, glenohumeral and acromioclavicular joints and hips. The synovial articulations of the axial skeleton may also be affected, especially the apophyseal and atlantoaxial joints of the cervical spine. Less commonly the sacroiliac and temporomandibular joints are involved.
2. Cartilaginous joints, e.g. discovertebral junctions outside the cervical spine, symphysis pubis and manubriosternal joints, and entheses are less frequently and less severely involved (cf. seronegative spondyloarthropathies).
3. The sequence of pathological/radiological changes at synovial joints is:
   (a) Synovial inflammation and effusion → soft-tissue swelling and widened joint space.
   (b) Hyperaemia and disuse → juxta-articular osteoporosis; later generalized.
   (c) Destruction of cartilage by pannus → joint-space narrowing.
   (d) Pannus destruction of unprotected bone at the insertion of the joint capsule → periarticular erosions.
   (e) Pannus destruction of subchondral bone → widespread erosions and subchondral cysts.
   (f) Capsular and ligamentous laxity → subluxation, dislocation and deformity.
   (g) Fibrous and bony ankylosis.
4. Periosteal reaction — uncommon.
5. Secondary degenerative arthritis in the major weight-bearing joints.

COMPLICATIONS

1. Joint complications:
   (a) Deformity and subluxation.
   (b) Pyogenic arthritis.
   (c) Tendon rupture.
   (d) Baker's cyst — which may rupture.
   (e) Cord or root compression due to cervical subluxation.
   (f) Hoarseness — due to involvement of the cricoarytenoid joints.

2. Subcutaneous nodules.
3. Anaemia.
4. Pulmonary complications:
   (a) Pleural effusion.
   (b) Rheumatoid nodules.
   (c) Fibrosing alveolitis.
   (d) Caplan's syndrome.
5. Cardiac complications:
   (a) Pericarditis ± effusion.
6. Ocular complications:
   (a) Episcleritis.
   (b) Uveitis.
   (c) Sjögren's syndrome.
7. Arteritis:
   (a) Raynaud's phenomenon.
   (b) Leg ulcers.
   (c) Visceral ischaemia.
8. Felty's syndrome (splenomegaly, leukopenia and rheumatoid arthritis).
9. Peripheral and autonomic neuropathy.
10. Amyloidosis.
11. Complications of therapy.

RICKETS

Increased uncalcified osteoid in the immature skeleton.

CHANGES AT THE GROWTH PLATE AND CORTEX

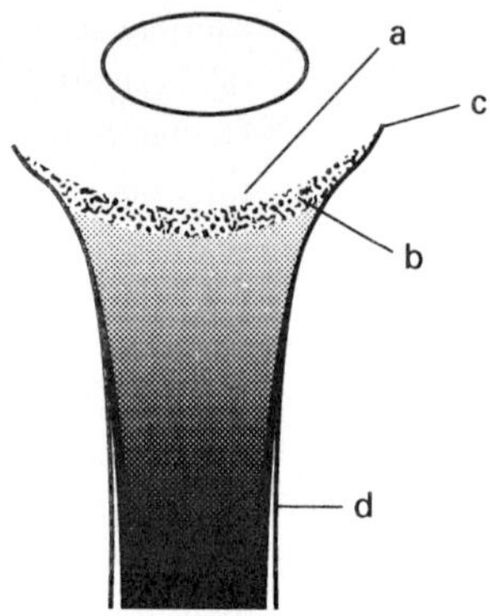

1. Widened growth plate (a).
2. Fraying, splaying and cupping of the metaphysis, which is of reduced density (b).
3. Thin bony spur extending from the metaphysis to surround the uncalcified growth plate (c).
4. Indistinct cortex because of uncalcified subperiosteal osteoid (d).
5. Rickety rosary — cupping of the anterior ends of the ribs and, on palpation, abnormally large costochondral junctions.
6. Looser's zones uncommon in children.

CHANGES DUE TO BONE SOFTENING (DEFORMITIES)

1. Bowing of long bones.
2. Triradiate pelvis.
3. Harrison's sulcus — indrawing of the lower part of the chest wall because of soft ribs.
4. Scoliosis.
5. Biconcave vertebral bodies.
6. Basilar invagination.
7. Craniotabes — flattening of the occiput and accumulating osteoid in the frontal and parietal regions.

GENERAL CHANGES

1. Retarded bone maturation and growth.
2. Decreased bone density — uncommon.

Further Reading

Pitt M.J. (1991) Rickets and osteomalacia are still around. *Radiol. Clin. North Am.*, 29(1): 97–118.

SAPHO

1. Acronym for **S**ynovitis, **A**cne, **P**ustulosis, **H**yperostosis, **O**steitis.
2. A spectrum of conditions related to chronic recurrent multifocal osteomyelitis. Histologically, bone shows chronic inflammation and osteonecrosis. Aetiology not confirmed but the micro-organism, *Propionibacterium acnes*, has been identified by some.
3. Sites — sternoclavicular joints > flat bones > long bones.
4. Bone scintigraphy — buffalo sign caused by increased activity in the manubrium sternum (head) and medial clavicles (horns).

Further Reading

Boutin R.D. & Resnick D. (1998) The SAPHO syndrome: an evolving concept for unifying severa

SARCOIDOSIS

A multisystem granulomatous disorder of unknown aetiology.
Commonest presentations are:

Erythema nodosum	30%
Incidental finding on CXR	25%
Respiratory symptoms	20%
Ocular symptoms	8%
Other skin lesions	5%

INTRATHORACIC SARCOIDOSIS (in 90%)

The CXR at presentation may be:

Normal	8%
Bilateral hilar lymphadenopathy (BHL)	50%
Bilateral hilar lymphadenopathy + pulmonary infiltrate	30%
Pulmonary infiltrate ± fibrosis	12%

1. Lymphadenopathy — bilateral hilar ± unilateral or bilateral paratracheal lymphadenopathy. Anterior mediastinal lymph nodes are also involved in 16%. Unilateral hilar lymphadenopathy in 1–5%. 'Egg-shell' calcification occurs in 1–5% and takes about 6 years to develop.
2. Parenchymal shadowing includes:
   (a) Micronodular shadows < 2 mm
   (b) Larger shadows < 5 mm, ill-defined, mimicking consolidation or oedema
   } predominantly mid zones.

(c) Large nodules, 1–4 cm, ill-defined, multiple, bilateral and in any zone.
(d) Coarse fibrosis — typically in the mid and upper zones.

3. Pleural involvement in 5–7%. Effusion in 2%.
4. Pneumothorax — secondary to chronic lung fibrosis.
5. Bronchial stenosis in 1–2% — extrinsic compression or endobronchial granuloma.

SKIN SARCOIDOSIS

1. Erythema nodosum — almost always in association with bilateral hilar lymphadenopathy.
2. Lupus pernio, plaques, subcutaneous nodules and scar infiltration.

OCULAR SARCOIDOSIS

1. Most commonly manifests as acute uveitis + bilateral hilar lymphadenopathy + erythema nodosum.

HEPATIC AND GASTROINTESTINAL SARCOIDOSIS

1. Hepatic granulomas in 66%, but symptomatic hepatobiliary disease is rare.
2. Gastric and peritoneal granulomas occur but are asymptomatic.

NEUROLOGICAL SARCOIDOSIS

1. Neuropathies — especially bilateral lower motor neuron VIIth nerve palsies.
2. Cerebral sarcoidosis is evident in 14% of autopsies of patients dying of sarcoidosis, but in only 1–5% clinically. Most commonly it produces nodular granulomatous masses in the basal meninges or adhesive meningitis, which result in cranial nerve palsies and/or hydrocephalus. Granulomas in the brain parenchyma present as space-occupying lesions. (On CT scanning they have a high attenuation, are homogeneously enhancing and peripherally situated.)

JOINT SARCOIDOSIS

1. A transient, symmetrical arthropathy involving knees, ankles and, less commonly, the wrists and interphalangeal joints.

BONE SARCOIDOSIS

1. In 3% of patients and most frequently associated with skin lesions.
2. Hands and feet are most commonly affected:
   (a) Enlarged nutrient foramina in phalanges and, occasionally, metacarpals and metatarsals.
   (b) Coarse trabeculation, eventually assuming a lacework, reticulated pattern. Initially metaphyseal and eventually affecting the entire bone.
   (c) Larger, well-defined lucencies.
   (d) Resorption of distal phalanges.
   (e) Terminal phalangeal sclerosis.
   (f) Periarticular calcification.
   (g) Subperiosteal bone resorption — simulating hyperparathyroidism.
   (h) Periosteal reaction.
   (i) Soft-tissue swelling — dactylitis.
3. In the remainder of the skeleton:
   (a) Well-defined lucencies with a sclerotic margin.
   (b) Paraspinal masses with an extradural block at myelography.
   (c) Destructive lesions of the nasal and jaw bones.

SARCOIDOSIS ELSEWHERE

1. Peripheral lymphadenopathy in 15%.
2. Hypercalcaemia (10%) and hypercalciuria (60%).
3. Splenomegaly in 6%.
4. Uveoparotid fever (uveitis, cranial nerve palsy, fever and parotitis).

Further Reading

Miller B.H., Rosado-de-Christenson M.L., McAdams H.P. *et al.* (1995) Thoracic sarcoidosis: radiologic–patholoic correlation. *RadioGraphics*, 15: 421–37.

SCLERODERMA (PROGRESSIVE SYSTEMIC SCLEROSIS)

A multisystem connective tissue disorder, the course of which varies from acute and fulminating to mild and chronic.

SOFT TISSUES

1. Raynaud's phenomenon (60%).
2. Skin thickening — initially of the fingers (and less often the toes) and of the mouth; progresses to shiny taut skin.
3. Subcutaneous calcification — especially in the fingertips and over bony prominences.
4. Myopathy or myositis.

JOINTS

1. Eventually 50% of patients have articular involvement. Fingers, wrists and ankles are commonly affected.
2. Terminal phalangeal resorption is associated with soft-tissue atrophy.
3. Erosions at the distal interphalangeal, first carpometacarpal, metacarpophalangeal and metatarsophalangeal joints.

MANDIBLE

1. Thickening of the periodontal membrane ± loss of the lamina dura.

RIBS

1. Symmetrical erosions on the superior surfaces which predominate along the posterior aspects of the third–sixth ribs.

RESPIRATORY SYSTEM

1. Lung involvement in 10–25%.
2. Aspiration pneumonitis secondary to gastro-oesophageal reflux.
3. Interstitial lung disease and fibrosis, more marked in the lower zones.

GASTROINTESTINAL SYSTEM

1. Oesophageal abnormalities (50%) — dilatation, atonicity, poor or absent peristalsis and free gastro-oesophageal reflux through a widely open gastro-oesophageal junction.
2. Small bowel (75%) — dilated, atonic, thickened mucosal folds and pseudosacculation.
3. Colon (75%) — atonic with pseudosacculations on the antimesenteric border.

HEART

1. Cardiomegaly (30%) — due to myocardial ± pericardial involvement. ± Pericardial effusion.
2. Cor pulmonale may develop secondary to the interstitial lung disease.

SCURVY

The result of vitamin C deficiency.

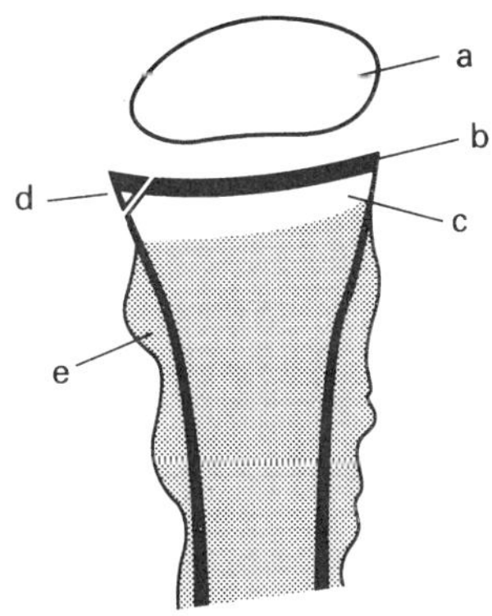

1. Onset at 6 months to 2 years. Rare in adults.
2. Earliest signs are seen at the knees.
3. Osteoporosis (usually the only sign seen in adults).
4. Loss of epiphyseal density with a pencil-thin cortex (Wimberger's sign) (a).
5. Dense zone of provisional calcification — due to excessive calcification of osteoid (b).
6. Metaphyseal lucency (Trümmerfeld zone) (c).
7. Metaphyseal corner fractures through the weakened lucent metaphysis (Pelkan spurs) resulting in cupping of the metaphysis (d).
8. Periosteal reaction due to subperiosteal haematoma (e).

SICKLE-CELL ANAEMIA

SKELETAL

1. Marrow hyperplasia produces widening of medullary cavities, decreased bone density, coarsening of the trabecular pattern, and cortical thinning and expansion. The changes are most marked in the axial skeleton.
   (a) Skull — coarse granular osteoporosis with widening of the diploë which spares the occiput below the internal occipital protuberance. 'Hair-on-end' appearance (5%). Focal lucencies (but probably due to infarcts).
   (b) Spine — osteoporosis, exaggerated vertical trabeculae and biconcave vertebral bodies (but see also 2(c) below).
2. Vascular occlusion due to sickling results in osteonecrosis.
   (a) Sickle-cell dactylitis (hand–foot syndrome) — in children aged 6 months to 2 years. Symmetrical soft-tissue swelling, patchy lucency and sclerosis of the shafts of metacarpals, metatarsals and phalanges, and periosteal reaction.
   (b) Long bones — diaphyseal or epiphyseal infarcts. The femoral head is affected in 12% of patients (60% in Hb SC disease).
   (c) Spine — square-shaped compression infarcts of the vertebral end-plates are virtually diagnostic.
3. Growth disturbances — retarded growth, delayed closure of epiphyses and tibiotalar slant.
4. Fractures.
5. Osteomyelitis and pyogenic arthritis — due to *Salmonella* in over 50% of cases. However, infarction is 50× more common than infection. There are no reliable imaging investigations which differentiate infection from infarction. Imaging can be used to guide biopsy.

EXTRASKELETAL

1. Extramedullary haemopoiesis — more common in thalassaemia.

THORAX

1. The acute chest syndrome is characterized by pleuritic chest pain, fever, rales and new infiltrates on CXR. Due to infection, infarction, fat embolism or any combination of these. Peak incidence at 2–4 years and decreases with age. CXR may be normal and may lag behind clinical symptoms. Two radiographic

patterns are seen: (a) lower lobe air space disease with rapid onset and resolution; and (b) bacterial pneumonia with slower resolution.
2. Defects in large and small vessels on radionuclide perfusion lung scanning; can mimic pulmonary embolism.
3. Some cases of acute chest pain are the result of rib infarcts.

SPLEEN

1. Splenomegaly is rare in adults with sickle-cell anaemia, but is common in other sickle haemoglobinopathies, e.g. Hb SC and Hb S beta thalassaemia.
2. Splenic hypofunction in 30% by 1 year and 90% by 6 years, increasing the risk of septicaemia (commonest cause of death in sickle-cell disease with peak at 1–3 years of age).
3. Splenic sequestration — severe anaemia and hypovolaemia due to sudden accumulation of blood in the spleen, usually before the age of 6 years.
4. Focal abnormalities in the spleen on ultrasound, CT and MRI have imaging characteristics of residual normal splenic tissue.

LIVER AND BILIARY SYSTEM

1. Gallstones in 10–55% of American children; incidence varies with age and geographical location.
2. Hepatobiliary syndromes:
   (a) Viral hepatitis.
   (b) Hepatic crisis.
   (c) Cirrhosis.
   (d) Cholelithiasis with cholecystitis.
   (e) Intrahepatic cholestasis.

RENAL DISEASE

1. Large kidneys, often with abnormal echogenicity; possibly related to glomerular hypertrophy and increased renal blood flow.
2. Papillary necrosis.
3. Primary nocturnal enuresis.
4. Proteinuria.
5. Priapism.
6. Renal medullary carcinoma — mostly in patients with sickle-cell trait.

CENTRAL NERVOUS SYSTEM DISEASE

1. Cerebrovascular accident is the commonest cause of death (12% of paediatric deaths).
2. Three patterns of vascular disease:
   (a) Proximal branch occlusion or stenosis.
   (b) Distal branch occlusion.
   (c) Aneurysm.

Further Reading

Crowley J.J. & Sarnaik S. (1999) Imaging of sickle cell disease. *Pediatr. Radiol.*, 29: 646–61.

Howlett D.C., Hatrick A.G., Jarosz J.M. *et al.* (1997) Pictorial review: the role of CT and MR in imaging the complications of sickle cell disease. *Clin. Radiol.*, 52: 821–9.

Lonergan G.J., Cline D.B., & Abbondanzo S.L. (2001) Sickle cell anemia. *RadioGraphics*, 21: 971–94.

Moran C.J., Siegel M.J. & DeBaun M.R. (1998) Sickle cell disease: imaging of cerebrovascular complications. *Radiology*, 206: 311–21.

SILICOSIS

Occurs in miners, quarry workers, masons, pottery workers, sand blasters, foundry workers and boiler scalers. The duration and degree of exposure determine the time of onset of disease.

(a) Chronic silicosis — disease after 20–40 years of exposure.
(b) Accelerated silicosis — disease after 5–15 years of exposure.
(c) Acute silicoproteinosis — heavy exposure over a short period of time (several months to 5 years), e.g. in sand blasters.

SIMPLE

1. Nodular shadows, pin-point to pea-sized, which are first seen around the right hilum but are later disseminated throughout both lungs with relative sparing of the extreme bases and apices. Exceptionally, they may be restricted to the upper zones.

2. Inhalation of pure silica produces very sharp, dense nodules. Mixed dusts are less well defined and of lower density. Density increases with the size of the nodule. Gold miners have very dense nodular shadows.
3. Nodules may calcify, especially in gold miners.
4. Minor hilar lymph-node enlargement, but only obvious when calcification occurs (in 5%). Anterior and posterior mediastinal lymph nodes may also enlarge.
5. Kerley A and B lines — more pronounced with mixed dusts.
6. Silicoproteinosis presents as diffuse alveolar disease.

COMPLICATED, i.e. PROGRESSIVE MASSIVE FIBROSIS (PMF)

1. Superimposed on the changes of simple silicosis.
2. The rapid development of massive, ill-defined, dense, oval or round shadows. Usually bilateral and fairly symmetrical in the upper two-thirds of the lungs.
3. They begin peripherally and increase in size and density as they move towards the hilum, leaving emphysematous lung at the periphery.
4. May cavitate or calcify.

COMPLICATIONS

1. Infections — chronic bronchitis and tuberculosis.
2. Pneumothorax — but usually limited by thickened pleura.
3. Cor pulmonale — a common cause of death.
4. Caplan's syndrome — in patients with rheumatoid disease. Well-defined, peripheral nodules 0.5–5 cm in diameter. Calcification and cavitation may occur.

SIMPLE BONE CYST

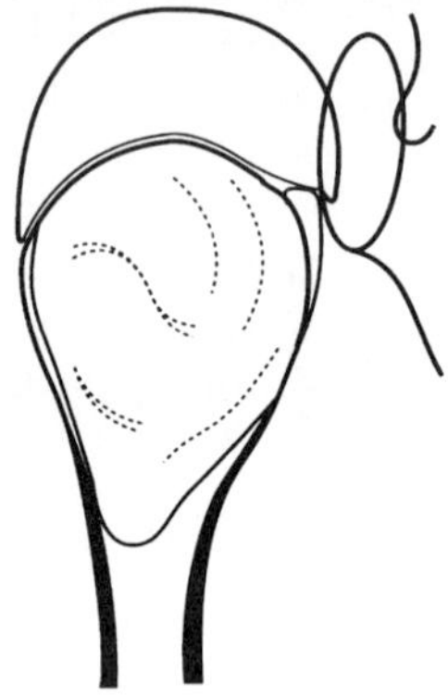

1. Age — 5–15 years.
2. Sites — proximal humerus and femur (75% of cases) and apophysis of the greater trochanter.
3. Frequently presents with a pathological fracture, especially proximal humerus.
4. Appearances:
   (a) Metaphyseal, extending to the epiphyseal plate. It migrates away from the metaphysis with time.
   (b) Well-defined lucency with a thin sclerotic rim.
   (c) Usually central.
   (d) Thinned cortex with slight expansion (never more than the width of the epiphyseal plate).
   (e) Thin internal septa.
   (f) Pathological fracture may be associated with the 'fallen fragment' sign — a small fragment of bone in the dependent part of the cyst.

SLIPPED CAPITAL FEMORAL EPIPHYSIS

1. Commonest hip abnormality in adolescence and a major cause of early osteoarthritis.
2. M > F. Black > White.
3. The child is often overweight.
4. Presentation with hip or knee pain. When it occurs before adolescence it may be associated with an underlying pathology such as malnutrition, endocrine disturbance or developmental dysplasia of the hip.
5. Radiology — AP and true lateral films. A frog lateral may exacerbate the slip. Initially widening of the physis is seen with or without demineralization. The femoral may then slip posteriorly so an early slip is best seen on a lateral view. With continued posterior slippage the femoral head may appear smaller with apparent narrowing of the physis. As the slip progresses the femoral head displaces medially and the Line of Klein becomes abnormal. The metaphyseal blanch sign may be seen before the slip itself is detected — it relates to an area of healing leading to a metaphyseal opacity.
6. Grading:
   (a) Mild slip = displacement of femoral head < 1/3 the metaphyseal diameter.
   (b) Moderate = displacement of femoral head 1/3–2/3 the metaphyseal diameter.
   (c) Severe = displacement of femoral head > 2/3 the metaphyseal diameter.
7. Complications:
   (a) Progression.
   (b) Chondrolysis — joint space less than 3 mm or loss of greater than 50% of the cartilage thickness. Occurs on both sides of the joint.
   (c) Avascular necrosis — causing the same appearance as seen in other causes of AVN.
   (d) Late complications leading to further radiographic changes including pistol grip deformity, (femoral neck broadening, shortening with varus angulation), osteoarthritis and differences in limb length.

Further Reading

Boles C.A. & el-Khoury G.Y. (1997) Slipped capital femoral epiphysis. *RadioGraphics*, 17: 809–23.

STEROIDS

See Cushing's syndrome.

SYSTEMIC LUPUS ERYTHEMATOSUS

MUSCULOSKELETAL

1. Polyarthritis — bilateral and symmetrical, involving the small joints of the hand, knee, wrist and shoulder. Soft-tissue swelling and periarticular osteoporosis of the proximal interphalangeal and metacarpophalangeal joints simulate rheumatoid arthritis, but periarticular erosions are not a usual feature.
2. Easily correctable deformities of the hand which cause little functional disability.
3. Osteonecrosis — most frequently of the femoral head.
4. Terminal phalangeal sclerosis and resorption.

CARDIORESPIRATORY

1. Pleural effusion (60%), which is often recurrent. Often accompanied by a pleurisy resulting in elevation of a hemidiaphragm and plate atelectasis at the base.
2. Uraemic pulmonary oedema.
3. Acute lupus pneumonitis.
4. Diffuse interstitial disease — uncommon.
5. Cardiomegaly — due to pericarditis with effusion, myocardial disease or fluid overload in renal failure.

ABDOMEN

1. Hepatosplenomegaly.
2. Renal disease eventually results in small, smooth, non-functioning kidneys.

THALASSAEMIA

SKELETAL

1. Marrow hyperplasia is more pronounced than in sickle-cell anaemia (q.v.). The changes in thalassaemia major are more severe than in thalassaemia minor. Initially both axial and appendicular skeleton are affected but as marrow regresses from the appendicular skeleton at puberty the changes in the latter diminish.
   (a) Skull — granular osteoporosis, widening of the diploë, thinning of the outer table and 'hair-on-end' appearance. Involvement of the facial bones produces obliteration of the paranasal sinuses, hypertelorism and malocclusion of the teeth. These changes are rarely a feature of other haemoglobinopathies and are important differentiating signs.
   (b) Spine — osteoporosis, exaggerated vertical trabeculae and fish-shaped vertebrae.
   (c) Ribs, clavicles and tubular bones of the hands and feet show the typical changes of marrow hyperplasia (see Sickle-cell anaemia).
2. Growth disturbances.
3. Fractures.

EXTRASKELETAL

1. Extramedullary haemopoiesis — including hepatosplenomegaly.
2. Cardiomegaly.

Further Reading

Tunaci M., Tunaci A., Engin G. *et al.* (1999) Imaging features of thalassaemia. *Eur. Radiol.*, 9: 1804–9.

TUBEROUS SCLEROSIS (see also 12.38)

AD with variable expression and a high incidence of fresh mutations (50%). Gene is located on the long arm of chromosome 11. Clinical features include seizures, mental retardation and skin lesions (adenoma sebaceum, hypomelanotic macules, fibrous plaques, shagreen patches and subungual fibromas). Café-au-lait spots are not more frequent in tuberous sclerosis (TS) than in the general population.

CENTRAL NERVOUS SYSTEM

1. Subependymal nodules — *CT:* calcified or non-calcified; increase in number and degree of calcification with time. *MRI:* low or intermediate signal ± high signal rim on T_2W ± enhancement with gadolinium.
2. Parenchymal tubers — *CT:* low attenuation, less commonly high attenuation, rarely calcified, non-enhancing; associated with gyral broadening; minimal progression with time. *MRI:* prolonged T_1 and T_2 signal; no enhancement. However, signal intensity changes with age:
   Newborn: T_1 hyperintense, T_2 hypointense.
   Young child: T_1 hypointense, T_2 hyperintense.
   Older child: T_1 isointense, T_2 hyperintense.
3. Hydrocephalus.
4. Cerebral neoplasms — giant cell astrocytoma, typically near the foramen of Monro. Marked enhancement on CT and MRI.
5. Retinal astrocytomas (phakomas) — an asymptomatic calcified retinal nodule(s).
6. Arterial ectasia and occlusion.

KIDNEYS

1. Angiomyolipomas (AML) — in 40–80% of patients with TS. 50% of patients with AML have TS. May be the only lesion of TS in some patients. Detected after infancy. Asymptomatic or causes haematuria. Multiple, bilateral and variable size. *US:* multiple echogenic nodules. *IVU:* stretching of calyces. *CT:* masses containing fat. *MRI:* high T_1W signal masses. *Angiography:* hypervascularity and irregular outpouchings from interlobar and interlobular arteries.
2. Cysts — in 50%. ± AML. May be present in the neonatal period. Similar appearance to dominant polycystic kidney disease.

3. Increased incidence of renal cell carcinoma and Wilms' tumour.
4. Intratumoral and perirenal haemorrhage.
5. Aneurysms of intrarenal arteries.

SKELETAL

1. Lesions are asymptomatic. Present in 1–50% of patients with TS.
2. Patchy, localized, sclerotic lesions in the skull, vertebrae, pelvis and long bones.
3. Irregular periosteal new bone formation.
4. Distal phalangeal erosion by subungual fibroma.
5. Cyst-like defects in phalanges, metacarpals and metatarsals.
6. Rib expansion and sclerosis.

LUNGS

1. In 0.1–1% of patients with TS. Majority are female. First respiratory symptoms at 18–34 years. Similar to lymphangiomyomatosis of lung but less pleural disease, especially chylothorax.
2. *CXR:* non-specific coarse generalized reticulonodular shadowing which progresses to honeycomb lung. *HRCT:* well-defined cystic spaces with thin walls, a few millimetres to 5 cm in diameter.

HEART

1. Cardiac rhabdomyomas are the earliest detectable lesions in TS. May be diagnosed as early as 22 weeks' gestation. Multiple tumours in 80–90%. At least 80% of those with cardiac rhabdomyomas have TS and 60% of patients with TS < 18 years have cardiac rhabdomyomas. Presentation with cardiac failure, murmur and/or arrhythmias. The tumours do not increase in size and most regress spontaneously (within weeks of birth). *CXR:* normal or non-specific cardiomegaly.

Further Reading

Bernauer T.A. (1999) The radial bands sign. *Radiology*, 212: 761–2.

Evans J.C. & Curtis J. (2000) The radiological appearances of tuberous sclerosis. *Br. J. Radiol.*, 73: 91–8.

Medley B.E., McLeod R.A. & Wayne Houser O. (1976) Tuberous sclerosis. *Semin. Roentgenol.*, 11: 35–54.

TURNER'S SYNDROME

Females with XO chromosome pattern.

1. Small stature with retarded bone maturation.
2. Mental retardation in 10%.
3. Osteoporosis.

CHEST

1. Cardiovascular abnormalities — present in 20%, and 70% are coarctation.
2. Broad chest, mild pectus excavatum; widely spaced nipples.

ABDOMEN

1. Ovarian dysgenesis.
2. Renal anomalies — 'horseshoe kidney' and bifid renal pelvis are the most common.

AXIAL SKELETON

1. Scoliosis and kyphosis.
2. Hypoplasia of the cervical spine.

APPENDICULAR SKELETON

1. Cubitus valgus in 70%.
2. Short fourth metacarpal and/or metatarsal in 50% ± short third and fifth metacarpals.
3. Madelung's deformity.
4. Enlargement of the medial tibial plateau ± small exostosis inferiorly.
5. Pes cavus.
6. Transient congenital oedema of the dorsum of the feet.

ULCERATIVE COLITIS

1. Diseased colon is affected in continuity with symmetrical involvement of the wall.
2. Rectum involved in 95%. The rectum may appear normal if steroid enemas have been administered.
3. Granular mucosa and mucosal ulcers.
4. 'Thumbprinting' due to mucosal oedema.
5. Blunting of haustral folds progresses to a narrowed, shortened and tubular colon if the disease becomes chronic.
6. Widening of the retrorectal space.
7. Inflammatory pseudopolyps due to regenerating mucosa. Found in 10–20% of ulcerative colitics and usually following a previous severe attack. Filiform polyps occur in quiescent phase.
8. Patulous ileocaecal valve with reflux ileitis (dilated terminal ileum).

COMPLICATIONS

1. Toxic megacolon — in 7–10%
2. Strictures — much less common than in Crohn's disease and must be differentiated from carcinoma.
3. Carcinoma of the colon — 20–30× increased incidence if extensive colitis has been present for more than 10 years.
4. Associated conditions:
   (a) Erythema nodosum, aphthous ulceration and pyoderma gangrenosum.
   (b) Arthritis — similar to Crohn's disease (q.v.).
   (c) Cirrhosis.
   (d) Chronic active hepatitis.
   (e) Pericholangitis.
   (f) Sclerosing cholangitis.
   (g) Bile duct carcinoma.
   (h) Oxalate urinary calculi.

Index